HPV-Vaccines

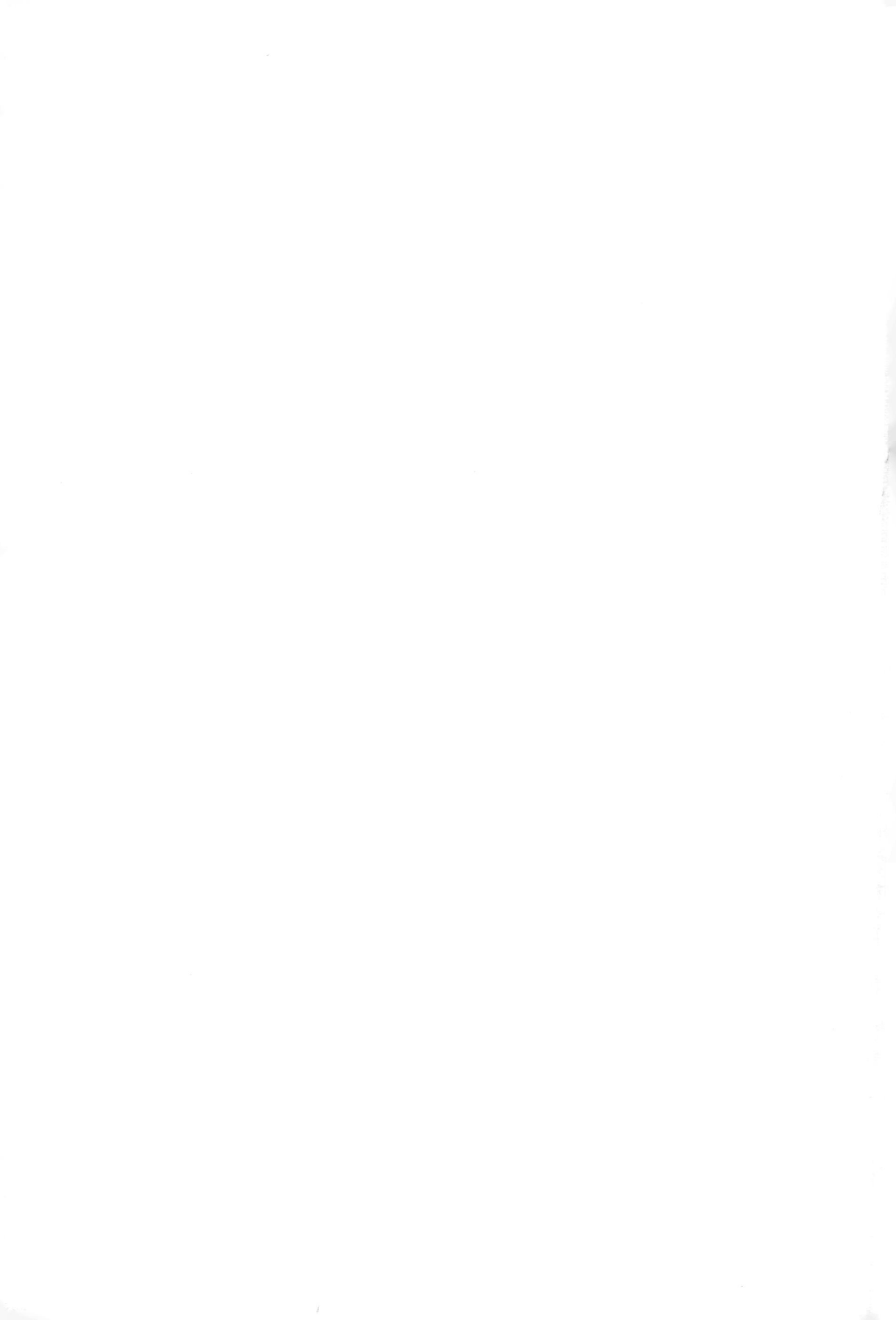

HPV-Vaccines

Editor

Gloria Calagna

MDPI • Basel • Beijing • Wuhan • Barcelona • Belgrade • Manchester • Tokyo • Cluj • Tianjin

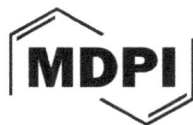

Editor
Gloria Calagna
University of Palermo
Italy

Editorial Office
MDPI
St. Alban-Anlage 66
4052 Basel, Switzerland

This is a reprint of articles from the Topical Collection published online in the open access journal *Vaccines* (ISSN 2076-393X) (available at: https://www.mdpi.com/journal/vaccines/topical_collections/HPV-Vaccines_vaccines).

For citation purposes, cite each article independently as indicated on the article page online and as indicated below:

LastName, A.A.; LastName, B.B.; LastName, C.C. Article Title. *Journal Name* **Year**, *Volume Number*, Page Range.

ISBN 978-3-0365-5917-9 (Hbk)
ISBN 978-3-0365-5918-6 (PDF)

© 2023 by the authors. Articles in this book are Open Access and distributed under the Creative Commons Attribution (CC BY) license, which allows users to download, copy and build upon published articles, as long as the author and publisher are properly credited, which ensures maximum dissemination and a wider impact of our publications.
The book as a whole is distributed by MDPI under the terms and conditions of the Creative Commons license CC BY-NC-ND.

Contents

Haruna Arakawa, Shohei Yokoyama, Takehiro Ohira, Dedong Kang, Kazuho Honda, Yoshihiko Ueda and Akihiro Tojo
Juvenile Membranous Nephropathy Developed after Human Papillomavirus (HPV) Vaccination
Reprinted from: *Vaccines* 2022, 10, 1442, doi:10.3390/vaccines10091442 1

Veronica Cordoba-Sanchez, Mariantonia Lemos, Diego Alfredo Tamayo-Lopera and Sherri Sheinfeld Gorin
HPV-Vaccine Hesitancy in Colombia: A Mixed-Methods Study
Reprinted from: *Vaccines* 2022, 10, 1187, doi:10.3390/ vaccines10081187 13

Gulzhanat Aimagambetova, Aisha Babi, Torgyn Issa and Alpamys Issanov
What Factors Are Associated with Attitudes towards HPV Vaccination among Kazakhstani Women? Exploratory Analysis of Cross-Sectional Survey Data
Reprinted from: *Vaccines* 2022, 10, 824, doi:10.3390/vaccines10050824 29

Dominik Pruski, Małgorzata Łagiedo-Żelazowska, Sonja Millert-Kalińska, Jan Sikora, Robert Jach and Marcin Przybylski
Immunity after HPV Vaccination in Patients after Sexual Initiation
Reprinted from: *Vaccines* 2022, 10, 728, doi:10.3390/vaccines10050728 45

Chinenye Lynette Ejezie, Ikponmwosa Osaghae, Sylvia Ayieko and Paula Cuccaro
Adherence to the Recommended HPV Vaccine Dosing Schedule among Adolescents Aged 13 to 17 Years: Findings from the National Immunization Survey-Teen, 2019–2020
Reprinted from: *Vaccines* 2022, 10, 577, doi:10.3390/vaccines10040577 55

Antonio Di Lorenzo, Paola Berardi, Andrea Martinelli, Francesco Paolo Bianchi, Silvio Tafuri and Pasquale Stefanizzi
Real-Life Safety Profile of the 9-Valent HPV Vaccine Based on Data from the Puglia Region of Southern Italy
Reprinted from: *Vaccines* 2022, 10, 419, doi:10.3390/vaccines10030419 71

Jill M. Maples, Nikki B. Zite, Oluwafemifola Oyedeji, Shauntá M. Chamberlin, Alicia M. Mastronardi, Samantha Gregory, et al.
Availability of the HPV Vaccine in Regional Pharmacies and Provider Perceptions Regarding HPV Vaccination in the Pharmacy Setting
Reprinted from: *Vaccines* 2022, 10, 351, doi:10.3390/vaccines10030351 81

Katarzyna Smolarczyk, Anna Duszewska, Slawomir Drozd and Slawomir Majewski
Parents' Knowledge and Attitude towards HPV and HPV Vaccination in Poland
Reprinted from: *Vaccines* 2022, 10, 228, doi:10.3390/vaccines10020228 93

Ayazhan Akhatova, Chee Kai Chan, Azliyati Azizan and Gulzhanat Aimagambetova
The Efficacy of Therapeutic DNA Vaccines Expressing the Human Papillomavirus E6 and E7 Oncoproteins for Treatment of Cervical Cancer: Systematic Review
Reprinted from: *Vaccines* 2022, 10, 53, doi:10.3390/vaccines10010053 111

Oluwafemifola Oyedeji, Jill M. Maples, Samantha Gregory, Shauntá M. Chamberlin, Justin D. Gatwood, Alexandria Q. Wilson, et al.
Pharmacists' Perceived Barriers to Human Papillomavirus (HPV) Vaccination: A Systematic Literature Review
Reprinted from: *Vaccines* 2021, 9, 1360, doi:10.3390/vaccines9111360 123

Zixin Wang, Yuan Fang, Paul Shing-fong Chan, Andrew Chidgey, Francois Fong, Mary Ip and Joseph T. F. Lau
Effectiveness of a Community-Based Organization—Private Clinic Service Model in Promoting Human Papillomavirus Vaccination among Chinese Men Who Have Sex with Men
Reprinted from: *Vaccines* **2021**, *9*, 1218, doi:10.3390/vaccines9111218 . . . . **137**

Akiyo Hineno and Shu-Ichi Ikeda
A Long-Term Observation on the Possible Adverse Effects in Japanese Adolescent Girls after Human Papillomavirus Vaccination
Reprinted from: *Vaccines* **2021**, *9*, 856, doi:10.3390/vaccines9080856 . . . . **153**

Edison J. Mavundza, Chinwe J. Iwu-Jaja, Alison B. Wiyeh, Blessings Gausi, Leila H. Abdullahi, Gregory Halle-Ekane and Charles S. Wiysonge
A Systematic Review of Interventions to Improve HPV Vaccination Coverage
Reprinted from: *Vaccines* **2021**, *9*, 687, doi:10.3390/vaccines9070687 . . . . **161**

Matthew Asare, Braden Popelsky, Emmanuel Akowuah, Beth A. Lanning and Jane R. Montealegre
Internal and External Validity of Social Media and Mobile Technology-Driven HPV Vaccination Interventions: Systematic Review Using the Reach, Effectiveness, Adoption, Implementation, Maintenance (RE-AIM) Framework
Reprinted from: *Vaccines* **2021**, *9*, 197, doi:10.3390/vaccines9030197 . . . . **191**

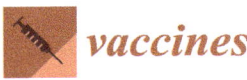

Case Report

Juvenile Membranous Nephropathy Developed after Human Papillomavirus (HPV) Vaccination

Haruna Arakawa [1], Shohei Yokoyama [1], Takehiro Ohira [1], Dedong Kang [2], Kazuho Honda [2], Yoshihiko Ueda [3] and Akihiro Tojo [1,*]

[1] Department of Nephrology & Hypertension, Dokkyo Medical University, Mibu 321-0293, Japan
[2] Department of Anatomy, Showa University School of Medicine, Tokyo 142-8555, Japan
[3] Department of Pathology, Dokkyo Medical University Saitama Medical Center, Saitama 343-8555, Japan
* Correspondence: akitojo@dokkyomed.ac.jp; Tel.: +81-282-86-1111

Abstract: A 16-year-old girl with no history of renal disease had a fever of 38 °C after her second HPV vaccination and was identified as positive for proteinuria. As she maintained urinary protein of 3.10 g/gCr and 5–9 urinary red blood cells/HPF, a renal biopsy was performed and small spikes on PAM staining with the granular deposition of IgG1++ and IgG3+ on the glomerular capillary wall were discovered by immunofluorescence, although PLA2R immunostaining was negative. Analysis by electron microscope showed electron density deposition in the form of fine particles under the epithelium. The diagnosis was secondary membranous nephropathy stage II. Immunostaining with the anti-p16 INK4a antibody was positive for glomerular cells, and Western blot analysis of urinary protein showed a positive band for p16 INK4a. However, laser-microdissection mass spectrometry analysis of a paraffin section of glomeruli failed to detect HPV proteins. It is possible that the patient was already infected with HPV and administration of the HPV vaccine may have caused secondary membranous nephropathy.

Keywords: human papillomavirus; vaccination; membranous nephropathy; p16 INK4a; mass spectrometry

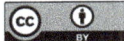

1. Introduction

SARS-CoV-2 vaccination was promoted during the COVID-19 pandemic; however, the effectiveness and side effects of the mRNA vaccines for SARS-CoV-2 were not fully elucidated. Gross hematuria in patients with IgA nephropathy and recurrence of nephrotic syndrome in patients with minimal change nephrotic syndrome (MCNS) were reported as side effects following SARS-CoV-2 vaccination [1–4]. Some young people are concerned about adverse reactions to the SARS-CoV-2 vaccination, especially in Japan, where young people have a distrust of the vaccine due to cases of side effects caused by the HPV vaccine [5].

Human papillomavirus HPV is a double-stranded DNA virus that can be divided into more than 100 types from the gene sequence of the surface capsid protein L1. High-risk HPV16, 18, 31, 33, 45, 51, 52, 56, 58, and 66 cause cervical cancer, and low-risk HPV6, 11, etc., cause condyloma acuminata [6–8]. In Japan, the recombinant divalent human papillomavirus vaccine Cervarix for high-risk HPV 16/18 was sold in 2009, and regular vaccination started in 2013 for 6th-grade elementary school to 1st-grade middle high school girls [8]. However, Cervarix was discontinued due to reports of adverse reactions, including chronic pain, motor impairment, and other symptoms after HPV vaccination. The recombinant precipitated 4-valent HPV-like particle vaccine has been on the market since 2011, and the recombinant precipitated 9-valent HPV-like particle vaccine has been on the market since 2021, although the Ministry of Health, Labor, and Welfare in Japan announced a suspension of the proactive recommendation for routine use of the HPV vaccine in the national immunization program in June 2013 [9] until November 2021. In Cervarix, the capsid protein of the recombinant precipitated divalent human papillomavirus is atomized and aluminum hydroxide and monophosphoryl lipid A (MPL) derived from the cell membrane of Salmonella are used as an adjuvant. These adjuvants destroy cells at the administration site, and the destroyed autologous cell DNA and proteins are recognized by the DAMPs in the innate immune response system [10] and cause not only fever and local swelling but also Guillain–Barré syndrome (GBS), systemic lupus erythematosus (SLE), autoimmune hepatitis, and cerebral vasculitis [11]. We experienced a case of secondary membranous nephropathy after the second injection of the divalent HPV vaccine Cervarix, and here we discuss the mechanism of membranous nephropathy after HPV vaccination.

2. Case Presentation

A 16-year-old girl had a fever of 39.0 °C for 4–5 days after the second HPV vaccination, even though she had no fever following the first HPV vaccination one month prior. She was prescribed acetaminophen, and she developed proteinuria for the first time 5 days after receiving the second vaccination. Her fever was resolved spontaneously, and proteinuria was not checked until the next school year in a urine checkup, which showed proteinuria 3+ and occult blood. She was hospitalized for examination by renal biopsy. She had a history of allergy to pollen. Her family history included cerebral hemorrhage in her maternal great-grandfather, multiple system atrophy in her grandfather, and hypertension in her grandmother. Physical findings on admission were blood pressure 120/82 mmHg, heart rate 115 bpm, body temperature 36.2 °C, SpO$_2$ 98% (room air) without tonsillitis, lymphadenopathy, or neurological dysfunction. A urinalysis showed urinary protein, 1.46 g/gCr, 5–9 RBC/HPF, 1–4 WBC/HPF, cast (-), NAG 2.7 U/L, and selectivity index 0.121. A blood test showed WBC 8100 × 10^6/L, (neutrophil 68.2%, eosinophil 1.7%, basophil 0.7%, monocyte 8.3%, lymphocyte 21.1%), Hb 11.9 g/dL, and platelet 39.8 × 10^{10}/L. Biochemistry data revealed TP 5.5 g/dL, Alb 3.5 g/dL, UN 11.0 mg/dL, Cr 0.47 mg/dL, eGFR 147.8 mL/min/1.73 m^2, and CRP 0.01 mg/dL. Immunological tests found ANA (-), anti-dsDNA antibody (-), anti-SM antibody (-), IgG 544 mg/dL, IgA 112.4 mg/dL, IgM 134.7 mg/dL, IgE 34.3 mg/dL, C$_3$ 141.9 mg/dL, C$_4$ 23.2 mg/dL, ASO 14 IU/mL, lupus anticoagulant negative, anti-CLβ2GP1 antibody 1.2 U/mL, anti-SS A/B antibody (−/−), MPO-ANCA (-), PR3-ANCA (-), anti-GBM antibody (-), HBs antigen (-), HCV antibody (-), and D dimer 0.3μg/mL. These data indicate that there were no possibilities of lupus nephritis, other autoimmune diseases, or antiphospholipid syndrome.

3. Renal Biopsy and Laser-Microdissection Mass Spectrometry

3.1. Renal Biopsy

Two samples of cortex were collected, including a total of 25 glomeruli without global sclerosis, mild mesangial cell proliferation in 10 glomeruli (40%), and normal tubulointerstitium and vascular system. PAM staining showed mild spikes with subepithelial immune complexes by AZAN staining, which were granularly stained along the capillary wall by fluorescent immunostaining for IgG (Figure 1).

Among the IgG subclasses, IgG1 was the strongest, IgG3 was mildly stained (Figure 2), and immunofluorescence for phospholipase A2 receptor (PLA2R) was negative (Figure 3A), suggesting secondary membranous nephropathy. Electron microscopy revealed an electron-dense deposit in the subepithelial membrane and partly in the basement membrane, indicating stage II–III membranous nephropathy (Figure 4).

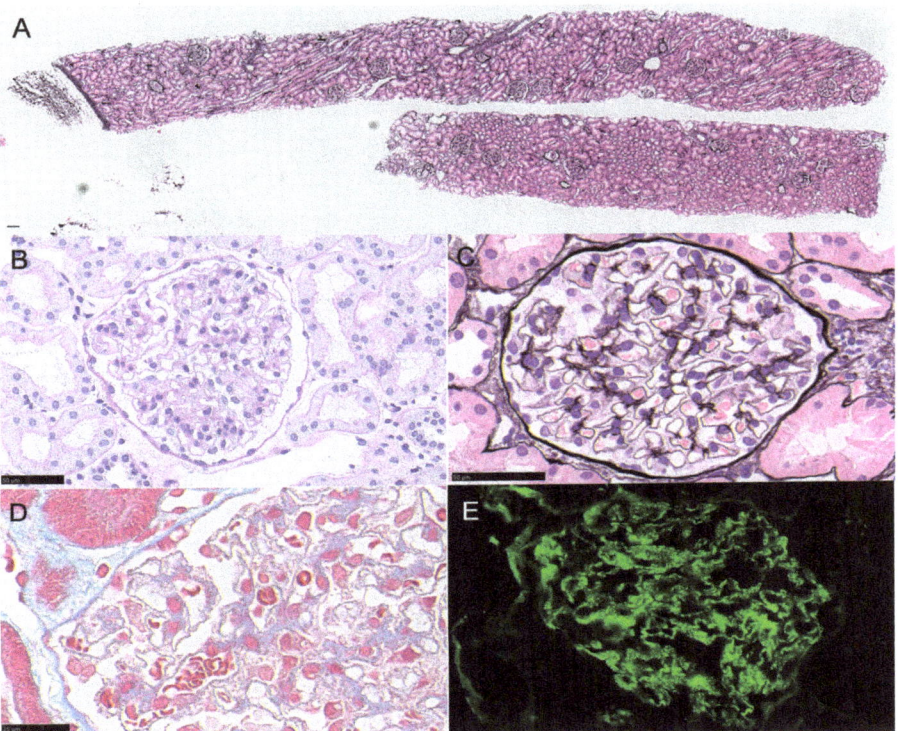

Figure 1. Renal biopsy. PAM staining (**A**,**C**), PAS staining (**B**), Azan staining (**D**), and immunofluorescence of IgG. The bars indicate 50 μm (**B**,**C**,**E**) and 25 μm (**D**).

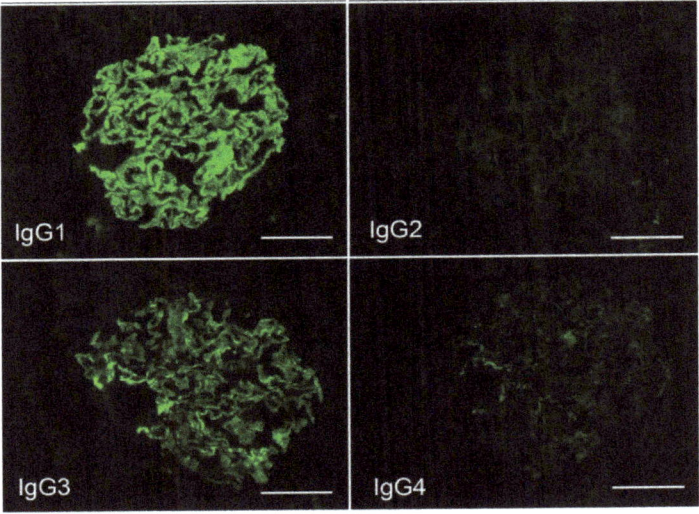

Figure 2. Immunofluorescence of IgG subclass staining. The bars indicate 50 μm.

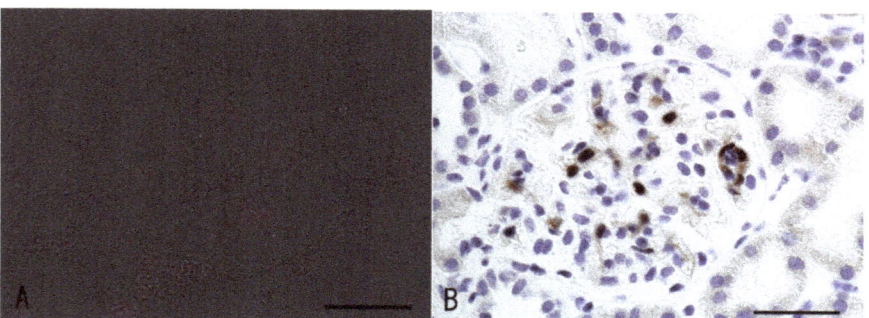

Figure 3. Immunofluorescence of PLA2R (**A**) and immunostaining for the p16-INK4a antibody (**B**). The bars indicate 50 μm.

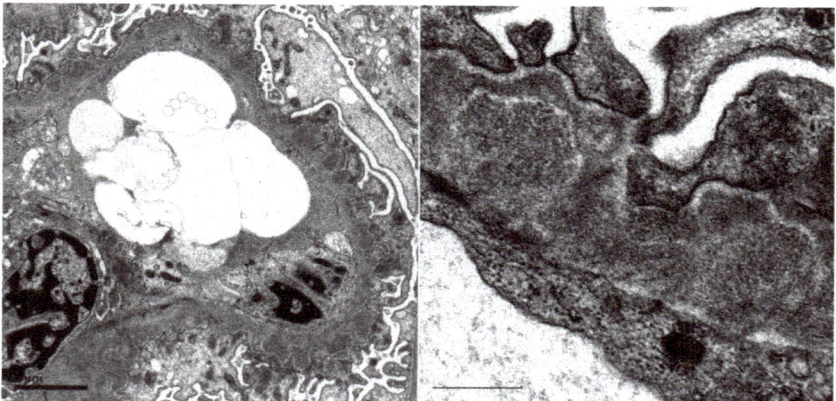

Figure 4. Electron microscopy. The bars indicate 2 μm and 0.5 μm.

3.2. Surrogate Marker for HPV Infection

Immunohistochemistry was performed with the Leica auto-immune stain system using the antibody against the anti-p16-INK4a antibody (CINtec® Histology, Roche Diagnostics KK, Tokyo, Japan), which is typically used as a surrogate marker of HPV infection in cervical cancer and oropharyngeal cancer [12,13]. The anti-p16-INK4a antibody showed significant staining in the intra-glomerular cells (Figure 3B).

Furthermore, Western blot analysis identified p16 protein in the urinary protein at the time of renal biopsy. On the other hand, it was not found in the urine of patients with secondary membranous nephropathy related to cancer or primary membranous nephropathy—it was specific to this case (Figure 5). Therefore, it was suggested that this case could have already been infected with HPV before the time of renal biopsy.

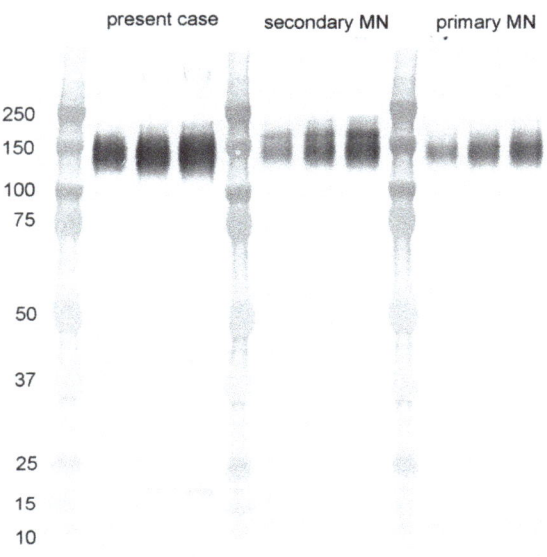

Figure 5. Western blot of the urinary protein at the time of renal biopsy for p16-INK4a. The urine of the present case showed a band at MW16kD, whereas the urine of other cases of membranous nephropathy did not show a band for p16-INK4a.

3.3. Laser Microdissection Mass Spectrometry

We performed laser microdissection mass spectrometry (LMD-MS), as mentioned previously [14], to detect HPV viral capsule proteins. LMD-MS failed to detect HPV protein or antigens for membranous nephropathy, including THSD7A, EXT1/2, NELL1, Sema 3B, PCDH7, HTRA1, Contactin 1 [15,16], which were negative, except for a small amount of PLA2R in one sample (Table 1). The cytokeratin-related proteins were increased, whereas podocyte proteins such as nephrin, podocin, and podocalyxin were decreased compared to the control glomeruli from the renal transplantation at 1 h biopsy (Table 1, Figure S1).

Table 1. Laser microdissection mass spectrometry analysis of glomeruli of this patient and glomeruli from the 1 h renal biopsy after renal transplantation as control.

MS/MS View: 899 Proteins in 665 Clusters	Alternate ID	Control	Pt. Glm1	Pt. Glm2	Pt. Glm3	Pt. Glm4	Pt. Mean	Fold (Pt./Control)
Increased proteins								
Desmoplakin	SDP	1	198	224	201	331	239	238.5
Keratin, type I cytoskeletal 24	KRT24	26	173	169	182	176	175	6.7
Keratin, type II cytoskeletal 78	KRT78	26	154	146	143	109	138	5.3
Junction plakoglobin	JUP	nd	93	95	97	121	102	∞
luster of Keratin, type II cytoskeletal 73	KRT73	8	89	80	90	62	80	10.0
Hornerin	HRNR	nd	43	53	55	101	63	∞
Keratin, type I cytoskeletal 23	KRT23	nd	57	59	50	50	54	∞
Desmoglein-1	DSG1	0	48	49	43	70	53	∞
Calmodulin-like protein 5	CALML5	nd	42	43	39	45	42	∞
Fatty acid-binding protein 5	FABP5	nd	42	43	39	45	42	∞
Galectin-7	LGALS7	nd	20	18	22	34	24	∞
Cystatin-A	CSTA	nd	17	22	18	25	21	∞
Plakophilin-1	PKP1	1	15	18	21	36	23	22.5
Serpin B12	SERPIN	nd	15	19	12	27	18	∞
Protein-glutamine gamma-glutamyltransferase E	TGM3	nd	12	14	9	24	15	∞
Filaggrin-2	FLG2	1	10	12	6	18	12	11.5
Arginase-1	ARG1	nd	7	9	9	15	10	∞

Table 1. Cont.

MS/MS View: 899 Proteins in 665 Clusters	Alternate ID	Control	Pt. Glm1	Pt. Glm2	Pt. Glm3	Pt. Glm4	Pt. Mean	Fold (Pt./Control)
Complement C3	C3	3	48	55	64	108	69	22.9
Cluster of Keratin, type II cytoskeletal 6A	KRT6A	236	2584	2466	2588	3111	2687	11.4
Cluster of Keratin, type I cytoskeletal 16	KRT16	158	2548	2420	2509	2754	2558	16.2
Keratin, type II cytoskeletal 1	KRT1	403	2078	1946	2049	2205	2070	5.1
Keratin, type I cytoskeletal 9	KRT9	311	1395	1269	1324	1416	1351	4.3
Deceased proteins								
Cluster of Vimentin	VIM	622	233	239	220	257	237	0.4
Cluster of Actin, cytoplasmic 2	ACTG1	500	249	230	234	227	235	0.5
Cluster of Alpha-actinin-4	ACTN4	264	84	92	80	153	102	0.4
Myosin-9	MYH9	213	78	85	93	185	110	0.5
Cluster of Tubulin beta chain	TUBB	103	36	36	34	59	41	0.4
Laminin subunit alpha-5	LAMA5	77	25	30	31	54	35	0.5
Cluster of Histone H2B type 1-M	H2BC14	101	47	40	46	61	49	0.5
basement membrane-specific heparan sulfate proteoglycan core pr.	HSPG2	26	13	14	11	46	21	0.8
Vinculin	VCL	51	13	13	15	40	20	0.4
Podocin	NPHS2	14	7	2	3	7	5	0.3
Podocalyxin	PODXL	9	5	4	4	8	5	0.6
Membranous nephropathy antigens								
Secretory phospholipase A2 receptor	PLA2R1	nd	nd	0	nd	5	1	
Thrombospondin-type -1 domain-containing 7A	THSD7A	nd	nd	nd	nd	nd	nd	
Exostosin 1 and exostosin 2	EXT1/2	nd	nd	nd	nd	nd	nd	
Protein kinase C-binding protein NELL1	NELL1	nd	nd	nd	nd	1	0.25	
Semaphorin 3b	Sema 3B	nd	nd	nd	nd	nd	nd	
Protocadherin 7	PCDH7	nd	nd	nd	nd	nd	nd	
Human high-temperature requirement A1	HTRA1	nd	nd	nd	nd	nd	nd	
Contactin 1		nd	nd	nd	nd	nd	nd	

3.4. Clinical Course

The angiotensin receptor blocker losartan 25 mg was administered to reduce the urinary protein, decreasing it from 3.1 g /gCr to 0.19 to 0.65 g /gCr. When the dose of losartan was reduced to 12.5 mg after 6 months, urinary protein increased slightly to 0.41 g/gCr (Figure 6).

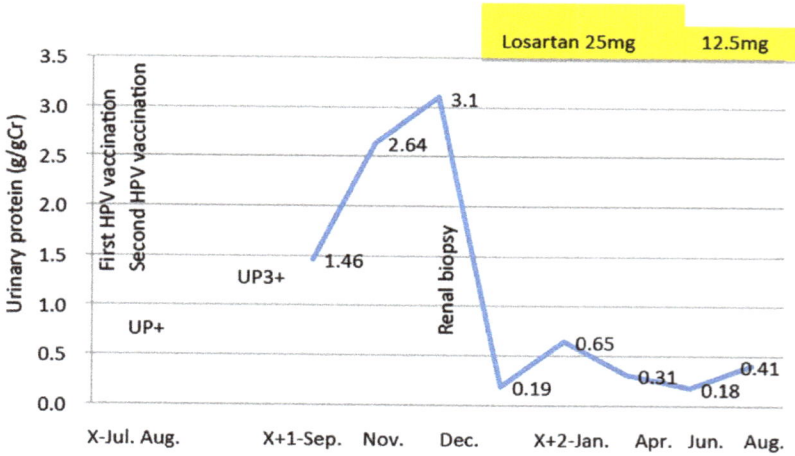

Figure 6. Time course of urinary protein after HPV vaccination and treatment with an angiotensin receptor blocker, losartan, as indicated by the yellow bar.

4. Discussion

This study focuses on a report of membranous nephropathy in an adolescent girl after HPV vaccination, and the pathogenic mechanism is investigated.

4.1. Characteristics of Adolescent Membranous Nephropathy

Membranous nephropathy is a major cause of nephrotic syndrome in middle-aged and elderly people but is rare in adolescents (1–2% of renal biopsies) [17]. Histopathologically, adolescent membranous nephropathy is found in a relatively early phase of Ehrenreich–Churg classification stages 1 and 2, in which patients are frequently positive for IgA, IgM, and C1q, in addition to IgG and C3 [18]. In the IgG subclass, IgG4 was 87.5%, whereas IgG1 was 46.9% and IgG3 was 56.3% were positive in half of the cases [19], and the frequency of PLA2R positivity was slightly lower than that in adults [20]. These data indicate that it is important to investigate secondary membranous nephropathy, such as SLE and HBV infection, in adolescent cases [18]. The present case was secondary membranous nephropathy with predominant IgG1 and IgG3 deposition but was negative for PLA2R. Most of the well-known causes of secondary membranous nephropathy were ruled out from clinical findings and laboratory tests. Therefore, HPV vaccination is presumed to be the cause of membranous nephropathy.

4.2. HPV Virus Infection and Kidney Disease

HPV is a sexually transmitted disease that is persistently transmitted locally to the cervix, and high-risk HPV types 16 and 18 cause about 70% of cervical cancers [8]. Interestingly, mother-to-child transmission can occur at birth [21], and 22.8% of newborns have HPV detected in the oral cavity at birth [22]. It is possible that even young people who have never had sexual intercourse have already been infected with HPV. In addition, 30.3% of 122 patients with renal cell carcinoma were found to be positive for HPV-DNA in the renal cell carcinoma site of the paraffin specimens by PCR method, 20.3% were found to be positive by immunostaining for p16-INK4a, and 45% were found to be positive for HPV by the in situ hybridization method [23]. This indicates that HPV was infected and latent in the kidney. In this case, p16-INK4a protein, a surrogate marker of HPV infection [12,13], was found in glomerular cells (Figure 4B) by immunohistochemistry and also in the urinary protein by Western blotting analysis (Figure 5). Therefore, it is possible that the patient was infected with HPV, having an antibody against it, and administration of viral protein as a vaccine formed circulating immune complexes and developed proteinuria soon after vaccination. The p16-INK4a is also detected in the glomerulus and tubules of the aging kidney and in kidneys with chronic allograft rejection [24,25], even though this was not the case with this young patient. HPV envelope proteins, such as E1 proteins, induce overexpression of a set of genes associated with proliferation and differentiation processes and downregulation of immune response genes [26]. LMD-MS, in this case, showed an increase in cytoskeletal proteins and epithelial junctional proteins as well, as downregulation of nephrin, podocin, and podocalyxin may reflect HPV infection in the podocytes. Unfortunately, we could not detect HPV envelope proteins by LMD-MS analysis. The possibility of primary membranous nephropathy still remains, as LMD-MS analysis detected a small amount of PLA2R protein in one glomerular sample.

4.3. Kidney Disease associated with Vaccination

In this study, the urinary protein was observed with a fever of 39 °C after two doses of a recombinant precipitated divalent HPV-like particle vaccine.

As shown in Table 2, a case of acute kidney injury and nephrotic syndrome due to membranous nephropathy was reported after influenza vaccination [27]. It has been reported that nephrotic syndrome could be caused by the HBV vaccine [28], pneumococcal vaccine [29], and COVID-19 vaccine [1,30]. However, there has never been a report of nephrotic syndrome caused by the HPV vaccine, and to the best of our knowledge, this study presents the first report of such a case.

Table 2. Nephrotic syndrome and nephritis associated with vaccination.

Reference	Age Sex	Vaccine	Onset after Injection	Proteinuria	Renal Function	Renal Biopsy	Treatment	Prognosis
Patel [27]	60 F	Influenza	2 weeks	20.5 g/day	AKI	MN stage 1, AIN	HD, PSL	CR with relapse
Kutlucan [31]	56 M	Influenza	20 days	7.3 g/day	Cr 1.2 mg/dL	MN IgG, C3	PSL1 mg/kg	CR
Kao [32]	72 M	Influenza	<2 weeks	5.7 g/day	ND	ND	mPSL pulse PEX	GBS UP decreased after 10 M
Kielstein [33]	65 F	Influenza	4 days	10.8 g/day	Ccr 65 mL/min	MCNS	Conservative	CR
Gutiérrez [34]	44 M	Influenza	18 days	4 g/day	Cr 4.4 mg/dL	MCNS	PSL60 mg	CR
Mader [35]	86 F	Influenza				HSP		CR
Patel [36]	77 M	Influenza	10 days	ND	Cr2.31 mg/dL	Mesangial proliferative GN, HSP	PSL60 mg	CR
Yanai-Berar [37]	63 M	Influenza	11 days	1.5 g/day	Cr 1.8 mg/dL	Pauci-immune crescentic GN	PSL60 mg	CR
Islek [28]	4 M	HBV	8 days	2 g/m^2/day	ND	ND	PSL	CR
Kikuchi [29]	67 F	Polyvalent pneumococcal polysaccharide	1 week	10.4 g/day	Cr 1.33 mg/dL	MCNS with TIN	mPSL pulse	CR
Claujus [38]	82 F	Tetanus–diphtheria–poliomyelitis	6 weeks	12 g/day	Cr 0.84 mg/dL	MCNS	PSL75 mg	CR
Anupama [30]	19 F	hAdOx1 nCoV-19	8 days	3.18 g/gCr	Cr1.09 mg/dL	MCNS	PSL1 mg/kg	CR
Lebedev [1]	50 M	BNT162b2 COVID-19	10 days	6.9 g/day	Cr 2.31 mg/dL	MCNS AIN	PSL	CR
Maas [39]	80 M	BNT162b2 COVID-19	7 days	15.3 g/gCr	Cr 1.43 mg/dL	MCNS	PSL80 mg	PR1
Present case	16 F	HPV	5 days	1.46 g/gCr	Cr 0.47 mg/dL	MN	ARB	PR1

The HPV vaccine Cervarix contains added aluminum hydroxide and monophosphoryl lipid A (MPL) derived from the cell membrane of Salmonella as an adjuvant. Aluminum oxyhydroxide (alum) binds to viral DNA fragments and lipid A derivatives to form alum-nanoparticles, which are taken up by macrophages and form a granulomatous lesion called macrophagic myofasciitis (MMF) [40,41]. MMF in the vaccine injection site induces cell death, and adjuvants conjugate with degraded nuclear DNA and proteins, producing autoantibodies, which may cause Guillain–Barré syndrome, SLE, autologous immune hepatitis, and cerebrovascular inflammation. These are so-called adjuvant diseases, an autoimmune/autoinflammatory syndrome induced by adjuvant (ASIA) [40,42,43]. In this case, the possibility of lupus was ruled out from clinical findings and immunological data.

5. Conclusions

We reported a case of young-onset IgG1-dominant and PLA2R-negative secondary membranous nephropathy after HPV vaccination. Since p16-INK4a was positive in glomerular and urinary proteins, she may have been infected with HPV, and administration of HPV envelop protein vaccines could be implicated in the development of secondary membranous nephropathy.

6. Take-Home Message and Lessons Learned

It is important to check proteinuria after HPV vaccination. Secondary membranous nephropathy could occur after HPV vaccination with viral proteins. If it is possible to check the plasma antibody titers for HPV before vaccination, this may help to prevent the occurrence of membranous nephropathy.

Supplementary Materials: The following supporting information can be downloaded at: https://www.mdpi.com/article/10.3390/vaccines10091442/s1, Figure S1 shows the whole proteins identified by LMD-MS analysis.

Author Contributions: Conceptualization, A.T.; methodology, A.T., Y.U., D.K. and K.H.; software, S.Y.; validation, Y.U., K.H. and A.T.; formal analysis, A.T.; investigation, H.A., S.Y. and D.K.; resources, A.T., Y.U. and K.H.; data curation, A.T. and D.K.; writing—original draft preparation, H.A., T.O. and A.T.; writing—review and editing, A.T. and K.H.; visualization, H.A., D.K. and A.T.; supervision, A.T., K.H. and Y.U.; project administration, A.T., K.H. and Y.U.; funding acquisition, A.T. and K.H. All authors have read and agreed to the published version of the manuscript.

Funding: This work was partially supported by a research donation from Naohiko Kobayashi, Director of Kobayashi Medical Clinic in Yasuzuka, Mibu, Japan (#2020-9, #2022-7).

Institutional Review Board Statement: The renal biopsy and sample analysis were performed with the approval of the research ethics committee of Dokkyo Medical University (R-2-1).

Informed Consent Statement: Written informed consent was obtained from the patient at the renal biopsy to use samples and data in anonymized reports or publications.

Data Availability Statement: A table showing all of the data from the LMD-MS analysis is available upon Supplementary Material.

Acknowledgments: We thank Kinichi Matsuyama and Mihoko Ishikawa from the Department of Pathology, Dokkyo Medical University, for their excellent technical help concerning immunohistochemistry and electron microscopy. We also thank Yasuko Mamada from the Clinical Research Support Center for assistance with the Western blotting.

Conflicts of Interest: The authors declare no conflict of interest.

References

1. Lebedev, L.; Sapojnikov, M.; Wechsler, A.; Varadi-Levi, R.; Zamir, D.; Tobar, A.; Levin-Iaina, N.; Fytlovich, S.; Yagil, Y. Minimal Change Disease Following the Pfizer-BioNTech COVID-19 Vaccine. *Am. J. Kidney Dis.* **2021**, *78*, 142–145. [CrossRef] [PubMed]
2. Lim, J.H.; Han, M.H.; Kim, Y.J.; Kim, M.S.; Jung, H.Y.; Choi, J.Y.; Cho, J.H.; Kim, C.D.; Kim, Y.L.; Park, S.H. New-onset Nephrotic Syndrome after Janssen COVID-19 Vaccination: A Case Report and Literature Review. *J. Korean Med. Sci.* **2021**, *36*, e218. [CrossRef] [PubMed]
3. Mancianti, N.; Guarnieri, A.; Tripodi, S.; Salvo, D.P.; Garosi, G. Minimal change disease following vaccination for SARS-CoV-2. *J. Nephrol.* **2021**, *34*, 1039–1040. [CrossRef] [PubMed]
4. Negrea, L.; Rovin, B.H. Gross hematuria following vaccination for severe acute respiratory syndrome coronavirus 2 in 2 patients with IgA nephropathy. *Kidney Int.* **2021**, *99*, 1487. [CrossRef]
5. Okuhara, T.; Ishikawa, H.; Okada, M.; Kato, M.; Kiuchi, T. Contents of Japanese pro- and anti-HPV vaccination websites: A text mining analysis. *Patient Educ. Couns.* **2018**, *101*, 406–413. [CrossRef]
6. Cutts, F.T.; Franceschi, S.; Goldie, S.; Castellsague, X.; de Sanjose, S.; Garnett, G.; Edmunds, W.J.; Claeys, P.; Goldenthal, K.L.; Harper, D.M.; et al. Human papillomavirus and HPV vaccines: A review. *Bull. World Health Organ.* **2007**, *85*, 719–726. [CrossRef]
7. Egawa, N.; Egawa, K.; Griffin, H.; Doorbar, J. Human Papillomaviruses; Epithelial Tropisms, and the Development of Neoplasia. *Viruses* **2015**, *7*, 3863–3890. [CrossRef]
8. Onuki, M.; Matsumoto, K.; Iwata, T.; Yamamoto, K.; Aoki, Y.; Maenohara, S.; Tsuda, N.; Kamiura, S.; Takehara, K.; Horie, K.; et al. Human papillomavirus genotype contribution to cervical cancer and precancer: Implications for screening and vaccination in Japan. *Cancer Sci.* **2020**, *111*, 2546–2557. [CrossRef]
9. Ikeda, S.; Ueda, Y.; Yagi, A.; Matsuzaki, S.; Kobayashi, E.; Kimura, T.; Miyagi, E.; Sekine, M.; Enomoto, T.; Kudoh, K. HPV vaccination in Japan: What is happening in Japan? *Expert Rev. Vaccines* **2019**, *18*, 323–325. [CrossRef]
10. Nakayama, T. An inflammatory response is essential for the development of adaptive immunity-immunogenicity and immunotoxicity. *Vaccine* **2016**, *34*, 5815–5818. [CrossRef]
11. Kashiwagi, Y.; Maeda, M.; Kawashima, H.; Nakayama, T. Inflammatory responses following intramuscular and subcutaneous immunization with aluminum-adjuvanted or non-adjuvanted vaccines. *Vaccine* **2014**, *32*, 3393–3401. [CrossRef] [PubMed]
12. Carozzi, F.; Confortini, M.; Dalla Palma, P.; Del Mistro, A.; Gillio-Tos, A.; De Marco, L.; Giorgi-Rossi, P.; Pontenani, G.; Rosso, S.; Sani, C.; et al. Use of p16-INK4A overexpression to increase the specificity of human papillomavirus testing: A nested substudy of the NTCC randomised controlled trial. *Lancet Oncol.* **2008**, *9*, 937–945. [CrossRef]

13. Rischin, D.; Young, R.J.; Fisher, R.; Fox, S.B.; Le, Q.T.; Peters, L.J.; Solomon, B.; Choi, J.; O'Sullivan, B.; Kenny, L.M.; et al. Prognostic significance of p16INK4A and human papillomavirus in patients with oropharyngeal cancer treated on TROG 02.02 phase III trial. *J. clin. Oncol. Off. J. Am. Soc. Clin. Oncol.* **2010**, *28*, 4142–4148. [CrossRef] [PubMed]
14. Ishimitsu, A.; Tojo, A.; Hirao, J.; Yokoyama, S.; Ohira, T.; Murayama, T.; Ishimitsu, T.; Kang, D.; Honda, K.; Ehara, T.; et al. AL-Kappa Primary Amyloidosis with Apolipoprotein A-IV Deposition. *Intern. Med.* **2022**, *61*, 871–876. [CrossRef]
15. Sethi, S. New 'Antigens' in Membranous Nephropathy. *J. Am. Soc. Nephrol. JASN* **2021**, *32*, 268–278. [CrossRef]
16. Caza, T.N.; Al-Rabadi, L.F.; Beck, L.H., Jr. How Times Have Changed! A Cornucopia of Antigens for Membranous Nephropathy. *Front. Immunol.* **2021**, *12*, 800242. [CrossRef]
17. International Study of Kidney Disease in Children. Nephrotic Syndrome in Children—Prediction of Histopathology from Clinical and Laboratory Characteristics at Time of Diagnosis. *Kidney Int.* **1978**, *13*, 159–165. [CrossRef]
18. Wang, Y.; Wang, G.P.; Li, B.M.; Chen, Q.K. Clinicopathological analysis of idiopathic membranous nephropathy in young adults. *Genet. Mol. Res.* **2015**, *14*, 4541–4548. [CrossRef]
19. Li, C.; Li, H.; Wen, Y.B.; Li, J.N.; Lin, W.F.; Cai, J.F.; Duan, L.; Li, Y.; Li, X.M.; Li, X.W. Clinicopathological Features of Idiopathic Membranous Nephropathy in 33 Adolescents. *Zhongguo Yi Xue Ke Xue Yuan Xue Bao Acta Acad. Med. Sin.* **2017**, *39*, 544–551.
20. Dettmar, A.K.; Wiech, T.; Kemper, M.J.; Soave, A.; Rink, M.; Oh, J.; Stahl, R.A.K.; Hoxha, E. Immunohistochemical and serological characterization of membranous nephropathy in children and adolescents. *Pediatric Nephrol.* **2018**, *33*, 463–472. [CrossRef]
21. Cason, J.; Kaye, J.N.; Jewers, R.J.; Kambo, P.K.; Bible, J.M.; Kell, B.; Shergill, B.; Pakarian, F.; Raju, K.S.; Best, J.M. Perinatal Infection and Persistence of Human Papillomavirus Type-16 and Type-18 in Infants. *J. Med. Virol* **1995**, *47*, 209–218. [CrossRef]
22. Syrjanen, S.; Rintala, M.; Sarkola, M.; Willberg, J.; Rautava, J.; Koskimaa, H.; Paaso, A.; Syrjanen, K.; Grenman, S.; Louvanto, K. Oral Human Papillomavirus Infection in Children during the First 6 Years of Life, Finland. *Emerg. Infect. Dis.* **2021**, *27*, 759–766. [CrossRef] [PubMed]
23. Farhadi, A.; Behzad-Behbahani, A.; Geramizadeh, B.; Sekawi, Z.; Rahsaz, M.; Sharifzadeh, S. High-risk human papillomavirus infection in different histological subtypes of renal cell carcinoma. *J. Med. Virol.* **2014**, *86*, 1134–1144. [CrossRef] [PubMed]
24. Chkhotua, A.B.; Gabusi, E.; Altimari, A.; D'Errico, A.; Yakubovich, M.; Vienken, J.; Stefoni, S.; Chieco, P.; Yussim, A.; Grigioni, W.F. Increased expression of p16(INK4a) and p27(Kip1) cyclin-dependent kinase inhibitor genes in aging human kidney and chronic allograft nephropathy. *Am. J. Kidney Dis.* **2003**, *41*, 1303–1313. [CrossRef]
25. Melk, A.; Schmidt, B.M.; Takeuchi, O.; Sawitzki, B.; Rayner, D.C.; Halloran, P.F. Expression of p16INK4a and other cell cycle regulator and senescence associated genes in aging human kidney. *Kidney Int.* **2004**, *65*, 510–520. [CrossRef] [PubMed]
26. Castro-Muñoz, L.J.; Manzo-Merino, J.; Muñoz-Bello, J.O.; Olmedo-Nieva, L.; Cedro-Tanda, A.; Alfaro-Ruiz, L.A.; Hidalgo-Miranda, A.; Madrid-Marina, V.; Lizano, M. The Human Papillomavirus (HPV) E1 protein regulates the expression of cellular genes involved in immune response. *Sci. Rep.* **2019**, *9*, 13620. [CrossRef] [PubMed]
27. Patel, C.; Shah, H.H. Membranous nephropathy and severe acute kidney injury following influenza vaccination. *Saudi J. Kidney Dis. Transplant. Off. Publ. Saudi Cent. Organ Transplant. Saudi Arabia* **2015**, *26*, 1289–1293.
28. Işlek, I.; Cengiz, K.; Cakir, M.; Küçüködük, S. Nephrotic syndrome following hepatitis B vaccination. *Pediatric Nephrol.* **2000**, *14*, 89–90.
29. Kikuchi, Y.; Imakiire, T.; Hyodo, T.; Higashi, K.; Henmi, N.; Suzuki, S.; Miura, S. Minimal change nephrotic syndrome, lymphadenopathy and hyperimmunoglobulinemia after immunization with a pneumococcal vaccine. *Clin. Nephrol.* **2002**, *58*, 68–72. [CrossRef]
30. Anupama, Y.J.; Patel, R.G.N.; Vankalakunti, M. Nephrotic Syndrome Following ChAdOx1 nCoV-19 Vaccine Against SARScoV-2. *Kidney Int. Rep.* **2021**, *6*, 2248. [CrossRef]
31. Kutlucan, A.; Gonen, I.; Yildizhan, E.; Aydin, Y.; Sav, T.; Yildirim, U. Can influenza H1N1 vaccination lead to the membranous glomerulonephritis? *Indian J. Pathol. Microbiol.* **2012**, *55*, 239–241. [PubMed]
32. Kao, C.D.; Chen, J.T.; Lin, K.P.; Shan, D.E.; Wu, Z.A.; Liao, K.K. Guillain-Barré syndrome coexisting with pericarditis or nephrotic syndrome after influenza vaccination. *Clin. Neurol. Neurosurg.* **2004**, *106*, 136–138. [CrossRef] [PubMed]
33. Kielstein, J.T.; Termühlen, L.; Sohn, J.; Kliem, V. Minimal change nephrotic syndrome in a 65-year-old patient following influenza vaccination. *Clin. Nephrol.* **2000**, *54*, 246–248. [PubMed]
34. Gutiérrez, S.; Dotto, B.; Petitti, J.P.; De Paul, A.L.; Dionisio de Cabalier, M.E.; Torres, A.I.; Mukdsi, J.H. Minimal change disease following influenza vaccination and acute renal failure: Just a coincidence? *Nefrol. Publ. Off. Soc. Esp. Nefrol.* **2012**, *32*, 414–415.
35. Mader, R.; Narendran, A.; Lewtas, J.; Bykerk, V.; Goodman, R.C.; Dickson, J.R.; Keystone, E.C. Systemic vasculitis following influenza vaccination–report of 3 cases and literature review. *J. Rheumatol.* **1993**, *20*, 1429–1431.
36. Patel, U.; Bradley, J.R.; Hamilton, D.V. Henoch-Schonlein Purpura after Influenza Vaccination. *Br. Med. J.* **1988**, *296*, 1800. [CrossRef]
37. Yanai-Berar, N.; Ben-Itzhak, O.; Gree, J.; Nakhoul, F. Influenza vaccination induced leukocytoclastic vasculitis and pauci-immune crescentic glomerulonephritis. *Clin. Nephrol.* **2002**, *58*, 220–223. [CrossRef]
38. Clajus, C.; Spiegel, J.; Bröcker, V.; Chatzikyrkou, C.; Kielstein, J.T. Minimal change nephrotic syndrome in an 82 year old patient following a tetanus-diphteria-poliomyelitis-vaccination. *BMC Nephrol.* **2009**, *10*, 21. [CrossRef]
39. Maas, R.J.; Gianotten, S.; van der Meijden, W.A.G. An Additional Case of Minimal Change Disease Following the Pfizer-BioNTech COVID-19 Vaccine. *Am. J. Kidney Dis.* **2021**, *78*, 312. [CrossRef]
40. Gherardi, R.K.; Authier, F.J. Macrophagic myofasciitis: Characterization and pathophysiology. *Lupus* **2012**, *21*, 184–189. [CrossRef]

41. Gherardi, R.K.; Coquet, M.; Cherin, P.; Authier, F.J.; Laforet, P.; Belec, L.; Figarella-Branger, D.; Mussini, J.M.; Pellissier, J.F.; Fardeau, M.; et al. Macrophagic myofasciitis: An emerging entity. *Lancet* **1998**, *352*, 347–352. [CrossRef]
42. Agmon-Levin, N.; Paz, Z.; Israeli, E.; Shoenfeld, Y. Vaccines and autoimmunity. *Nat. Rev. Rheumatol.* **2009**, *5*, 648–652. [CrossRef] [PubMed]
43. Shoenfeld, Y.; Agmon-Levin, N. 'ASIA'—Autoimmune/inflammatory syndrome induced by adjuvants. *J. Autoimmun.* **2011**, *36*, 4–8. [CrossRef] [PubMed]

Article

HPV-Vaccine Hesitancy in Colombia: A Mixed-Methods Study

Veronica Cordoba-Sanchez [1,*], Mariantonia Lemos [2], Diego Alfredo Tamayo-Lopera [1] and Sherri Sheinfeld Gorin [3,*]

1 Department of Psychology, School of Social Sciences, Institucion Universitaria de Envigado, Envigado 055422, Colombia; datamayo@correo.iue.edu.co
2 Department of Psychology, School of Arts and Social Sciences, Universidad EAFIT, Medellín 050022, Colombia; mlemosh@eafit.edu.co
3 School of Medicine, University of Michigan, Ann Arbor, MI 48109, USA
* Correspondence: vcordobas@correo.iue.edu.co (V.C.-S.); ssgorin@med.umich.edu (S.S.G.)

Abstract: In Colombia, the uptake rate of the HPV vaccine dropped from 96.7% after its introduction in 2013 to 9% in 2020. To identify the behavioural components of HPV-vaccine hesitancy in females aged 15 and under and their families, we conducted a convergent mixed-methods study in which 196 parents/caregivers responded to an online questionnaire and 10 focus groups were held with 13 of these parents/caregivers, and 50 age-eligible girls. The study is novel as it is the first to explore the factors influencing HPV-vaccine hesitancy alongside the COVID vaccine within an integrative model of behaviour change, the capability-opportunity-motivation-behaviour (COM-B) model. We found that COVID-19 has had an impact on the awareness of HPV and HPV vaccination. Lack of information about the vaccination programs, concerns about vaccine safety and the relationship between HPV and sexuality could be related to vaccine hesitancy. Trust in medical recommendations and campaigns focused on the idea that vaccination is a way of protecting daughters from cervical cancer could improve HPV vaccine uptake.

Keywords: vaccination; human papilloma virus; health behaviour; vaccine hesitancy; cervical cancer

1. Introduction

Cervical cancer is the fourth-most-common cancer among women worldwide. In 2020, there were an estimated of 604,127 new cases and 341,831 deaths [1]. In less-developed countries, its incidence is higher and it ranks second for mortality, after breast cancer [2]. In Colombia, cervical cancer has a crude incidence rate of 18.3 per 100,000 women per year (95% UI: 4.311–5.216) and a mortality rate of 9.61 (95% UI: 2.316–2.677) [3]. In 2020, 7.9% of all new cancer cases in Colombian women were of cervical cancer, the equivalent of 4742 new cases [4]. Population-based studies in this country report that women diagnosed with cervical cancer are younger, of lower incomes, and more often live in non-metropolitan/rural areas than those diagnosed with breast cancer [5]. The highest mortality rates are observed in the most deprived regions (along the main rivers, harbours, and cities along the country's borders). The low impact of cervical cancer screening programs in the country is attributed to the poor quality of pap smears; low coverage, especially of women at high risk; and a lack of or partial follow-up of women with abnormal cytology [6].

Almost all cervical cancers are caused by persistent infections with oncogenic, or high-risk, types of human papillomavirus [7,8]. Rates of cervical cancer have declined worldwide in countries with successful HPV-vaccination strategies, cervical cancer screening programs, and the treatment of cervical intraepithelial neoplasia (CIN) earlier in the pathogenesis pathway to invasive cervical cancer [9–21]. By contrast, countries without cervical cancer prevention and control strategies—or where the strategies are not effective—have seen a rapid increase in early mortality due to this pathology [2], especially in low- and middle-income countries [22]. To encourage wider implementation of successful cervical cancer prevention and control strategies worldwide, on 17 November 2020, after the closure of the 73rd World Health Assembly, the WHO Global Strategy for Cervical Cancer Elimination was formalized [23]. WHO set the following goals for 2030: 90% of girls fully vaccinated with the HPV vaccine by the age of 15, 70% of women screened using a high-performance test by the age of 35, and again by the age of 45, and 90% of women diagnosed with pre-cancer and invasive cancer treated [24].

While HPV vaccines are effective against many of the oncogenic types of HPV, vaccination uptake and completion are low among young Colombian females. In 2012, Colombia was among the first countries in South America to implement HPV vaccination among age-eligible girls, reaching 97.5% uptake of first doses and 96.7% uptake of second doses. In 2013, Colombia's HPV vaccination rate was one of the highest in the world [25]. In 2014, however, a group of young women in a Colombian coastal town who had been vaccinated experienced a mass psychogenic response including fainting spells, weakness, limb paraesthesia, chest pain, tachycardia, and headaches (the "Carmen de Bolivar" event). The purported vaccine side effects were videoed by various media outlets and shared widely on social networks [26]. While the Instituto Nacional de Salud Colombiano (Colombian National Health Institute) conducted a rigorous epidemiological study of this event and did not find any organic association between the vaccine and symptoms described [27], the lingering effects of the event continued to lower HPV vaccine rates in 2016 to 14% for first doses and 5% for the second. By 2021, however, the rate of HPV uptake had risen to 39.4% for first doses and 11.8% for second doses, according to the Colombia Health Ministry [28].

This crisis was similar to others in countries such as Denmark, Japan, and Austria. Denmark experienced a rapid decline in vaccination in 2014 following negative public attention coinciding with increased suspected adverse event reporting to the Danish Medicines Agency. This negative public attention included stories of the supposedly harmful effects of HPV vaccination that were widely shared on social media [29,30]. In Japan, active recommendations for HPV vaccination were suspended in June 2013 following media reports of girls having various symptoms such as chronic pain and motor impairment after vaccination [31]. The suspension remained until November 2021, despite large-scale epidemiologic studies showing the effectiveness and safety of the vaccine in Japan and worldwide, and the scientific community repeatedly calling for the resumption of active recommendations by the Japanese government [31]. In Austria, the HPV vaccine was licensed in 2006, comparatively early relative to other countries, but was not free of debate in a nation with a historical scepticism towards vaccination. To retain the HPV vaccine, policy makers and scientific experts disassociated the vaccine from gender, vaccine manufacturers, and youth sexuality, ultimately making the vaccine a strength of the Austrian Immunization Program [32].

These crises have led to lowering the rates of HPV vaccination worldwide, with the current rate of HPV vaccination far below the 90% goal proposed by the WHO [23]. Factors associated with vaccine hesitancy in South America are a lack of information and doubts about its safety and effectiveness [33]. These results were similar to those found in a qualitative study of young females in Colombia that highlighted that parents/caregivers of girls eligible for the first dose of the HPV vaccine had little knowledge about the aetiology of cervical cancer, had not received information about vaccination benefits, and feared its adverse events [34].

Since HPV vaccination requires parental consent, parental hesitancy may be one of the strongest influences on uptake among adolescent females [35]. Parental HPV-vaccine hesitancy is a complex phenomenon that is influenced by lack of information, the opinions of important others, the attitudes/beliefs of healthcare providers, news about adverse effects, religious beliefs, and, as HPV is a sexually-transmitted infection, attitudes towards adolescent sexual behaviour [36].

The aim of this study is to identify the behavioural components of HPV-vaccine hesitancy among girls aged 15 and under and their families at educational institutions in

Colombia. These factors are best understood within an integrative model of behaviour change. This study relies on the capability-opportunity-motivation-behaviour (COM-B) model of behaviour [37]. To our knowledge, the study is the first to explore the factors influencing HPV-vaccine hesitancy alongside the COVID vaccine in Colombia within an integrative model of behaviour change.

In accord with a phased approach to behavioural research [38], the findings from this study are intended to undergird a subsequent efficacy trial of a behavioural intervention to decrease HPV-vaccine hesitancy.

2. Materials and Methods

2.1. Study Design

This study used a convergent mixed-methods design with multiple data collection strategies to ensure completeness and integration of results, and to describe the perspectives of participants at different levels in a system (Figure 1).

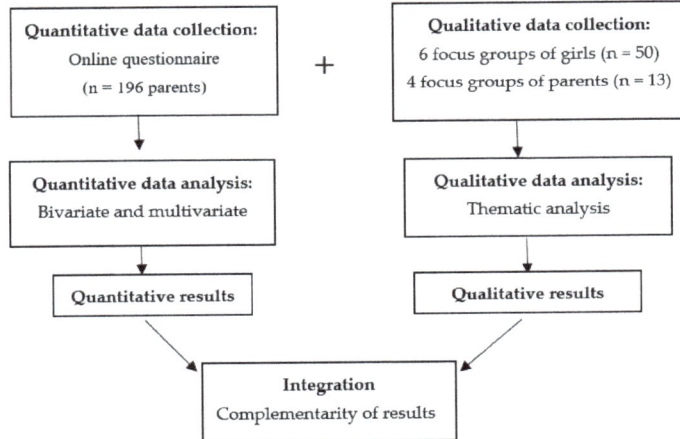

Figure 1. Convergent mixed-methods design.

2.2. Setting

Medellín is in the Metropolitan Area of the Aburra Valley; this is the second-largest urban area of Colombia with more than four million people. The city has 229 public schools (from first to eleventh grade of basic education) and 337 private (with tuition) schools (including kindergarten only) [39]. Healthcare in Colombia is both private, or contributory, and public, with a government subsidy, depending on household income levels. The HPV-vaccine is administered in schools, hospitals, and health centres in a two-dose series (0, 6 months) with no cost for girls between 9 and 17 years old and a three-doses series (0, 6, 60 months) for women 18 years and older [40].

2.3. Study Model

We used the COM-B model (capability, opportunity, motivation, and behaviour [38]), to select the study's quantitative measures and for qualitative data collection, and as a guide for analysing the data. COM-B posits that behaviour change is influenced by three factors: (1) capability, having the physical and psychological abilities to engage in the behaviour; (2) opportunity, having the physical or social opportunities to engage in the behaviour; and (3) motivation, psychological processes that energise and direct behaviour such as the belief that a behaviour is important and/or socially desirable [41].

2.4. Participants

All age-eligible female students (9–15 years) with an incomplete vaccination schedule (0 or 1 dose) and their parents from schools in Medellín and surrounding cities were recruited to participate in the study. The convenience sample was comprised of 196 parents who consented to participate in the online questionnaire and 50 girls who participated in the focus groups after their parents' consent was given.

2.5. Study Measures

Based on the COM-B model, we developed an online questionnaire that was administered to the sample of parents (see items in Appendix A). The quantitative measures were: perceived susceptibility, vaccine awareness, trust, beliefs about vaccine safety and efficacy, likelihood of vaccinating, factors influencing the decision to vaccinate or to complete the vaccination schedule, and intention to complete the vaccination schedule.

The same questions were asked of both the parents and the young women who participated in 10 focus groups, alongside prompts to encourage them to explain their responses more fully, to gain a deeper understanding of their thinking patterns within their social contexts [42]. An example is: "If you are worried about the safety of the HPV vaccine, tell us—what are your concerns?" By matching the qualitative focus-group questions to the quantitative survey items, we were able to integrate and interpret findings from the two approaches in a joint display.

2.6. Procedure

A convenience sample of three public and one private school was recruited; within each school, invitations were sent to parents to complete the online questionnaire and to participate in focus groups. In addition, to reach the largest possible number of participants in the defined geographical area, the online questionnaire was also shared in the social-media and instant-messaging groups of parents from different schools. Parents/caregivers who attended the focus groups were also asked for permission for us to contact their daughters to participate in focus groups with other girls from their own school and of the same approximate age. Groups with parents/caregivers were conducted using video-call platforms (Microsoft Teams and Google Meet) and lasted an average of 34.7 min. They were coordinated by a male psychologist and two research assistants. The girls' groups lasted an average of 28 min and were coordinated by a female psychologist and two research assistants using a room and schedule provided by the schools.

2.7. Ethics

Before starting, both parents and girls gave their consent and assent, respectively, in writing. All focus groups were recorded and then transcribed verbatim for subsequent analysis. Data were collected between September and November 2021. This project was approved by the Universidad EAFIT Ethics Board.

2.8. Data Analysis

The sample was characterized by descriptive statistics. Associations were established between categorical variables using Fisher's chi-square, and correlations were established using Spearman's rho. A binary logistic regression analysis of the probability of HPV vaccination was conducted, with the following independent variables: socioeconomic position, religion, factors associated with vaccination uptake such as cost, and medical recommendation, in accord with the COM-B model.

The qualitative data were analysed with thematic analysis [43], using AtlasTi version 7.5.4 for data management. Thematic analysis included: (1) Familiarization: Transcribing the entire dataset, and reading it twice to gain familiarity with the data; (2) Coding: generating initial codes, attaching codes to significant quotes, refining codes through two rounds to collate or split them if necessary; (3) Generating initial themes: examining the codes and looking for patterns and connections to cluster similar codes and create candidate themes; (4) Developing and reviewing themes, using visual maps and reading the codes of each theme; (5) Refining and naming themes; and (6) Writing the synthesis of each theme and attaching illustrative quotes.

The data were integrated by assessing the concordance between the quantitative and qualitative results according to the components of the COM-B model. As is common in mixed-methods analyses, quantitative data were elaborated and further explained with the qualitative data through a joint display table, a strategy to organize and integrate the data and show how they were mixed [44]. Our joint display showed both the quantitative factors influencing HPV-vaccine hesitancy for parents/caregivers and daughters based on the COM-B model and the qualitative information to support each component.

3. Results

3.1. Description of the Sample

One hundred and ninety-six adults, with an average age of 42.2 years (SD = 6.39), 89.3% of whom were female, responded to the online questionnaire (see Table 1). Of the respondents, 13 parents/caregivers agreed to participate in the focus groups. Fifty girls aged 9–15 (average age of 11.5 years, SD = 1.9) who were students from schools in Medellín and surrounding cities, with an incomplete vaccination schedule (0 or 1 dose), participated in the focus groups (see Table 2).

Table 1. Sociodemographic characteristics of online questionnaire participants (N = 196).

Adults	%	N
Sex		
Female	89.3%	175
Male	10.7%	21
Socioeconomic status		
Low	15.8%	31
Medium	23.5%	46
High	60.7%	119
Daughter's school type		
Private	71.4%	140
Public	28.6%	56
Doses		
0	57.1%	112
1	42.9%	84
Religious practice		
Yes	82.7	162
No	17.3	34
Healthcare-system affiliation		
Contributory plan	96.9%	190
Subsidized plan	3.1%	6

3.2. Analysis Based on the COM-B Model

In the sections that follow, we present both quantitative and qualitative findings aligned with the COM-B model. Qualitative themes were determined by matching content of the focus groups with constructs from the model after analysis (see Table 3). In the COM-B component capability, the themes that we established were 'lack of information' and 'the relationship between HPV and cervical cancer.' The only theme describing opportunity was trust in traditional institutions. The association of HPV with sexuality and the vaccine as an act of care was related to automatic motivation, while respect for the personal decision to be vaccinated was related to reflective motivation. One theme that was transversal to each component was the impact of COVID-19 on the conception of HPV.

Table 2. Sociodemographic characteristics of girls and adolescents in focus groups (N = 50).

Girls and Adolescents	%	N
Education level		
Primary	60%	30
Secondary	40%	20
Type of school		
Private	48%	24
Public	52%	26
School location		
Urban	74%	37
Rural	26%	13
Doses		
0	42%	21
1	58%	29

Table 3. A joint display of factors influencing HPV-vaccine hesitancy to parents/caregivers and daughters based on the COM-B model.

Source of Behaviour	Quantitative Data from the Online Questionnaire	Themes from the Focus Groups
Capability	11.7% did not perceive that their daughter would be susceptible to contracting HPV. Relationship between likelihood of vaccinating daughter and perceived susceptibility to HPV; Spearman $r = 0.309$, $p < 0.001$. 84.7% perceived that their daughter was susceptible to cervical cancer. 96.9% were aware that they should get their daughter vaccinated. 69.4% did not receive any information about HPV vaccination for their daughter. 87.8% trusted the information they received about vaccines. Relationship between likelihood of getting vaccinated and receiving positive information about the vaccine; Spearman $r = 0.338$, $p < 0.001$	Lack of information Relationship between HPV and cervical cancer
Opportunity	Relationship between likelihood of getting vaccinated and medical recommendation; Spearman $r = 0.221$, $p < 0.01$ Relationship between likelihood of getting vaccinated and seeing others get vaccinated; Spearman $r = 0.158$, $p < 0.05$	Trust in traditional institutions
Motivation	30.1% were concerned about vaccine effectiveness 32.7% were concerned because vaccines may have adverse effects 31.6% were concerned about vaccine safety Relationship between likelihood of getting vaccinated and vaccine safety; Spearman $r = 0.277$, $p < 0.001$.	Association of HPV with sexuality The vaccine as an act of care Respect for the personal decision to be vaccinated

3.2.1. Capability

Most participants perceived a susceptibility to cervical cancer and HPV, and were aware that their daughters should be vaccinated, but 69.4% stated they had not received any information about the vaccine. Likewise, there was a relationship between the likelihood of getting their daughter vaccinated and perceived susceptibility to HPV, as well as receiving positive information about the vaccine. Qualitative analyses confirmed that parents did not have enough information about the vaccine and vaccine programs, and some cited misinformation about the Carmen de Bolivar event. Additionally, there is a recognition that cancer is a severe disease that could be treatable if it is diagnosed early. However, participants were not completely aware of the link between HPV and cancer because they thought that, given the age of the girls, they were not at risk.

Lack of Information

Participants reported a lack of information about HPV; further, many still remembered the images of the women and girls who fainted en masse in Carmen de Bolivar. For example, one of the parents said: *"I saw on the news when the girls from the coast were vaccinated and they fainted, so there is no one in my family who has received those vaccines"* (mother of unvaccinated girl, 45 years old, private school). The legacy of this event has been distorted, with misinformation highly prevalent. Participants stated that the correct information needs to be provided to individual parents by doctors, but this approach is limited to one parent at a time. Thus, the larger responsibility for increasing public awareness and public education rests with the health and educational systems.

"I think that there has been a need for an education campaign, that is, promulgation of what papilloma is and what the vaccine does, because normally when a vaccine is talked about repeatedly by many media and people get educated, people have more awareness and then they do it conscientiously, but I have not heard that there has been much of a campaign or education on the subject". (mother of unvaccinated girl, 51 years old, private school)

For some parents, however, the first mention of the HPV vaccine is as a requirement for school: *"In my home we realized, first at school because they were asking about the vaccination card, and then with the prepaid healthcare provider; there the doctor talked about the vaccine"* (mother of girl with one dose, 41 years old, private school).

Some parents had gained limited and biased knowledge from their physicians, only in the context of their own diagnoses.

"I was diagnosed with HPV 10 or 12 years ago (…) they explained to me that even the nuns get it [HPV], even if they haven't had sex. I am in this meeting because I have many gaps [in my knowledge] and ignorance on the subject". (mother of unvaccinated girl, 45 years old, private school)

Relationship between HPV and Cervical Cancer

Among all the focus groups of girls, cancer meant severe disease, with difficult treatments, and death as a possible outcome. However, this was not specific to cervical cancer but to the concept of cancer. *"For me, the worst thing that can happen to a person is the treatments they have to do, because they need quick treatment or they can die, because it is a very serious cancer, and it affects women".* (girl, one dose, 10 years old, public school).

For parents, cervical cancer is treatable when detected early. *"They do a surgery on that, don't they? If it is detected in time, they operate on it, then people do not metastasize or something like that. That's the only thing I know"* (mother of girl with one dose, 41 years old, private school).

Girls recognize the value of the vaccine for reducing HPV susceptibility and severity. The participants imagine (incorrectly) that the vaccine puts a little bit of the virus into the body; thus, if they get the disease, it will not be serious. They know that several doses are required for it to be effective, and one of them believed that the effect of the vaccine gets lost over time. *"They put bits of the virus into the vaccine so that when the virus reaches your body the virus doesn't hit you so hard, so that's what I know about vaccines"* (girl, one dose, 10 years old, public school).

3.2.2. Opportunity

In focus groups of parents, participants mentioned that healthcare providers and schools were trusted information sources. Girls tended to trust their families, especially their mothers.

Trust in Traditional Institutions

The family and the health system are most trusted sources from which to receive information about the vaccine, and to make recommendations. For example, one of the girls said, *"If your mother tells you [to get vaccinated] it is because you mother wants the best for your life"* (unvaccinated girl, 9 years old, private school).

These two institutions are so important that they can alter previous negative attitudes and beliefs toward the vaccine. The healthcare provider can influence HPV vaccine uptake, particularly when other vaccines are routinely administered. Paradoxically, even in a country like Ecuador, which has higher reported rates of HPV vaccination than Colombia according to the WHO [45], one participant stated that she had never heard of the vaccine.

"I wanted to say that my ignorance is even bigger because my children were born in Ecuador and there nobody talks about HPV (. . .). I was one of those mothers who said that I would not give my daughter that vaccine, until recently, when I went to get a booster for my other 10-year-old son and I spoke with a doctor who explained to me that it was absolutely safe, so I began to think differently". (mother of unvaccinated girl, 45 years old, private school)

Parents tend to trust in their doctors even when they have doubts about the vaccine. There is little reported discomfort with the vaccination-card requirement at school or with vaccination campaigns at schools, supporting the idea that institutions take care of people.

Quantitative data corroborated this finding, since 87.8% of respondent trusted the information they received about vaccines. We also found a bivariate relationship between the likelihood of getting vaccinated and receiving positive information about the vaccine (Spearman r = 0.338, $p < 0.001$). For parents, a binary logistic regression showed that the recommendation of the doctor was the most important factor related to the probability of the daughter getting vaccinated (See Table 4).

Table 4. Logistic regression results for predicting the reasons to vaccinate daughters using socioeconomic position (SEP), religion, and other influences as independent variables.

Step	Variable Entered	B	Wald	Sig	Exp (B)	C.I for Exp (B)	
						Lower	Upper
1	SEP medium	−0.575	0.616	0.432	0.562	0.134	2.366
	SEP high	−0.736	1.424	0.233	0.479	0.143	1.604
	Religion	−0.532	0.828	0.363	0.587	0.187	1.847
2	Cost	−0.065	0.045	0.832	0.937	0.514	1.709
	Easy access to vaccine	0.142	0.245	0.620	1.153	0.657	2.025
	Social norms	−0.053	0.017	0.896	0.949	0.431	2.088
	Medical recommendation	−0.713	5.167	0.023	0.490	0.265	0.906
	Others' recommendations	−0.593	2.408	0.121	0.553	0.261	1.169
	Safety	0.873	3.200	0.074	2.394	0.920	6.233
	Susceptibility	−0.584	3.617	0.057	0.558	0.306	1.018
	Positive information	−0.460	2.365	0.124	0.631	0.351	1.135

Note. SEP = Socioeconomic position.

3.2.3. Motivation

Regarding motivation, survey data revealed that some parents were concerned about the effectiveness, adverse effects, and safety of the vaccines. In focus groups, parents also revealed a conflict between their desire to protect their daughters from the harmful virus and their concerns about encouraging early sexual activity through vaccination. Often, this led to parents avoiding talking about the HPV vaccine.

The Vaccine as an Act of Care

Most parents considered that vaccination is a form of protection and care for their daughters, which leads them to demand clear information about its effectiveness and safety. *"I did it [vaccinate the daughter] first of all, to protect my daughter's life"* (mother of girl with one dose, 41 years old, public school).

"It is a matter of avoiding the disease; one does not know when it could happen, God willing it does not happen, but it is a way of caring for and protecting them". (mother of girl with one dose, 41 years old, private school)

Often, parents would mention the adverse event at Carmen de Bolívar, leading to uncertainty about the impact of the vaccine.

"I have heard many mothers who did not want to vaccinate their daughters; I do not know why. A long time ago there was a problem with some vaccine, after which many mothers believe in these things, and they are scared to vaccinate their daughters". (mother of unvaccinated girl, 43 years old, private school)

Respect for the Personal Decision to Be Vaccinated

Some of the participants reported that vaccination is an individual act and at the same time, an act of collective responsibility. The decision cannot be forced, however. *"I think there must be free will there. Not only from parents, since at a certain age, young people make decisions regarding their bodies, and I think that it should not be mandatory"* (father of girl with one dose, 53 years old, private school).

Girls understood that to access to the vaccine they must go through two gatekeepers: first their parents and then their healthcare provider, acknowledging that, as minors, the decision rests with the parents. Some of the girls think that the vaccination is their decision; however, most of them think that this is a parental decision. *"Well, it depends, my mom talks about it with me; I tell her there is this vaccine, then she tells me yes, and the decision is mine, as she says: your body is yours"* (girl, one dose, 10 years old, public school).

"I never had the power to decide if I wanted to get vaccinated or not; it was not a subject that I could get into". (Girl, one dose, 15 years old, public rural school)

Association of HPV with Sexuality

As HPV is a sexually transmitted infection, some parents state that prevention can be conducted through education in values, not talking about sexuality openly.

"I consider that in the subject of the infection with the human papilloma virus, it is possible to take a look from the biological point of view as the subject of the disease; let's say that it is detached from the subject of sexuality and that is perfectly well because one can approach the subject with one's daughter like that". (Father of girl with one dose, 53 years old, private school)

Some parents stated that HPV infection occurred because people start sexual life early; they considered it an adult issue and did not consider their daughters susceptible to infection at their young ages. *"I have an acquaintance who had this cancer because she began her sexual life very young. That person passed away. She always warned us about the dangers of such a crazy sex life"* (mother of girl with one dose, 40 years old, public school).

This is also perceived by the girls, who state that their parents delegate the issue of sexuality to others, and that at school the information is provided superficially or not at all. *"Because it is a sexually transmitted disease, people avoid talking about it"* (girl with one dose, 15 years old, private school).

3.2.4. The Impact of COVID-19 on HPV Hesitancy

As a result of the pandemic, people understand more about how vaccines work and what happens with a virus, and the analogy with COVID-19 allows them to understand that to be fully protected, they need several doses of a vaccine. Some of the young participants incorrectly think that the vaccines contain live viruses, however. In Colombia, greater understanding of COVID has allowed certain anti-vaccine discourses to be demystified (relatives of participants who were anti-vaccine but were now vaccinated) and negative ideas about vaccines to be discredited.

"I don't know exactly how the virus spreads, but I suppose that, like a normal virus, like when you get vaccinated against the coronavirus, you prevent yourself and others, that you don't spread it, nor are you infected". (girl with one dose, 15 years old, public school)

Yet, especially in younger girls, different forms of HPV and COVID transmission, prevention, vaccination components and dosage, and side effects can be confused. *"Well, I think it is transmitted like when you cough on someone or if you are with that person a lot, the virus passes to you or something like that"* (unvaccinated girl, 9 years old, private school).

Importantly, regarding opportunities, the pandemic further limited access to the HPV vaccines and reduced the importance of health campaigns focused on HPV vaccines.

4. Discussion

The aim of this study was to understand the psychological predictors of HPV vaccine hesitancy in girls aged 15 and under and their parents/caregivers who live in and around Medellín. In this sample, more than half (57.1%) of participants have not initiated vaccination despite quantitative data showing that parents and caregivers who participated in the study perceived a high level of susceptibility to HPV and cervical cancer in girls and adolescents. They also had high awareness of the need for the vaccine. However, qualitative data revealed some unrealistic parental views of their daughters' susceptibility to HPV; many parents thought that since their daughters are young, they were far from starting their sexual life. There is limited information about organized HPV vaccination programs in this sample, nor does it reveal how physical and social opportunities affect access to vaccines. Additionally, despite Colombia Health Ministry-led public health communications about the safety of the HPV vaccine, some participants remained concerned about the vaccine's effectiveness and safety, and the side effects that the vaccine might cause.

Parents also were not especially aware of the vaccine's benefits. This finding was also reported in an earlier study in a Colombian population [34]. Limited information and low vaccination rates are clear challenges for public health, given the prevalence of cervical cancer in Colombia and worldwide [2,5]. These findings point to the need for interventions that provide information about HPV, its relationship to cervical cancer, and the country's national vaccination program to increase the public's vaccine uptake. However, simply providing information does not cause a change in vaccination behaviour [46]. Perceived susceptibility to HPV is a fruitful target for future intervention approaches. Multiple studies have reported that perceived susceptibility is associated with a greater likelihood of getting vaccinated [47]. Educational interventions that also focus on susceptibility, by pointing out that HPV causes genital warts and that vaccination prevents diseases attributable to this virus have demonstrated effectiveness [48,49]. The WHO communication guidelines include educational interventions designed to increase HPV-vaccine uptake to increase the perception of susceptibility and the consequences of HPV infection [50].

The COVID-19 pandemic has highlighted the threat of an infectious disease and has increased awareness of the vaccine-development process, since many parents had never seen the devastating consequences of an infectious disease before 2020 [51]. This creates an opportunity to generate awareness about HPV and its relationship with cervical cancer, but also to promote the use of the vaccine as the best way of preventing future complications.

This study also showed how physical and social opportunities have an influence on vaccine-access behaviour. It is crucial that barriers to vaccine access be reduced, by offering inoculations at schools [52], at times when parents can give consent, since that is needed for vaccination. Educational institutions may be optimal settings for HPV-vaccine interventions, as natural gathering sites for students, parents, healthcare professionals, and teachers. School-based interventions may help to change attitudes and beliefs, as well as increase knowledge to increase HPV-vaccine uptake [53].

We found that people trust their healthcare professionals (HCPs) and the information they provide. This element is crucial when we consider that HCPs can promote vaccination by sharing accurate information and offering counselling to parents to facilitate decision making. Nonetheless, previous studies have found that the percentage of HCPs who speak with parents about HPV vaccines for their children is very low [54]. However, HCPs are critical to HPV-vaccine uptake, so provider-based interventions also offer considerable promise [55]. A provider-focus has also been recommended by the HPV Prevention and Control Board of Colombia, so broader implementation is a next step [56].

Lastly, it is important to remember the motivational component of this behaviour. Paradoxically, although most participants in this study trusted the vaccine information received and the healthcare system providing it, some of them were distrustful about vaccine safety, efficacy, and potential adverse effects. This aligns with studies in other countries, in which fears about side effects and vaccine safety, distrust in the vaccine, fear of the possibility of death, and negative comments from neighbours or acquaintances about the HPV vaccine were paramount in parents who did not want to vaccinate their children [57]. In Colombia, these fears were enhanced with the widespread coverage of the 2014 mass psychogenic response [26] that still remains in the public's memories.

The thematic analysis showed that although the act of vaccine is seen as an individual decision, mothers have a crucial influence on their daughters. Generally, parents' motivation was to protect and take care of their daughters. To increase the vaccination rates, parents should be involved, as has been suggested in other studies [36,48].

As HPV is primarily a sexually transmitted disease, the HPV vaccine is different from other vaccines for children. In Colombia, it is intended especially for girls [58], although HPV-vaccination should be gender neutral. Both men and women can develop cancer caused by HPV; further, it is easier to ensure a high coverage to achieve herd immunity when both sexes are vaccinated [59].

Several studies have reported that parents and caregivers may associate the vaccine with fears of compromising fertility [60] or giving children permission to become sexually active [61]. While the perceived risks are nearer term, the potential benefits of HPV vaccination are much longer term, since it takes 15 to 20 years for cervical cancer to develop in women with normal immune systems [62] and the estimated median time from HPV acquisition to cancer detection ranges from 17.5 to 26 years [63]. Educational interventions could highlight both the near-term and longer-term benefits of the HPV vaccine.

Creating opportunities for public discussion, led by trusted healthcare providers, for example, could help to allay these parental fears and increase HPV-vaccine uptake. Parents and educational institutions should be involved in the co-design of these public forums. Currently, governments should take clear actions to improve vaccination rates. Denmark shows how a nation grappled with negative media coverage of HPV vaccination with a parent information campaign designed to boost confidence in the safety of the vaccine [64]. Austria launched a renewed national discourse on vaccination, changing the message of vaccination from "save women's lives" to "save lives" to disassociate the vaccine from gender [32].

The US Centers for Disease Control and Prevention (CDC) has recommended ten strategies for healthcare providers to increase the HPV vaccine. These range from giving active recommendations, recommending the HPV vaccine the same day and the same way as all other vaccines, preparing to answer more common questions, learning the reasons for vaccine refusal, and implementing systems to ensure that an opportunity to vaccinate is never missed [65].

Before concluding, we want to highlight the limitations of the study. It was conducted in the middle of the COVID-19-pandemic health emergency. This meant that all parent focus groups were remote, and their participation was limited by connection capability and speed. However, remote data-collection strategies may increase participation among those who may not otherwise be able to participate due to logistical or time constraints [66,67]. Use of a convenience sample from a geographically-limited set of participants may bias the findings and limit generalizability. For the quantitative analysis, we did not include variables that have predicted HPV-vaccine hesitancy in other studies, such as the level of parental education [68], so the findings may be confounded. Importantly, the use of mixed methods combines the strengths of both quantitative and qualitative research, by allowing the researcher to add insights that could be omitted when only a single method is adopted [69].

5. Conclusions

To summarize, this study improves the understanding of the capabilities, opportunities, and motivations associated with the HPV vaccine to reduce HPV-vaccine hesitancy for parents, girls, and adolescents in Medellín and nearby cities. It is important to provide information about the national vaccination program and HPV's association with cervical cancer. Likewise, it is important to make vaccination access easier by returning to the strategy developed in 2012 to bring the program to schools, thereby reducing barriers to access. Lastly, parents' concerns about vaccine safety and side effects should be acknowledged; healthcare leaders should create spaces for discussion so that the ideas behind the distrust can be dismantled.

Author Contributions: Conceptualization, V.C.-S. and M.L.; Data curation, S.S.G.; Formal analysis, V.C.-S. and M.L.; Funding acquisition, V.C.-S., M.L., D.A.T.-L. and S.S.G.; Investigation, V.C.-S., M.L., D.A.T.-L. and S.S.G.; Methodology, V.C.-S., M.L. and D.A.T.-L.; Project administration, D.A.T.-L.; Supervision, S.S.G.; Writing—original draft, V.C.-S., M.L. and D.A.T.-L.; Writing—review and editing, S.S.G. All authors have read and agreed to the published version of the manuscript.

Funding: This research was funded by Institucion Universitaria de Envigado (V.C.-S. and D.A.T.-L.), COD_00-202 and Universidad EAFIT (M.L.). S.S.G. was supported in part by Michigan Institute for Clinical and Health Research grant UL1TR002240. The study sponsors had no role in the design of the study.

Institutional Review Board Statement: The study was conducted in accordance with the Declaration of Helsinki, and approved by the Ethics Committee of Universidad EAFIT on 21 August 2021.

Informed Consent Statement: Informed consent was obtained from all subjects involved in the study.

Data Availability Statement: The data supporting reported results can be found at https://osf.io/n396v/?view_only=6f04d370460a419bbeceba5600ce91c3 (accessed on 31 May 2022).

Acknowledgments: We thank the IBTN for introducing us during IBTN Summer School 2021 and the Colombian schools that helped us to recruit participants. Thanks also to Melissa Dejonckheere and Tim Guetterman for their helpful comments on the paper.

Conflicts of Interest: The authors declare no conflict of interest and the funders had no role in the design of the study; in the collection, analyses, or interpretation of data; in the writing of the manuscript, or in the decision to publish the results.

Appendix A. Online Questionnaire

Perceived susceptibility, vaccine awareness, and intention to complete the vaccination schedule:

- Do you think your daughter may get cervical cancer at some point in her life? Yes/No
- Do you think your daughter could get HPV? Yes/No
- Have you heard of the HPV vaccine? Yes/No
- Has anyone told you that your daughter needs to be vaccinated against HPV? Yes/No
- Is your daughter going to complete the vaccination schedule? Yes/No

Trust, beliefs about vaccine safety and efficacy:

These items were answered on a Likert scale ranging from 0 (Not at all concerned) to 3 (Very concerned).

- How concerned are you that your daughter might have a serious side effect from a shot?
- How concerned are you that anyone of the childhood shots might not be safe?
- How concerned are you that a shot might not prevent the disease?

These items were from the Parent Attitudes about Childhood Vaccines (PACV) questionnaire, developed by Opel et al. (2011) and adapted into Spanish by Cunningham et al. (2019). This questionnaire has a Cronbach's alpha of 0.74 for the safety and efficacy domain, 0.84 for the general attitudes domain, and 0.74 for the behaviour domain [59].

Factors influencing the decision to vaccinate or to complete the vaccination schedule:

- "If a vaccine against HPV was available for your daughter, how likely is it that she would have it?" 0 (Extremely likely) to 3 (Not at all likely).

The following questions covered factors related to the vaccination decision from previous literature [60], which were answered on a Likert scale ranging from 0 (Very much) to 3 (Not at all).

- Cost
- Ease
- Knowing that other people have put it on
- Doctor's recommendation
- Someone else's recommendation
- Knowing that the vaccine is safe
- Thinking that my daughter is at higher risk for HPV
- Listening to positive opinions about the vaccine.

References

1. Bruni, L.; Albero, G.; Serrano, B.; Mena, M.; Collado, J.J.; Gómez, D.; Muñoz, J.; Bosch, X.; de Sanjosé, S. *Human Papillomavirus and Related Diseases Report WORLD*; Barcelona, Spain, 2021. Available online: https://hpvcentre.net/statistics/reports/XWX.pdf (accessed on 4 June 2022).
2. Bray, F.; Ferlay, J.; Soerjomataram, I.; Siegel, R.L.; Torre, L.A.; Jemal, A. Global cancer statistics 2018: GLOBOCAN estimates of incidence and mortality worldwide for 36 cancers in 185 countries. *CA Cancer J. Clin.* **2018**, *68*, 394–424. [CrossRef] [PubMed]
3. Bruni, L.; Albero, G.; Serrano, B.; Mena, M.; Collado, J.J.; Gómez, D.; Muñoz, J.; Bosch, X.; de Sanjosé, S. *Human Papillomavirus and Related Diseases Report COLOMBIA*; Barcelona, Spain, 2021. Available online: https://hpvcentre.net/statistics/reports/COL.pdf?t=1624248056406 (accessed on 4 June 2022).
4. IARC [International Agency for Cancer Research]. *Colombia Facts Sheet*; UNHCR: Geneva, Switzerland, 2020.
5. Hernández Vargas, J.A.; Ramírez Barbosa, P.X.; Gil Quijano, A.M.; Valbuena, A.M.; Acuña, L.; González, J.A. Patterns of breast, prostate and cervical cancer incidence and mortality in Colombia: An administrative registry data analysis. *BMC Cancer* **2020**, *20*, 1097. [CrossRef] [PubMed]
6. Muñoz, N.; Bravo, L.E. Epidemiology of cervical cancer in Colombia. *Colomb. Med.* **2012**, *43*, 298–304. [CrossRef]
7. Walboomers, J.M.M.; Jacobs, M.V.; Manos, M.M.; Bosch, F.X.; Kummer, J.A.; Shah, K.V.; Snijders, P.J.F.; Peto, J.; Meijer, C.J.L.M.; Muñoz, N. Human papillomavirus is a necessary cause of invasive cervical cancer worldwide. *J. Pathol.* **1999**, *189*, 12–19. [CrossRef]
8. Muñoz, N.; Bosch, F.X.; de Sanjosé, S.; Herrero, R.; Castellsagué, X.; Shah, K.V.; Snijders, P.J.F.; Meijer, C.J.L.M. Epidemiologic classification of human papillomavirus types associated with cervical cancer. *N. Engl. J. Med.* **2003**, *348*, 518–527. [CrossRef] [PubMed]
9. Jones, B.A.; Davey, D.D. Quality management in gynecologic cytology using interlaboratory comparison. *Arch. Pathol. Lab. Med.* **2000**, *124*, 672–681. [CrossRef]
10. De Rijke, J.M.; Van der Putten, H.W.H.M.; Lutgens, L.C.H.W.; Voogd, A.C.; Kruitwagen, R.F.P.M.; Van Dijck, J.A.A.M.; Schouten, L.J. Age-specific differences in treatment and survival of patients with cervical cancer in the southeast of The Netherlands, 1986–1996. *Eur. J. Cancer* **2002**, *38*, 2041–2047. [CrossRef]
11. Smith, M.A.; Liu, B.; McIntyre, P.; Menzies, R.; Dey, A.; Canfell, K. Fall in genital warts diagnoses in the general and indigenous Australian population following implementation of a national human papillomavirus vaccination program: Analysis of routinely collected national hospital data. *J. Infect. Dis.* **2015**, *211*, 91–99. [CrossRef]
12. Robertson, G.; Robson, S.J. Excisional Treatment of Cervical Dysplasia in Australia 2004–2013: A Population-Based Study. *J. Oncol.* **2016**, *2016*, 3056407. [CrossRef]
13. Australian Institute of Health and Welfare. *Cervical Screening in Australia 2014–2015*; Australian Institute of Health and Welfare: Canberra, Australia, 2017.
14. Goldie, S.J.; Kohli, M.; Grima, D.; Weinstein, M.C.; Wright, T.C.; Xavier Bosch, F.; Franco, E. Projected clinical benefits and cost-effectiveness of a human papillomavirus 16/18 vaccine. *J. Natl. Cancer Inst.* **2004**, *96*, 604–615. [CrossRef]
15. Watson, M.; Benard, V.; Flagg, E.W. Assessment of trends in cervical cancer screening rates using healthcare claims data: United States, 2003–2014. *Prev. Med. Rep.* **2018**, *9*, 124–130. [CrossRef] [PubMed]

16. U.S. Cancer Statistics Working Group. U.S. Cancer Statistics Data Visualizations Tool. The Centers for Disease Control and Prevention (CDC) and the National Cancer Institute (NCI); 2016. Available online: https://www.cdc.gov/cancer/uscs/dataviz/index.htm (accessed on 24 March 2022).
17. Quinn, M.; Babb, P.; Jones, J.; Allen, E. Effect of screening on incidence of and mortality from cancer of cervix in England: Evaluation based on routinely collected statistics. *BMJ* **1999**, *318*, 904. [CrossRef] [PubMed]
18. Arbyn, M.; Xu, L.; Simoens, C.; Martin-Hirsch, P.P.L. Prophylactic vaccination against human papillomaviruses to prevent cervical cancer and its precursors. *Cochrane Database Syst. Rev.* **2018**, *5*, 1. [CrossRef] [PubMed]
19. Arbyn, M.; Ronco, G.; Anttila, A.; Chris, C.J.L.; Poljak, M.; Ogilvie, G.; Koliopoulos, G.; Naucler, P.; Sankaranarayanan, R.; Peto, J. Evidence regarding human papillomavirus testing in secondary prevention of cervical cancer. *Vaccine* **2012**, *30* (Suppl. S5), F88–F99. [CrossRef]
20. Ronco, G.; Dillner, J.; Elfström, K.M.; Tunesi, S.; Snijders, P.J.F.; Arbyn, M.; Kitchener, H.; Segnan, N.; Gilham, C.; Giorgi-Rossi, P.; et al. Efficacy of HPV-based screening for prevention of invasive cervical cancer: Follow-up of four European randomised controlled trials. *Lancet* **2014**, *383*, 524–532. [CrossRef]
21. Machalek, D.A.; Garland, S.M.; Brotherton, J.M.L.; Bateson, D.; McNamee, K.; Stewart, M.; Rachel Skinner, S.; Liu, B.; Cornall, A.M.; Kaldor, J.M.; et al. Very Low Prevalence of Vaccine Human Papillomavirus Types Among 18- to 35-Year Old Australian Women 9 Years Following Implementation of Vaccination. *J. Infect. Dis.* **2018**, *217*, 1590–1600. [CrossRef]
22. Chesson, H.W.; Mayaud, P.; Aral, S.O. Sexually Transmitted Infections: Impact and Cost-Effectiveness of Prevention. In *Disease Control Priorities, Third Edition: Major Infectious Diseases*; World Bank: Washington DC, USA, 2017; Volume 6, pp. 203–232. [CrossRef]
23. World Health Organization. *Global Strategy to Accelerate the Elimination of Cervical Cancer as a Public Health Problem*; WHO: Geneva, Switzerland, 2020.
24. OMS [Organización Mundial de la Salud]. Por un Futuro sin Cáncer del Cuello Uterino: Por Primera vez el Mundo se ha Comprometido a Eliminar un Cáncer—OPS/OMS | Organización Panamericana de la Salud. 2020. Available online: https://www.who.int/es/news/item/17-11-2020-a-cervical-cancer-free-future-first-ever-global-commitment-to-eliminate-a-cancer (accessed on 1 December 2021).
25. Ministerio de Salud y Protección Social República de Colombia. Colombia Cuenta con las Mejores Coberturas de Vacunación Contra VPH del Mundo 2014. Available online: https://www.minsalud.gov.co/Paginas/Colombia-cuenta-con-las-mejores-coberturas-de-vacunacion.aspx (accessed on 2 December 2021).
26. Simas, C.; Munoz, N.; Arregoces, L.; Larson, H.J. HPV vaccine confidence and cases of mass psychogenic illness following immunization in Carmen de Bolivar, Colombia. *Hum. Vaccines Immunother.* **2019**, *15*, 163–166. [CrossRef]
27. Martinez, M.; Estevez, A.; Quijada, H.; Walteros, D.; Tolosa, N.; Paredes, A.; Alvarez, C.; Armenta, A.; Osorio, L.; Castillo, O.; et al. Brote de evento de etiología desconocida en el municipio de El Carmen de Bolívar, Bolívar, 2014. *Inf. Quinc. Epidemiol. Nac.* **2015**, *20*, 41–76.
28. Silva Numa, S. ¿Quién salvará la vacunación contra el VPH en Colombia? *El Espectador*, 16 December 2021.
29. Suppli, C.H.; Hansen, N.D.; Rasmussen, M.; Valentiner-Branth, P.; Krause, T.G.; Mølbak, K. Decline in HPV-vaccination uptake in Denmark—The association between HPV-related media coverage and HPV-vaccination. *BMC Public Health* **2018**, *18*, 1360. [CrossRef]
30. Baandrup, L.; Valentiner-Branth, P.; Kjaer, S.K. HPV vaccination crisis and recovery: The Danish case. *HPV World Newsl.* **2021**, 1–5. Available online: https://www.hpvworld.com/articles/hpv-vaccination-crisis-and-recovery-the-danish-case (accessed on 4 June 2022).
31. Haruyama, R.; Obara, H.; Fujita, N. What is the current status of Japan's efforts to meet global goals and targets to eliminate cervical cancer? *Glob. Health Med.* **2021**, *3*, 44. [CrossRef]
32. Paul, K.T. "Saving lives": Adapting and adopting Human Papilloma Virus (HPV) vaccination in Austria. *Soc. Sci. Med.* **2016**, *153*, 193–200. [CrossRef] [PubMed]
33. Notejane, M.; Zunino, C.; Aguirre, D.; Méndez, P.; García, L.; Pérez, W.; Notejane, M.; Zunino, C.; Aguirre, D.; Méndez, P.; et al. Estado vacunal y motivos de no vacunación contra el virus del papiloma humano en adolescentes admitidas en el Hospital Pediátrico del Centro Hospitalario Pereira Rossell. *Rev. Méd. Urug.* **2018**, *34*, 10–28. [CrossRef]
34. Cordoba-Sanchez, V.; Tovar-Aguirre, O.L.; Franco, S.; Arias Ortiz, N.E.; Louie, K.; Sanchez, G.I.; Garces-Palacio, I.C. Perception about barriers and facilitators of the school-based HPV vaccine program of Manizales, Colombia: A qualitative study in school-enrolled girls and their parents. *Prev. Med. Rep.* **2019**, *16*, 100977. [CrossRef] [PubMed]
35. Patel, P.R.; Berenson, A.B. Sources of HPV vaccine hesitancy in parents. *Hum. Vaccines Immunother.* **2013**, *9*, 2649. [CrossRef] [PubMed]
36. Shapiro, G.K.; Head, K.J.; Rosberger, Z.; Zimet, G.D. Parents hesitancy about HPV vaccination. *HPV World* **2018**, *72*, 1–4.
37. Michie, S.; van Stralen, M.M.; West, R. The behaviour change wheel: A new method for characterising and designing behaviour change interventions. *Implement. Sci.* **2011**, *6*, 42. [CrossRef]
38. Czajkowski, S.M.; Powell, L.H.; Adler, N.; Naar-King, S.; Reynolds, K.D.; Hunter, C.M.; Laraia, B.; Olster, D.H.; Perna, F.M.; Peterson, J.C.; et al. From ideas to efficacy: The ORBIT model for developing behavioral treatments for chronic diseases. *Health Psychol.* **2015**, *34*, 971–982. [CrossRef]

39. Secretaría de Educación de Medellín. 66.8% de las Instituciones Públicas de Medellín ya Aplican la Alternancia ⋆ Secretaría de Educación 2021. Available online: https://www.medellin.edu.co/66-8-de-las-instituciones-publicas-de-medellin-ya-aplican-la-alternancia/ (accessed on 6 January 2022).
40. Ministerio de Salud y Protección Social República de Colombia. Vacuna Contra el Cáncer de Cuello Uterino n.d. Available online: https://www.minsalud.gov.co/salud/publica/Vacunacion/Paginas/ABC-de-la-vacuna-contra-el-cancer-cuello-uterino.aspx (accessed on 6 January 2022).
41. Vallis, M.; Bacon, S.; Corace, K.; Joyal-Desmarais, K.; Gorin, S.S.; Paduano, S.; Presseau, J.; Rash, J.; Yohannes, A.M.; Lavoie, K. Ending the Pandemic: How Behavioural Science Can Help Optimize Global COVID-19 Vaccine Uptake. *Vaccines* **2021**, *10*, 7. [CrossRef]
42. Winkinson, S. Using focus groups. Exploring the meanings of health and illness. In *A Handbook of Reseach Methods for Clinical and Health Psychology*; Miles, J., Gilbert, P., Eds.; Oxford University Press: New York, NY, USA, 2005; pp. 79–94.
43. Braun, V.; Clarke, V. Using thematic analysis in psychology. *Qual. Res. Psychol.* **2006**, *3*, 77–101. [CrossRef]
44. McCrudden, M.T.; Marchand, G.; Schutz, P.A. Joint displays for mixed methods research in psychology. *Methods Psychol.* **2021**, *5*, 100067. [CrossRef]
45. Bruni, L.; Saura-Lázaro, A.; Montoliu, A.; Brotons, M.; Alemany, L.; Diallo, M.S.; Afsar, O.Z.; LaMontagne, D.S.; Mosina, L.; Contreras, M.; et al. HPV vaccination introduction worldwide and WHO and UNICEF estimates of national HPV immunization coverage 2010–2019. *Prev. Med.* **2021**, *144*, 106399. [CrossRef] [PubMed]
46. Habersaat, K.B.; Jackson, C. Understanding vaccine acceptance and demand-and ways to increase them. *Bundesgesundheitsblatt Gesundh. Gesundh.* **2020**, *63*, 32–39. [CrossRef] [PubMed]
47. Ling, W.Y.; Razali, S.M.; Ren, C.K.; Omar, S.Z. Does the success of a school-based HPV vaccine programme depend on teachers' knowledge and religion?—A survey in a multicultural society. *Asian Pac. J. Cancer Prev.* **2012**, *13*, 4651–4654. [CrossRef] [PubMed]
48. Nwanodi, O.; Salisbury, H.; Bay, C. Multimodal Counseling Interventions: Effect on Human Papilloma Virus Vaccination Acceptance. *Healthcare* **2017**, *5*, 85S. [CrossRef]
49. Paskett, E.D.; Krok-Schoen, J.L.; Pennell, M.L.; Tatum, C.M.; Reiter, P.L.; Peng, J.; Bernardo, B.M.; Weier, R.C.; Richardson, M.S.; Katz, M.L. Results of a Multilevel Intervention Trial to Increase Human Papillomavirus (HPV) Vaccine Uptake among Adolescent Girls. *Cancer Epidemiol. Biomark. Prev.* **2016**, *25*, 593–602. [CrossRef]
50. WHO; HPV Vaccine Communication. Special Considerations for a Unique Vaccine. Who/Ivb/1312 2013:31–2. Available online: https://www.who.int/publications/i/item/10665250279 (accessed on 2 December 2021).
51. McNally, V.V.; Bernstein, H.H. The Effect of the COVID-19 Pandemic on Childhood Immunizations: Ways to Strengthen Routine Vaccination. *Pediatr. Ann.* **2020**, *49*, e516–e522. [CrossRef]
52. Gallagher, K.E.; Howard, N.; Kabakama, S.; Mounier-Jack, S.; Griffiths, U.K.; Feletto, M.; Burchett, H.E.D.; LaMontagne, D.S.; Watson-Jones, D. Lessons learnt from human papillomavirus (HPV) vaccination in 45 low- and middle-income countries. *PLoS ONE* **2017**, *12*, e0177773. [CrossRef]
53. Da Silva, P.M.C.; Silva, I.M.B.; da Conceição Souza Interaminense, I.N.; Linhares, F.M.P.; Serrano, S.Q.; Pontes, C.M. Knowledge and attitudes about human papillomavirus and vaccination. *Esc. Anna Nery* **2018**, *22*, 2018. [CrossRef]
54. Hendaus, M.A.; Hassan, M.; Alsulaiti, M.; Mohamed, T.; Mohamed, R.; Yasrab, D.; Mahjoob, H.; Alhammadi, A.H. Parents attitudes toward the human papilloma virus (HPV) vaccine: A new concept in the State of Qatar. *J. Fam. Med. Prim. Care* **2021**, *10*, 2488. [CrossRef]
55. Dolan, P.; Hallsworth, M.; Halpern, D.; King, D.; Metcalfe, R.; Vlaev, I. Influencing behaviour: The mindspace way. *J. Econ. Psychol.* **2012**, *33*, 264–277. [CrossRef]
56. Vorsters, A.; Bosch, F.X.; Bosch, F.X.; Bonanni, P.; Franco, E.L.; Baay, M.; Simas, C.; Waheed, D.E.N.; Castro, C.; Murillo, R.; et al. Prevention and control of HPV infection and HPV-related cancers in Colombia- a meeting report. *BMC Proc.* **2020**, *14*, 8. [CrossRef] [PubMed]
57. Aquino Rojas, E.; Aquino Rojas, W.A.; Soto Flores, R.; Soto Flores, O. Tácticas de fortalecimiento para la prevención del cáncer cervico uterino a través de la vacunación contra el virus del papiloma humano, agosto de 2017 a marzo de 2018. *Gac. Méd. Boliv.* **2019**, *42*, 52–58. [CrossRef]
58. Congreso de Colombia. Ley 1626, por Medio de la Cual se Garantiza la Vacunación Gratuita y Obligatoria a la Población Colombiana Objeto de la Misma, se Adoptan Medidas Integrales para la Prevención del Cáncer Cérvico Uterino y se Dictan otras Disposiciones. 2013. Available online: http://www.secretariasenado.gov.co/senado/basedoc/ley_1626_2013.html (accessed on 4 June 2022).
59. Hintze, J.M.; O'Neill, J.P. Strengthening the case for gender-neutral and the nonavalent HPV vaccine. *Eur. Arch. Otorhinolaryngol.* **2018**, *275*, 857–865. [CrossRef] [PubMed]
60. Friedman, A.L.; Oruko, K.O.; Habel, M.A.; Ford, J.; Kinsey, J.; Odhiambo, F.; Phillips-Howard, P.A.; Wang, S.A.; Collins, T.; Laserson, K.F.; et al. Preparing for human papillomavirus vaccine introduction in Kenya: Implications from focus-group and interview discussions with caregivers and opinion leaders in Western Kenya. *BMC Public Health* **2014**, *14*, 855. [CrossRef]
61. Morales-Campos, D.Y.; Snipes, S.A.; Villarreal, E.K.; Crocker, L.C.; Guerrero, A.; Fernandez, M.E. Cervical cancer, human papillomavirus (HPV), and HPV vaccination: Exploring gendered perspectives, knowledge, attitudes, and cultural taboos among Mexican American adults. *Ethn. Health* **2021**, *26*, 206–224. [CrossRef]

62. World Health Organization. Cervical Cancer. Cerv Cancer Fact Sheets 2022. Available online: https://www.who.int/news-room/fact-sheets/detail/cervical-cancer (accessed on 6 July 2022).
63. Burger, E.A.; De Kok, I.M.C.M.; Groene, E.; Killen, J.; Canfell, K.; Kulasingam, S.; Kuntz, K.M.; Matthijsse, S.; Regan, C.; Simms, K.T.; et al. Estimating the Natural History of Cervical Carcinogenesis Using Simulation Models: A CISNET Comparative Analysis. *J. Natl. Cancer Inst.* **2020**, *112*, 955–963. [CrossRef]
64. Hansen, P.R.; Schmidtblaicher, M.; Brewer, N.T. Resilience of HPV vaccine uptake in Denmark: Decline and recovery. *Vaccine* **2020**, *38*, 1842–1848. [CrossRef]
65. Centers for Disease Control and Prevention. Top 10 Tips to Improve HPV Vaccine Rates | CDC 2018. Available online: https://www.cdc.gov/hpv/hcp/2-dose/top-10-vaxsuccess.html (accessed on 4 June 2022).
66. Gray, L.M.; Wong-Wylie, G.; Rempel, G.R.; Cook, K. Expanding Qualitative Research Interviewing Strategies: Zoom Video Communications. *Qual. Rep.* **2020**, *25*, 1292–1301. [CrossRef]
67. Hensen, B.; Mackworth-Young, C.R.S.; Simwinga, M.; Abdelmagid, N.; Banda, J.; Mavodza, C.; Doyle, A.M.; Bonell, C.; Weiss, H.A. Remote data collection for public health research in a COVID-19 era: Ethical implications, challenges and opportunities. *Health Policy Plan.* **2021**, *36*, 360–368. [CrossRef]
68. Nguyen, K.H.; Santibanez, T.A.; Stokley, S.; Lindley, M.C.; Fisher, A.; Kim, D.; Greby, S.; Srivastav, A.; Singleton, J. Parental vaccine hesitancy and its association with adolescent HPV vaccination. *Vaccine* **2021**, *39*, 2416. [CrossRef]
69. Fetters, M.D.; Freshwater, D. The 1 + 1 = 3 Integration Challenge. *J. Mix. Methods Res.* **2015**, *9*, 115–117. [CrossRef]

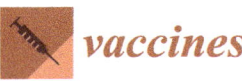

Article

What Factors Are Associated with Attitudes towards HPV Vaccination among Kazakhstani Women? Exploratory Analysis of Cross-Sectional Survey Data

Gulzhanat Aimagambetova [1,*], Aisha Babi [1], Torgyn Issa [1] and Alpamys Issanov [2,3]

[1] Department of Biomedical Sciences, School of Medicine, Nazarbayev University, Nur-Sultan 010000, Kazakhstan; aisha.mukushova@nu.edu.kz (A.B.); tshokanbaeva@nu.edu.kz (T.I.)
[2] Department of Medicine, School of Medicine, Nazarbayev University, Nur-Sultan 010000, Kazakhstan; alpamys.issanov@nu.edu.kz
[3] School of Population and Public Health, The University of British Columbia, Vancouver, BC V6T1Z8, Canada
* Correspondence: gulzhanat.aimagambetova@nu.edu.kz

Abstract: Background. The high prevalence of HPV infection among Kazakhstani women and the absence of an HPV vaccination program are directly reflected in increasing rates of cervical cancer incidence and mortality. Kazakhstan made its first attempt at introducing the HPV vaccine in 2013, but was unsuccessful due to complications and low public acceptance. The attitudes of Kazakhstani women towards the vaccine were never measured. Therefore, this study aims to investigate the attitudes of women towards the HPV vaccine and determine factors associated with positive, negative, or neutral attitudes. **Methods.** A 29-item survey consisting of 21 demographic and contextual questions and 8 Likert-scale questions was distributed among women attending gynecological offices in four major cities of Kazakhstan from December 2021 until February 2022. Attitudes of women were measured based on their answers to the eight Likert-scale questions. Ordinal logistic regression was built to find associations between demographic characteristics and attitudes of women. **Results.** Two hundred thirty-three women were included in the final analysis. A total of 54% of women had positive attitudes towards the vaccine. The majority of women did not trust or had a neutral attitude towards the government, pharmaceutical industry, and traditional and alternative media. However, the trust of women was high in medical workers and scientific researchers. Women's age, education, number of children, effect of the 2013 HPV program, and trust in alternative medicine were included in the ordinal logistic model. Women with a low level of education, a high number of children, who believe in alternative medicine, and who were affected by the failed 2013 vaccination program were less likely to have a positive attitude towards the vaccine. **Conclusions.** Contrary attitudes towards HPV vaccination exist among Kazakhstani women, with approximately half having positive and almost half having negative or neutral attitudes towards the vaccine. An informational campaign that takes into consideration women's levels of trust in different agencies, as well as targets those who are the most uninformed, might help in a successful relaunch of the HPV vaccination program. However, more studies that cover a higher number of women are required.

Keywords: HPV; HPV vaccine; HPV vaccine knowledge; HPV vaccine awareness; Kazakhstan; cervical cancer prevention

Citation: Aimagambetova, G.; Babi, A.; Issa, T.; Issanov, A. What Factors Are Associated with Attitudes towards HPV Vaccination among Kazakhstani Women? Exploratory Analysis of Cross-Sectional Survey Data. *Vaccines* **2022**, *10*, 824. https://doi.org/10.3390/vaccines10050824

Academic Editor: Gloria Calagna

Received: 26 March 2022
Accepted: 5 May 2022
Published: 23 May 2022

Publisher's Note: MDPI stays neutral with regard to jurisdictional claims in published maps and institutional affiliations.

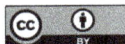

Copyright: © 2022 by the authors. Licensee MDPI, Basel, Switzerland. This article is an open access article distributed under the terms and conditions of the Creative Commons Attribution (CC BY) license (https://creativecommons.org/licenses/by/4.0/).

1. Introduction

High-risk human papillomavirus (HR-HPV) infections cause a wide variety of benign and malignant conditions, including cervical cancer [1–4]. More than 90% of cervical cancer cases are attributed to HR-HPV infections, with HPV-16 and HPV-18 being reported to cause 70–75% of cases [3,4]. The knowledge that persistent HR-HPV infection is causally associated with cervical cancer has resulted in the development of prophylactic vaccines to prevent HPV infection and, thus, decrease the rates of HPV-related diseases [4]. HPV vaccination programs have been implemented successfully in many high-income countries and have led to a decline in cervical cancer incidence rates [5–7]. However, the situation in low-income countries remains deplorable—cervical cancer is the leading cause of cancer-related death in women, as primary and secondary prevention interventions are insufficient or lacking [4].

The association of HPV infection with anal, penile, head, and neck cancers is also well documented [8–10]. Therefore, immunization with the HPV vaccine can protect from the development of other HPV-related cancers.

The prevalence of HPV infection varies among countries worldwide, with the highest prevalence of HR-HPV infection among women in the developing regions of Southern and Eastern Asia (44.4% and 36.3%, respectively) [11]. A high prevalence of HPV infection was also identified among Northern American and Eastern European populations (41.1% and 28.9%, respectively) [11]. The lowest prevalence of HPV infection is reported in Middle Eastern and North African countries (7–16%) [12]. According to the available epidemiological data, HR-HPV prevalence in Kazakhstan is high among women attending gynecological offices, ranging from 39% to 43% [13–15].

The high prevalence of HR-HPV strains in Kazakhstan is contributing to increasing cervical cancer rates. Over the past 10 years (2009–2018), the crude rate of cervical cancer incidence in Kazakhstan has increased from 16.3 ± 0.4 to 19.5 ± 0.5 per 100,000 female population ($p < 0.001$) [16]. The national cervical cancer screening program was updated in 2017 [17], and eligible women received the screening free of charge. However, according to reports, the state-funded coverage reached only 50% of the target population [18]; thus, the screening coverage was low (around 46%) [18–20].

In 2013, the HPV vaccination campaign was introduced in Kazakhstan as a pilot program in four large regions [21]. Bivalent and tetravalent HPV vaccines were approved for the campaign, targeting 11–12-year-old girls [18]. However, the lack of an HPV vaccination awareness campaign that should have preceded and accompanied the vaccination program and the influence of social media's negative content on the program have led to a negative public reaction and unwillingness of parents to vaccinate their children against HPV [18,21,22]. Parents refused to vaccinate their daughters due to concerns about the HPV vaccine's safety and efficacy [23]. The vaccination program was discontinued in 2015 indefinitely. In 2020, the Ministry of Healthcare of the Republic of Kazakhstan announced the intention to relaunch the HPV vaccination program; however, due to the COVID-19 pandemic, it has been postponed.

Given the importance of the reintroduction of HPV immunization to prevent new cervical cancer cases, it is essential to understand what factors are associated with parents' willingness to vaccinate their children. Studies have shown that attitudes towards HPV vaccination are associated with HPV vaccination uptake [24]. Multiple factors play a role in shaping attitudes towards vaccination [25,26]. Education, social status, income, and cultural and religious preferences have a substantial impact on people's beliefs, thus affecting their understanding of different aspects of HPV as a sexually transmitted infection (STI) and its related diseases [26]. As reported by studies, attitudes and intentions to receive HPV vaccination vary from 15% to 95% in different societies, depending on the multiple factors involved [26–28].

As one of the tasks announced by the World Health Organization (WHO) in the Global Strategy to Accelerate the Elimination of Cervical Cancer [29,30] is to increase HPV vaccination coverage up to 90% among the target group, it is very important to investigate HPV knowledge, awareness, and attitudes towards HPV vaccination. For the successful relaunching and implementation of the HPV vaccination program in Kazakhstan, the investigation of attitudes to HPV vaccination among the general population has become even more essential, especially among women, the population most affected by HPV-related cancers. Thus, by surveying Kazakhstani women across the country, this pilot study aimed to evaluate attitudes towards HPV vaccination and explore factors potentially associated with differing attitudes towards the vaccine.

2. Materials and Methods

2.1. Study Design and Subjects

This is a cross-sectional study, which was conducted from December 2021 until February 2022 in four major cities (Nur-Sultan, Almaty, Aktobe, Oskemen, Kazakhstan) representing the central, southern, western, and eastern regions of Kazakhstan. Women aged from 18 to 70 years old visiting gynecological offices were recruited for the study. A total of 399 women agreed to participate in the study, and 347 reported full demographic characteristics. Out of those 347 women, 321 (80.45%) fully answered the HPV vaccine attitude questions. Almost 27% were excluded due to incomplete answers to the contextual questions. In total, 233 women were included in the complete-case analysis (Figure 1).

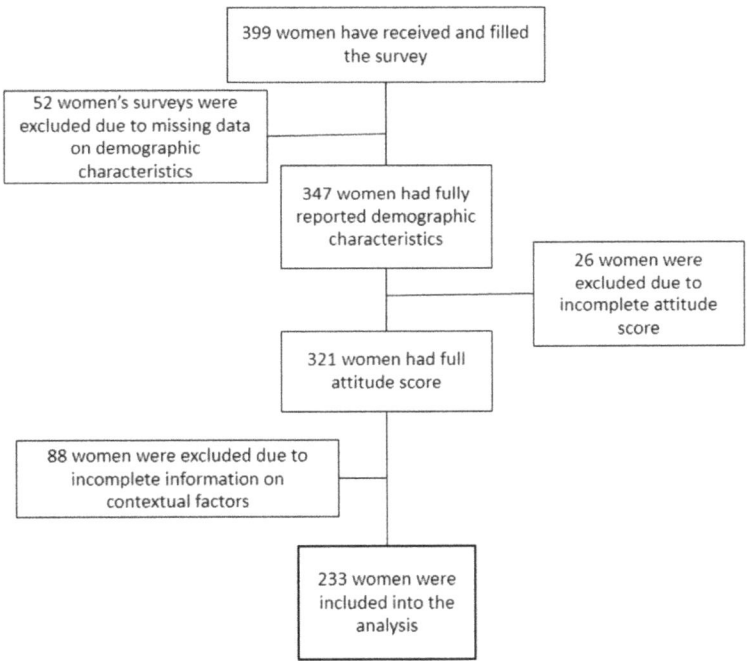

Figure 1. Flow chart on participants' inclusion.

2.2. Study Instrument

Two questionnaires were used in the study. The first collected data on demographic characteristics of women. The second questionnaire was adapted from the French Survey Questionnaire for the Determinants of HPV Vaccine Hesitancy (FSQD-HPVH) [31]. The questionnaire was adapted to the context of Kazakhstan (Supplementary Material). Based on experts' opinions, some questions were removed due to being irrelevant, and equivalent questions were added. For example, statements such as "Most of my friends get their daughters vaccinated against HPV" were removed, as the HPV vaccine is not readily available in Kazakhstan. The statement "Since the controversy over the H1N1 flu vaccination, I have less confidence in the French vaccination recommendations" was replaced with a statement of COVID-19, as it fits the context. All questions were translated and back-translated to Kazakh and Russian languages (official languages of the country) by experienced independent bilingual translators. The questionnaire included 29 items asking about contextual factors (historical factors, policies, and mandates), trust in different agencies, and beliefs and attitudes towards HPV vaccination.

2.3. Study Variables

2.3.1. Independent Variables

Independent variables were socio-economic and demographic characteristics such as age, ethnicity, level of education, city, family income, marital status, and number of children. According to age, women were categorized into four major groups: 18–27 years old, 28–33 years old, 34–43 years old, and 44 years old and older. Age of women was categorized according to the quartiles. Ethnicity was categorized into 2 groups: Kazakh and other ethnic groups. There were three levels of education: high school or below, college, and university. In January 2022, the average income in Kazakhstan was 269 149 tenge (USD ≈ 520) [32]. Income lower and higher than the average was categorized as lower and upper income, while average income was categorized as middle income.

In addition, contextual factors such as historical factors, policies, and mandates were used as independent variables. This section consisted of 6 Likert-scale questions. The major topics of the questions were the impact of COVID-19 vaccination on trust in HPV vaccine recommendations (COVID-19 effect), the 2013 HPV vaccination program in Kazakhstan (2013 HPV program), the relationship of HPV vaccination with sexual promiscuity, compulsory vaccine mandated by the government, freedom of vaccine choice for children, and alternative medicine strengthening body immune system (alternative medicine beliefs). Statements about trust in different agencies were also used as independent variables. The Likert scale was used to measure trust in agencies and health systems such as the pharmaceutical industry, government, medical workers, scientific researchers, traditional media, and alternative media.

2.3.2. Outcome Variable

The attitude of the participants was measured using 3 positive statements and 5 negative statement items on the Likert scale. Negative statements were reversed, and the mean attitude score of the participants was calculated. The attitude of the women was categorized as <3—negative attitude, 3—neutral attitude, and >3—positive attitude to separate women who have a positive or negative opinion about the vaccine from those who are hesitant. It is important to differentiate those who refuse vaccination from those who do not have an opinion and lack confidence in vaccination [33].

2.4. Statistical Analysis

Statistical analysis was performed using STATA 16 [34]. Cronbach's alpha was calculated for attitude items to measure internal reliability. The scale included both positive and negative items. Positive items had a Cronbach's alpha coefficient of 0.82. Negative statements had a Cronbach's alpha coefficient of 0.75, and the overall Cronbach's alpha was 0.79. Factor analysis was performed to test the questionnaire's consistency and validity. The Kaiser–Meyer–Olkin measure of sampling adequacy (0.752) and the Bartlett test of sphericity ($p < 0.001$) were performed before the factor analysis. All factors had a uniqueness lower than 0.6, except for the statement "Majority of my friends vaccinate their daughters from HPV", which had a uniqueness of 0.81. The item was dropped from the attitude scale, as it was not relevant to the Kazakhstan context due to the HPV vaccine not being readily available in the country.

Descriptive statistics consisting of mean values, standard deviations, and frequencies were obtained using univariable and bivariable analysis. Chi-square and Fisher's exact tests with a significance value of <0.005 were used to analyze the relationships between categorical variables.

Ordinal logistic regression was performed to explore factors associated with attitude towards HPV vaccination among women. Variables that showed significance in the bivariable analysis and were important as epidemiological factors were included in the final model. Among participants' characteristics, variables such as age, education, and number of children were included in the final model. Although participants' age was not a statistically significant factor, it was included in the final model due to its importance for the epidemiological picture. Two contextual factors such as distrust in the healthcare system due to complications of the HPV vaccination program in Kazakhstan in 2013 and trust in alternative medicine (alternative medicine strengthening the body's defenses) were considered for the final model. The model assumptions were checked. The goodness of fit of the model was checked with Hosmer–Lemeshow, Pulkstenis–Robinson Chi-square, and deviance tests, as well as the Lipsitz likelihood-ratio test.

2.5. Ethical Considerations

The study was conducted in compliance with the Declaration of Helsinki and was approved by the Institutional Research Ethics Committee of Nazarbayev University (NU IREC) on 23 April 2019 (IREC Number: 146/4042019). Before inclusion in the study, all potential participants were informed about the aims, methods, risks, and benefits of the study. Verbal consent was received from participants after an explanation of the voluntary and anonymous nature of the study.

3. Results

3.1. Participants' Characteristics

The social and demographic characteristics of women are shown in Table 1. The mean age of the study participants was 36.46 ± 11.18 years. More than 80% of women represented the Kazakh ethnicity. Most women (55%) had a university degree, which is in line with the official government statistics that reported the gross enrollment rate in higher education in Kazakhstan in 2020 to be 64.07%, of which 70.5% were women [32]. The majority were either married or were in a committed relationship (80%) and had one to three children (69%). There was almost an equal distribution of the place of residence among the participants, except for Aktobe city, where the number of participants was 29%. Almost half of women (48%) reported a family income lower than the national average level.

Table 1. Social and demographic characteristics of the study participants (N = 347).

Variables	Total N = 347 (%)
Age, Mean 36.46 ± 11.18	
19–27	74 (21%)
28–33	94 (27%)
34–43	86 (25%)
44+	93 (27%)
Ethnicity	
Kazakh	284 (82%)
Other	63 (18%)
Education	
Unfinished/finished school	38 (11%)
College	117 (34%)
University	192 (55%)
City	
Nur-Sultan	86 (25%)
Almaty	80 (23%)
Aktobe	100 (29%)
Oskemen	81 (23%)

Table 1. *Cont.*

Variables	Total N = 347 (%)
Income *	
Low	166 (48%)
Middle	84 (24%)
Upper	97 (28%)
Marital status	
Single	71 (20%)
Not single	276 (80%)
Children	
No children	73 (21%)
1–3 children	239 (69%)
4 or more children	35 (10%)

* Agency for Strategic Planning and Reforms of the Republic of Kazakhstan. Bureau of National Statistics.

3.2. Contextual Factors

Table 2 demonstrates to which extent women agreed with the statements about contextual factors. Most women (48%) were neutral about COVID-19's effect on trust in the HPV vaccine and about the 2013 HPV program's effect on their trust in the healthcare system. More than half of women (56%) disagreed with the statement that vaccinating teenage girls against HPV encourages them to have sex. The majority of women (42%) were not in favor of the compulsory vaccines for children mandated by the government of Kazakhstan. The majority of women (44%) were neutral to the statement that everyone should be able to decide which vaccines are needed for their children. More than half of women (61%) agreed that alternative medicines strengthen the body's defenses, thus leading to a complete cure.

Table 2. Contextual factors, N = 233.

Questions	Disagree N (%)	Neutral N (%)	Agree N (%)
Since the controversy over the COVID-19 vaccination, I have less confidence in the HPV vaccination recommendations	88 (38%)	112 (48%)	33 (14%)
Since HPV vaccination program started in Kazakhstan in 2013, had led to complications in few cases, I have less confidence in the health care system	83 (36%)	112 (48%)	38 (16%)
I think vaccinating teenage girls against HPV encourages them to have sex	130 (56%)	80 (34%)	23 (10%)
I am in favor of the compulsory vaccines for children mandated by the government of Kazakhstan	98 (42%)	59 (25%)	76 (33%)
Everyone should be able to decide which vaccines are needed for their children	45 (19%)	103 (44%)	85 (37%)
Alternative medicines strengthen the body's defenses, thus leading to a complete cure	45 (19%)	47 (20%)	141 (61%)

3.3. Trust in Sources about Vaccination

The least trusted information sources among women were alternative media, the government, and the pharmaceutical industry. The most trusted were scientific researchers, closely followed by medical workers (Figure 2).

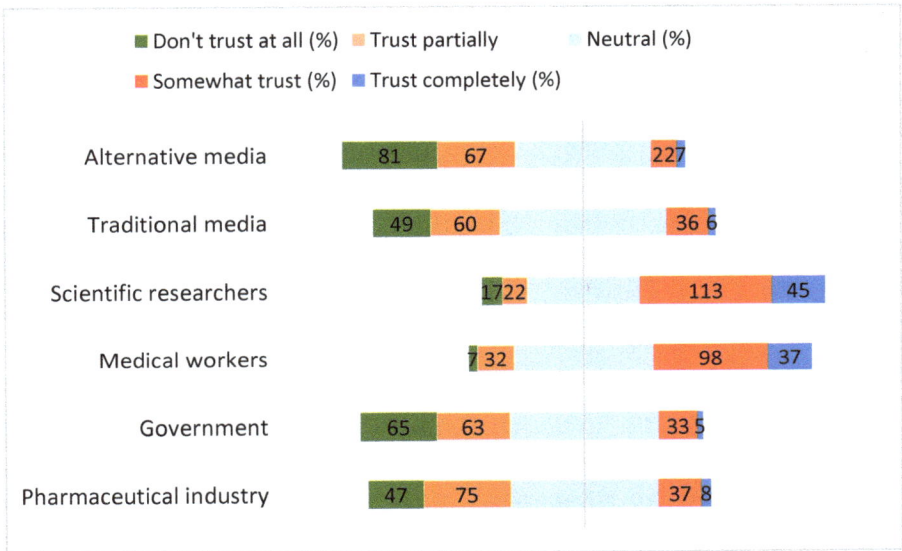

Figure 2. Respondents' trust to information providers.

Table 3 demonstrates the extent to which women trust the sources to tell the truth about the vaccine. The most trusted sources to tell the truth about the vaccine, associated with a positive attitude towards vaccination, were healthcare professionals (60%) and scientific researchers (61%). The high level of distrust of the pharmaceutical industry was associated with a positive attitude towards HPV vaccination (58%). The government was also not viewed as a trustworthy source and was associated with a positive attitude towards HPV vaccination (61%). Both alternative (WhatsApp Messenger, Instagram, Telegram, YouTube, etc.) and traditional media (TV, newspapers) had lower trust levels among the participants with both negative and positive attitudes towards HPV vaccination. All the sources were statistically significantly associated with attitude towards HPV vaccination.

Table 3. Association between attitude towards HPV vaccination and the trust to the sources, N = 218.

Variables	Attitude towards HPV Vaccination N (%)			p Value
	Low 45 (21%)	Middle 63 (29%)	High 110 (50%)	
Pharmaceutical industry				$p = 0.002$ *
Distrust	24 (26%)	15 (16%)	53 (58%)	
Neutral	12 (13%)	39 (43%)	40 (44%)	
Trust	9 (26%)	9 (26%)	17 (48%)	

Table 3. Cont.

Variables	Attitude towards HPV Vaccination N (%)			p Value
	Low 45 (21%)	Middle 63 (29%)	High 110 (50%)	
Government				p < 0.001 *
Distrust	25 (26%)	12 (13%)	58 (61%)	
Neutral	12 (12%)	46 (48%)	58 (40%)	
Trust	8 (30%)	5 (18%)	14 (52%)	
Healthcare professional				p = 0.004 **
Distrust	8 (36%)	3 (14%)	11 (50%)	
Neutral	17 (19%)	38 (41%)	37 (40%)	
Trust	20 (19%)	22 (21%)	62 (60%)	
Scientific researchers				p < 0.001 *
Distrust	4 (15%)	5 (19%)	17 (66%)	
Neutral	17 (24%)	35 (50%)	18 (26%)	
Trust	24 (20%)	23 (19%)	75 (61%)	
Traditional media				p < 0.001 *
Distrust	19 (24%)	10 (12%)	52 (64%)	
Neutral	17 (15%)	48 (42%)	48 (43%)	
Trust	9 (37%)	5 (21%)	10 (42%)	
Alternative media				p < 0.001 **
Distrust	24 (22%)	17 (15%)	71 (63%)	
Neutral	15 (16%)	44 (48%)	33 (36%)	
Trust	6 (43%)	2 (14%)	6 (42%)	

* p value < 0.05, Chi-square test. ** p value < 0.05, Fisher's exact test.

3.4. Attitude towards HPV Vaccination

3.4.1. Bivariable Analysis

Bivariable analysis between attitude towards HPV vaccination and patient characteristics and contextual factors is shown in Table 4. A positive attitude towards HPV vaccination was reported by 52% of the respondents, with the highest proportion in the youngest age group and the lowest in the oldest age group. There was no statistical difference in ethnicities regarding attitude towards HPV vaccination. The highest proportion of positive attitudes (58%) was observed among women with a university degree and the lowest (14%) among women with only high school or unfinished high school education. Negative attitude was the lowest among women with middle income (7%) and highest among women with low income (27%), while women with an upper level of income had the highest proportion of positive attitudes (62%). The majority of women without children (72%) had a positive attitude towards the vaccine, while only 16% of women with 4 and more children had the same attitude.

The Chi-square test showed that all contextual factors were statistically significantly associated with the level of attitude towards HPV vaccination. Among women who had no prejudice that HPV vaccination encourages teenage girls to have sex, 65% had a positive attitude. Among those who disagreed with compulsory vaccination, a majority (54%) had a positive attitude to the HPV vaccine, and among those who agreed with compulsory vaccination, a majority (58%) had a positive attitude to the HPV vaccine. Similarly, a majority of women who agreed (52%) or disagreed (71%) with freedom of vaccine choice for their children were women with a positive attitude towards the HPV vaccine. The majority of women (73%) who disagree with the statement that alternative medicine strengthens the body's defenses had a positive attitude towards the HPV vaccine.

Table 4. Attitude towards HPV vaccination among women including social and demographic characteristics and contextual factors, (N = 233).

Variables	Attitude Prevalence N (%)			p Value	Attitude COR (95%)	Attitude AOR (95%) ***
	Negative 43 (18%)	Neutral 70 (30%)	Positive 120 (52%)			
Age						
19–27	7 (14%)	11 (23%)	31 (63%)	p = 0.377	1	1
28–33	16 (24%)	18 (26%)	34 (50%)		0.55 (0.27–1.15)	0.80 (0.36–1.76)
34–43	8 (14%)	20 (35%)	29 (51%)		0.67 (0.32–1.42)	1.23 (0.52–2.93)
44+	12 (20%)	21 (36%)	26 (44%)		0.50 (0.24–1.05)	0.88 (0.37–2.08)
Ethnicity						
Kazakh	33 (18%)	60 (32%)	94 (50%)	p = 0.381		
Other	10 (22%)	10 (22%)	26 (56%)			
Education						
Unfinished/finished school	5 (24%)	13 (62%)	3 (14%)	p = 0.001 *	1	1
College	17 (24%)	19 (26%)	36 (50%)		2.29 (0.98–5.34)	1.81 (0.73–4.48)
University	21 (15%)	38 (27%)	81 (58%)		3.40 (1.53–7.56)	2.38 (1.01–5.65)
City						
Nur-Sultan	4 (7%)	17 (30%)	35 (63%)	p = 0.003 **	1	
Almaty	15 (24%)	13 (21%)	35 (56)		0.60 (0.29–1.23)	
Aktobe	8 (12%)	27 (41%)	31 (47%)		0.57 (0.29–1.14)	
Oskemen	16 (33%)	13 (27%)	19 (40%)			
Family income						
Low	26 (27%)	30 (32%)	39 (41%)	p = 0.004 **	1	
Middle	5 (7%)	25 (37%)	37 (55%)		2.13 (1.18–3.85)	
Upper	12 (17%)	15 (21%)	44 (62%)		2.29 (1.25–4.21)	
Marital status						
Single	11 (22%)	12 (25%)	26 (53%)	p = 0.548		
Not single	32 (17%)	58 (32%)	94 (51%)			
Children						
No children	7 (12%)	9 (16%)	42 (72%)	p < 0.001 **	1	1
1–3 children	31 (21%)	45 (30%)	74 (49%)		0.38 (0.20–0.73)	0.45 (0.21–0.94)
4 or more children	5 (20%)	16 (64%)	4 (16%)		0.18 (0.07–0.43)	0.26 (0.10–0.73)
Effect of COVID-19 vaccination on HPV vaccine perception						
Disagree	10 (12%)	16 (19%)	57 (69%)	p = 0.001 **	1	
Neutral	21 (19%)	43 (38%)	48 (43%)		0.39 (0.22–0.69)	
Agree	12 (32%)	11 (29%)	15 (39%)		0.27 (0.13–0.58)	

Table 4. Cont.

Variables	Attitude Prevalence N (%)			p Value	Attitude COR (95%)	Attitude AOR (95%) ***
	Negative 43 (18%)	Neutral 70 (30%)	Positive1 20 (52%)			
The 2013 HPV vaccination program in Kazakhstan						
Disagree	9 (10%)	16 (18%)	63 (72%)	$p < 0.001$ **	1	1
Neutral	21 (19%)	45 (40%)	46 (41%)		0.31 (0.18–0.56)	0.34 (0.19–0.62)
Agree	13 (40%)	9 (27%)	11(33%)		0.16 (0.07–0.37)	0.21 (0.09–0.50)
Relation of HPV vaccination to sexual promiscuity						
Disagree	21 (16%)	25 (19%)	84 (65%)	$p < 0.001$ **	1	
Neutral	14 (18%)	37 (46%)	29 (36%)		0.42 (0.25–0.71)	
Agree	8 (35%)	8 (35%)	7 (30%)		0.25 (0.22–0.59)	
Compulsory vaccine mandated by the government						
Disagree	18 (18%)	27 (28%)	53 (54%)	$p = 0.037$ **	1	
Neutral	9 (15%)	27 (46%)	23 (39%)		0.70 (0.39–1.27)	
Agree	16 (21%)	16 (21%)	44 (58%)		1.08 (0.60–1.94)	
Freedom of vaccine choice for their children						
Disagree	4 (9%)	9 (20%)	32 (71%)	$p < 0.001$ **	1	
Neutral	4 (8%)	29 (62%)	14 (30%)		0.29 (0.13–0.66)	
Agree	35 (25%)	32 (23%)	74 (52%)		0.39 (0.19–0.80)	
Alternative medicine strengthening the body's defenses						
Disagree	4 (9%)	8 (18%)	33 (73%)	$p = 0.015$ **	1	1
Neutral	50 (19%)	38 (37%)	45 (44%)		0.31 (0.14–0.65)	0.48 (0.21–1.10)
Agree	19 (22%)	24 (28%)	42 (50%)		0.34 (0.16–0.74)	0.41 (0.18–0.94)

* p value < 0.05, Fisher's exact test. ** p value < 0.05, Chi-square test. *** OR adjusted for age, education, number of children, the 2013 HPV vaccination program in Kazakhstan, alternative medicine strengthening the body's defenses.

3.4.2. Ordinal Logistic Regression

Women aged between 34 and 43 were 1.23 times more likely to have a positive (in relation to neutral or negative) attitude towards HPV vaccination in comparison to women aged between 19 and 27 years, adjusting for other variables (Table 4). Having a college or university degree increased the odds of a positive attitude by 1.81-fold and 2.38-fold, respectively, compared to incomplete/complete high school education, holding other variables constant. Women with 1–3 children or 4+ children were 0.45 and 0.26 times the odds of a positive attitude towards HPV vaccination in comparison with women with no children, adjusting for other factors.

Women who were neutral about their confidence in the healthcare system were 0.34 times the odds of a positive attitude towards HPV vaccination. Agreeing that alternative medicines strengthen the body's defenses or being neutral about the statement decreased the odds of a positive attitude by 0.41-fold and by 0.48-fold compared with women who disagreed with the statement, adjusting for other variables (Table 4).

4. Discussion

To date, there are no published studies investigating attitudes toward the HPV vaccine among Kazakhstani women. Thus, this is the first study that aimed to examine attitudes toward HPV vaccination and explore factors associated with a positive attitude toward HPV vaccination in Kazakhstani women. Since HR-HPV prevalence is high among women in

Kazakhstan [13–15,21], and cervical cancer incidence has increased in the past decade [16], becoming the fourth leading cause of death from cancer among women [35], it is important to implement primary prevention of HPV infection and its related diseases in the country. However, the successful relaunching of the HPV vaccination program largely depends on HPV vaccine attitudes; therefore, studies investigating society's attitudes towards the vaccine are an essential part of facilitating the process.

Some historical contextual factors were taken into consideration in this study, such as previous HPV vaccination program complications/failure in Kazakhstan. The situation in Japan closely resembles the failure of the HPV vaccination program in Kazakhstan. Reports of side effects in mass media and prompt cancellation of the program had a long-lasting effect in Japan, causing the vaccine coverage to fall to less than 1% [36]. In Kazakhstan, the pushback intensified after media coverage of two 11–12-year-old girls having trouble breathing, hallucinations, and being hospitalized in the ICU immediately after administration of the HPV vaccine. As was later clarified, such a reaction resulted from inappropriate actions of medical personnel, who panicked at an allergic rash to the vaccine and administered a mixture of sedatives and painkiller medications. Nevertheless, the damage was done. The media quoted government officials and medical workers saying "73 percent of participants in [HPV] vaccine trials acquired new diseases—similar facts have been recorded around the world" and "Who knows what will happen to the reproductive function of [HPV] vaccinated girls in ten years?" [37].

Among our respondents, those who were affected by the failed 2013 HPV vaccination program had a 79% lower likelihood of having a positive attitude towards the vaccine, adjusting for other variables. Overall, 16% of women indicated that the failure of the 2013 HPV vaccination program in Kazakhstan had affected their confidence in the healthcare system, and the majority of them (40%) had a negative attitude towards the HPV vaccine. Thus, an unsuccessful attempt to implement the HPV vaccination program in Kazakhstan in 2013 had a significant impact. This finding is similar to the study reporting data from Romania and France, where the initial HPV vaccination program coverage reported a poor response and required specific action plans to improve the situation [38,39].

Rapid introduction of the COVID-19 vaccine is another factor considered in this study, as it has been reported previously that the level of COVID-19 hesitancy is high in Kazakhstan [40,41], and the media coverage of the vaccine is politicized worldwide [42,43], which might carry over to other domains in healthcare, such as the HPV vaccine [44].

The ongoing debates around the COVID-19 vaccine, however, did not have the same effect. Among women who disagreed with having less confidence in HPV vaccination recommendations since the controversy over the COVID-19 vaccination, 69% still had a positive level of attitude towards HPV vaccination. Overall, 14% of women indicated that COVID-19 controversies have affected their trust in HPV vaccination, and their distribution among the attitude groups was even. This finding falls in line with previous studies that show a lack of hesitancy overlap between HPV and COVID-19 vaccines [45].

Unfortunately, this study revealed a low trust of the respondents in the government (including the Ministry of Healthcare) as the main policymaker in Kazakhstan and in pharmaceutical companies. The majority of the respondents (44%) did not trust the government; only 13% did, the rest remaining neutral. This evidence shows that the Ministry of Healthcare and other governmental agencies in Kazakhstan should reinforce the information campaign in trustworthy ways. Similarly, participants had low levels of trust in alternative media and mostly low or neutral levels of trust in traditional media. At the same time, the fact that in our study, researchers and healthcare professionals are the most trusted source of information about the vaccine gives hope and identifies directions that the Ministry of Healthcare can employ to increase HPV vaccine awareness and improve attitudes. Engaging and strengthening the relevant healthcare workforce in preparation for HPV vaccine introduction could be achieved through training/seminars, information about the evidence and necessity of HPV vaccination and cervical cancer, and communication training to address parents' concerns and make recommendations. Our findings of trust are comparable with studies in European countries (Sweden, Hungary, France, and the UK), where mistrust of health authorities was reported by 47% to 55% of the respondents [46]. On the other hand, the results of one Italian study showed high trust in doctors (85.3%) and teachers (90.4%) [47]. Similar to our finding, the study by Karafillakis et al. (2019) also revealed mistrust of pharmaceutical companies due to their underlying profit-making motives reported in many other European countries (Bulgaria, Romania, Sweden, Ireland, the Netherlands, Spain, and the UK) [46]. The results are also somewhat comparable to those in the USA, where levels of trust were generally high for healthcare providers and low for pharmaceutical companies. The trust for governmental organizations, however, showed mixed results in varying studies. Unlike in our study, the factor of ethnicity was significant for trust levels in the USA [48]. This could be explained by a more homogenous ethnical composition of Kazakhstan.

In this study, a positive attitude towards HPV vaccination was reported by 52% of the respondents. Education, place of residence, level of income, and number of children were the factors that were found to be significantly associated with the level of attitude towards HPV vaccination. Women with high income levels had the highest proportion of positive attitudes toward the HPV vaccine (62%). On the other hand, among women with high-school-level education and those who did not finish high school, 62% were neutral towards HPV vaccination. Thus, the level of education directly correlates with positive attitudes toward the HPV vaccine. Similar results were obtained in an Italian study, where 49.7% of the respondents had a positive attitude toward the HPV vaccine [47], and in a Romanian study, where 50.7% of women have a positive attitude toward the vaccine [38]. Both cited studies, and our study, confirmed that level of awareness and attitudes were directly linked to education [38,47]. This was also confirmed in the study by Özdemir et al. (2020), where positive attitudes towards HPV and the HPV vaccine increased in employed women and those who had high education and economic levels [49].

However, having such a huge proportion of neutral respondents in our study indicates the direction of further actions. Informational interventions to increase awareness of the HPV vaccine and the advantages of being vaccinated should be developed, as a positive attitude toward the HPV vaccine is associated with a higher level of intention to receive the HPV vaccine [26,50].

Unfortunately, only 16% of mothers with four or more children had a positive attitude towards the HPV vaccine, and the majority (64%) had a neutral attitude. This is an important group of the population, who requires more information on the vaccine, as their attitude towards the vaccine has a direct impact on the HPV vaccination program coverage among the target group of 9–11 years old girls. The situation could be improved if relevant and effective informational programs are employed to explain the advantages of the HPV vaccine in HPV infection and cancer prevention, as has been demonstrated by a study among parents in Japan [51].

As was confirmed by many studies, a significant reduction in the incidence of pre-cancerous cervical lesions and cervical cancer was observed after the introduction of HPV vaccination programs [6,52–54]. Moreover, HPV vaccination is associated with a substantially reduced risk of invasive cervical cancer at the population level [52]. This knowledge, together with the knowledge of HPV as the most common STI, could improve the HPV infection spread [55]. However, very few studies have reported the association between knowledge of STI and sexual behavior and HPV status [56,57]. Thus, more research on HPV infection and HPV vaccine knowledge, behavior, and attitudes is required.

Study strengths and limitations. This was the first study to assess attitudes towards HPV vaccination among Kazakhstani women. Another strength of this study is covering the female population in the big cities of four Kazakhstani regions (central, southern, eastern, and western) and investigating the factors associated with attitudes towards HPV vaccination. However, since we approached only the population of big cities, but not these regions' rural areas, this study cannot fully represent the whole country's female population. Moreover, in this study, the proportions of participants with university-level and college-level education were 55% and 34%, respectively. These indicators could be different if we include participants from rural areas. These are the major limitations that we hope to overcome in our future studies to obtain a more precise picture in terms of participants' residence and education. Another limitation of this study is its cross-sectional nature and resulting lack of causality. The study employed convenience sampling with self-reporting methods. This limits the representativeness of our findings due to selection and nonresponse biases. The descriptive nature of our statistical model, as well as the low number of respondents, prompts for expansion of the study beyond the pilot investigation. Moreover, in future studies, we should investigate parents'/mothers' attitudes towards HPV vaccination further, as they are the main decision makers if the vaccination of the target group is planned.

There are many issues related to cervical cancer prevention that require solving in Kazakhstan in the near future [18]. Although it requires attention and effort from healthcare policymakers, social media could help to improve the situation with overall societal awareness. Evidence from recent studies has indicated that social media has good potential to reach adolescents and young adults with information about HPV [58], and instead of creating a negative view, it could help to promote the HPV vaccination campaign.

5. Conclusions

This study shows contrary attitudes toward HPV vaccination exist among Kazakhstani women, with approximately half of women having positive and almost half having negative or neutral attitudes towards the vaccine. We found that women's age, education, number of children, confidence in the healthcare system, and belief in alternative medicine were associated with attitudes towards HPV vaccination. These factors, as well as high levels of trust towards medical and science workers, should be taken into consideration when planning context-specific health educational interventions to form positive attitudes towards HPV vaccination in Kazakhstani women. In addition, sharing accurate information regarding the safety, effectiveness, and benefits of HPV vaccination to prevent HPV infection and related diseases could potentially improve women's attitudes. HPV educational interventions are warranted to successfully relaunch and include HPV vaccination in the national immunization program in Kazakhstan.

Supplementary Materials: The following supporting information can be downloaded at: https://www.mdpi.com/article/10.3390/vaccines10050824/s1, HPV vaccine questionnaire.

Author Contributions: Conceptualization, G.A.; data curation, A.B. and T.I.; formal analysis, T.I. and A.I.; funding acquisition, G.A.; methodology, G.A.; project administration, G.A.; software, A.I.; supervision, G.A.; validation, A.I.; visualization, A.B. and A.I.; writing—original draft, A.B. and T.I.; writing—review and editing, G.A. All authors have read and agreed to the published version of the manuscript.

Funding: This study was supported by the Faculty Development Research Grant Program 2019–2021 (Funder Project Reference: 110119FD4528, title: A molecular epidemiological study to determine the prevalence of oncogenic HPV strains for cervical cancer prevention in Kazakhstan). G.A. is the PI of the project.

Institutional Review Board Statement: The study was conducted according to the guidelines of the Declaration of Helsinki and was approved by the Institutional Research Ethics Committee of Nazarbayev University (NU IREC) on 23 April, 2019 (IREC number: 146/4042019).

Informed Consent Statement: Informed consent was obtained from all subjects involved in the study.

Data Availability Statement: The study questionnaires are available per resonable request form the study PI via email gulzhanat.aimagambetova@nu.edu.kz.

Acknowledgments: The authors thank the Nazarbayev University School of Medicine for the continuous support that enabled the completion of this study. The authors would like to express gratitude to Brett Craig, WHO, Regional Office for Europe, for comments that greatly improved the manuscript.

Conflicts of Interest: The authors declare no conflict of interest. The funders had no role in the design of the study; in the collection, analyses, or interpretation of data; in the writing of the manuscript, or in the decision to publish the results.

References

1. zur Hausen, H. Papillomaviruses and cancer: From basic studies to clinical application. *Nat. Rev. Cancer* **2002**, *2*, 342–350. [CrossRef] [PubMed]
2. Aimagambetova, G.; Azizan, A. Epidemiology of HPV Infection and HPV-Related Cancers in Kazakhstan: A Review. *Asian Pac. J. Cancer Prev. APJCP* **2018**, *19*, 1175–1180. [CrossRef] [PubMed]
3. Chan, C.K.; Aimagambetova, G.; Ukybassova, T.; Kongrtay, K.; Azizan, A. Human Papillomavirus Infection and Cervical Cancer: Epidemiology, Screening, and Vaccination-Review of Current Perspectives. *J. Oncol.* **2019**, *2019*, 3257939. [CrossRef] [PubMed]
4. Arbyn, M.; Weiderpass, E.; Bruni, L.; de Sanjosé, S.; Saraiya, M.; Ferlay, J.; Bray, F. Estimates of incidence and mortality of cervical cancer in 2018: A worldwide analysis. *Lancet Glob. Health* **2020**, *8*, e191–e203. [CrossRef]
5. Patel, C.; Brotherton, J.M.; Pillsbury, A.; Jayasinghe, S.; Donovan, B.; Macartney, K.; Marshall, H. The impact of 10 years of human papillomavirus (HPV) vaccination in Australia: What additional disease burden will a nonavalent vaccine prevent? *Euro Surveill. Bull. Eur. Sur Mal. Transm. Eur. Commun. Dis. Bull.* **2018**, *23*, 1700737. [CrossRef] [PubMed]
6. Falcaro, M.; Castañon, A.; Ndlela, B.; Checchi, M.; Soldan, K.; Lopez-Bernal, J.; Elliss-Brookes, L.; Sasieni, P. The effects of the national HPV vaccination programme in England, UK, on cervical cancer and grade 3 cervical intraepithelial neoplasia incidence: A register-based observational study. *Lancet* **2021**, *398*, 2084–2092. [CrossRef]
7. Jacot-Guillarmod, M.; Pasquier, J.; Greub, G.; Bongiovanni, M.; Achtari, C.; Sahli, R. Impact of HPV vaccination with Gardasil® in Switzerland. *BMC Infect. Dis.* **2017**, *17*, 790. [CrossRef]
8. Sand, L.; Jalouli, J. Viruses and oral cancer. Is there a link? *Microbes Infect.* **2014**, *16*, 371–378. [CrossRef]
9. Syrjänen, S. Oral manifestations of human papillomavirus infections. *Eur. J. Oral Sci.* **2018**, *126* (Suppl. 1), 49–66. [CrossRef]
10. Strycharz-Dudziak, M.; Fołtyn, S.; Dworzański, J.; Kiełczykowska, M.; Malm, M.; Drop, B.; Polz-Dacewicz, M. Glutathione Peroxidase (GPx) and Superoxide Dismutase (SOD) in Oropharyngeal Cancer Associated with EBV and HPV Coinfection. *Viruses* **2020**, *12*, 1008. [CrossRef]
11. Vinodhini, K.; Shanmughapriya, S.; Das, B.C.; Natarajaseenivasan, K. Prevalence and risk factors of HPV infection among women from various provinces of the world. *Arch. Gynecol. Obstet.* **2012**, *285*, 771–777. [CrossRef] [PubMed]
12. Obeid, D.A.; Almatrrouk, S.A.; Alfageeh, M.B.; Al-Ahdal, M.N.A.; Alhamlan, F.S. Human papillomavirus epidemiology in populations with normal or abnormal cervical cytology or cervical cancer in the Middle East and North Africa: A systematic review and meta-analysis. *J. Infect. Public Health* **2020**, *13*, 1304–1313. [CrossRef] [PubMed]
13. Niyazmetova, L.; Aimagambetova, G.; Stambekova, N.; Abugalieva, Z.; Seksembayeva, K.; Ali, S.; Azizan, A. Application of molecular genotyping to determine prevalence of HPV strains in Pap smears of Kazakhstan women. *Int. J. Infect. Dis. IJID Off. Publ. Int. Soc. Infect. Dis.* **2017**, *54*, 85–88. [CrossRef] [PubMed]
14. Babi, A.; Issa, T.; Issanov, A.; Akilzhanova, A.; Nurgaliyeva, K.; Abugalieva, Z.; Ukybassova, T.; Daribay, Z.; Khan, S.A.; Chan, C.K.; et al. Prevalence of high-risk human papillomavirus infection among Kazakhstani women attending gynecological outpatient clinics. *Int. J. Infect. Dis. IJID Off. Publ. Int. Soc. Infect. Dis.* **2021**, *109*, 8–16. [CrossRef]
15. Aimagambetova, G.; Babi, A.; Issanov, A.; Akhanova, S.; Udalova, N.; Koktova, S.; Balykov, A.; Sattarkyzy, Z.; Abakasheva, Z.; Azizan, A.; et al. The Distribution and Prevalence of High-Risk HPV Genotypes Other than HPV-16 and HPV-18 among Women Attending Gynecologists' Offices in Kazakhstan. *Biology* **2021**, *10*, 794. [CrossRef]
16. Igissinov, N.; Igissinova, G.; Telmanova, Z.; Bilyalova, Z.; Kulmirzayeva, D.; Kozhakhmetova, Z.; Urazova, S.; Turebayev, D.; Nurtazinova, G.; Omarbekov, A.; et al. New Trends of Cervical Cancer Incidence in Kazakhstan. *Asian Pac. J. Cancer Prev. APJCP* **2021**, *22*, 1295–1304. [CrossRef]
17. Aimagambetova, G.; Chan, C.K.; Ukybassova, T.; Imankulova, B.; Balykov, A.; Kongrtay, K.; Azizan, A. Cervical cancer screening and prevention in Kazakhstan and Central Asia. *J. Med. Screen.* **2021**, *28*, 48–50. [CrossRef]
18. Balmagambetova, S.; Tinelli, A.; Mynbaev, O.A.; Koyshybaev, A.; Urazayev, O.; Kereyeva, N.; Ismagulova, E. Human Papillomavirus Selected Properties and Related Cervical Cancer Prevention Issues. *Curr. Pharm. Des.* **2020**, *26*, 2073–2086. [CrossRef]
19. Kaidarova, D. The Experience of Cervical Cancer Screening Program in Kazakhstan. In Proceedings of the Eurasian Cancer Screening Conference, Minsk, Belarus; 2018. Available online: https://onco.kz/wp-content/uploads/2018/05/Cervical_Minsk.ENG_.pdf (accessed on 25 March 2022).
20. Kaidarova, D.; Zhylkaidarova, A.; Dushimova, Z.; Bolatbekova, R. Screening for Cervical Cancer in Kazakhstan. *J. Glob. Oncol.* **2018**, *4*, 50s. [CrossRef]
21. Issa, T.; Babi, A.; Issanov, A.; Akilzhanova, A.; Nurgaliyeva, K.; Abugalieva, Z.; Azizan, A.; Khan, S.A.; Chan, C.K.; Alibekova, R.; et al. Knowledge and awareness of human papillomavirus infection and human papillomavirus vaccine among Kazakhstani women attending gynecological clinics. *PLoS ONE* **2021**, *16*, e0261203. [CrossRef]
22. Bray, F.; Lortet-Tieulent, J.; Znaor, A.; Brotons, M.; Poljak, M.; Arbyn, M. Patterns and Trends in Human Papillomavirus-Related Diseases in Central and Eastern Europe and Central Asia. *Vaccine* **2013**, *31*, H32–H45. [CrossRef] [PubMed]
23. Nasritdinova, N.Y.; Reznik, V.L.; Kuatbaieva, A.M.; Kairbaiev, M.R. The awareness and attitude of population of Kazakhstan to inoculation against human papilloma virus. *Probl Sotsialnoi Gig. Zdr. Istor. Med.* **2016**, *24*, 304–307.

24. Villanueva, S.; Mosteiro-Miguéns, D.G.; Domínguez-Martís, E.M.; López-Ares, D.; Novío, S. Knowledge, Attitudes, and Intentions towards Human Papillomavirus Vaccination among Nursing Students in Spain. *Int. J. Environ. Res. Public Health* **2019**, *16*, 4507. [CrossRef] [PubMed]
25. Browne, M.; Thomson, P.; Rockloff, M.J.; Pennycook, G. Going against the Herd: Psychological and Cultural Factors Underlying the 'Vaccination Confidence Gap'. *PLoS ONE* **2015**, *10*, e0132562. [CrossRef] [PubMed]
26. Sallam, M.; Al-Mahzoum, K.; Eid, H.; Assaf, A.M.; Abdaljaleel, M.; Al-Abbadi, M.; Mahafzah, A. Attitude towards HPV Vaccination and the Intention to Get Vaccinated among Female University Students in Health Schools in Jordan. *Vaccines* **2021**, *9*, 1432. [CrossRef]
27. Bal-Yılmaz, H.; Koniak-Griffin, D. Knowledge, Behaviors, and Attitudes about Human Papilloma Virus among Nursing Students in Izmir, Turkey. *J. Cancer Educ. Off. J. Am. Assoc. Cancer Educ.* **2018**, *33*, 814–820. [CrossRef]
28. Khatiwada, M.; Kartasasmita, C.; Mediani, H.S.; Delprat, C.; Van Hal, G.; Dochez, C. Knowledge, Attitude and Acceptability of the Human Papilloma Virus Vaccine and Vaccination among University Students in Indonesia. *Front. Public Health* **2021**, *9*, 607. [CrossRef]
29. World Health Organization. A Cervical Cancer-Free Future: First-Ever Global Commitment to Eliminate a Cancer [Internet]. 2020. Available online: https://www.who.int/news/item/17-11-2020-a-cervical-cancer-free-future-first-ever-global-commitment-to-eliminate-a-cancer (accessed on 7 February 2022).
30. Canfell, K. Towards the global elimination of cervical cancer. *Papillomavirus Res.* **2019**, *8*, 100170. [CrossRef]
31. Dib, F.; Mayaud, P.; Launay, O.; Chauvin, P.; FSQD-HPVH Study Group. Design and content validation of a survey questionnaire assessing the determinants of human papillomavirus (HPV) vaccine hesitancy in France: A reactive Delphi study. *Vaccine* **2020**, *38*, 6127–6140. [CrossRef]
32. Agency for Strategic Planning and Reforms of the Republic of Kazakhstan. Bureau of National Statistics. Available online: https://www.stat.gov.kz/ (accessed on 2 May 2022).
33. Dubé, E.; Laberge, C.; Guay, M.; Bramadat, P.; Roy, R.; Bettinger, J. Vaccine hesitancy: An overview. *Hum. Vaccines Immunother.* **2013**, *9*, 1763–1773. [CrossRef]
34. StataCorp LLC. Stata Statistical Software: Release 16. 2019. Available online: https://www.stata.com/support/faqs/resources/citing-software-documentation-faqs/#:~{}:text=2019.,Station%2CTX%3AStataCorpLLC.&text=StataCorp.,-2017 (accessed on 1 March 2022).
35. Bruni, L.; Albero, G.; Serrano, B.; Mena, M.; Collado, J.J.; Gómez, D.; Muñoz, J.; Bosch, F.X.; de Sanjosé, S. ICO/IARC Information Centre on HPV and Cancer (HPV Information Centre). In *Human Papillomavirus and Related Diseases in Kazakhstan*; Summary Report 22 October 2021; Institut Català d'Oncologia Avda: Barcelona, Spain; Available online: www.hpvcentre.net (accessed on 9 March 2022).
36. Hanley, S.J.; Yoshioka, E.; Ito, Y.; Kishi, R. HPV vaccination crisis in Japan. *Lancet* **2015**, *385*, 2571. [CrossRef]
37. Vaccine against Papilloma Virus. Salvation or Experiment? [Article in Russian]. Available online: https://www.caravan.kz/gazeta/vakcina-protiv-virusa-papillomy-spasenie-ili-ehksperiment-83376/ (accessed on 3 May 2022).
38. Grigore, M.; Teleman, S.I.; Pristavu, A.; Matei, M. Awareness and Knowledge about HPV and HPV Vaccine among Romanian Women. *J. Cancer Educ.* **2016**, *33*, 154–159. [CrossRef] [PubMed]
39. Lefèvre, H.; Schrimpf, C.; Moro, M.R.; Lachal, J. HPV vaccination rate in French adolescent girls: An example of vaccine distrust. *Arch. Dis. Child.* **2017**, *103*, 740–746. [CrossRef] [PubMed]
40. Issanov, A.; Akhmetzhanova, Z.; Riethmacher, D.; Aljofan, M. Knowledge, attitude, and practice toward COVID-19 vaccination in Kazakhstan: A cross-sectional study. *Hum. Vaccin Immunother.* **2021**, *17*, 3394–3400. [CrossRef]
41. World Helth Organization. Mid-Activity Report, 2021. WHO Country Office, Kazakhstan. Available online: https://apps.who.int/iris/bitstream/handle/10665/349205/WHO-EURO-2021-3196-42954-60020-eng.pdf?sequence=1 (accessed on 2 May 2022).
42. Jennings, W.; Stoker, G.; Bunting, H.; Valgarðsson, V.; Gaskell, J.; Devine, D.; McKay, L.; Mills, M. Lack of Trust, Conspiracy Beliefs, and Social Media Use Predict COVID-19 Vaccine Hesitancy. *Vaccines* **2021**, *9*, 593. [CrossRef]
43. Yakunin, K.; Mukhamediev, R.I.; Zaitseva, E.; Levashenko, V.; Yelis, M.; Symagulov, A.; Kuchin, Y.; Muhamedijeva, E.; Aubakirov, M.; Gopejenko, V. Mass Media as a Mirror of the COVID-19 Pandemic. *Computation* **2021**, *9*, 140. [CrossRef]
44. Fowler, E.F.; Nagler, R.H.; Banka, D.; Gollust, S.E. Effects of politicized media coverage: Experimental evidence from the HPV vaccine and COVID-19. *Prog. Mol. Biol. Transl. Sci.* **2022**, *188*, 101–134. [CrossRef]
45. Walker, K.K.; Head, K.J.; Owens, H.; Zimet, G.D. A qualitative study exploring the relationship between mothers' vaccine hesitancy and health beliefs with COVID-19 vaccination intention and prevention during the early pandemic months. *Hum. Vaccines Immunother.* **2021**, *17*, 3355–3364. [CrossRef]
46. Karafillakis, E.; Simas, C.; Jarrett, C.; Verger, P.; Peretti-Watel, P.; Dib, F.; De Angelis, S.; Takacs, J.; Ali, K.A.; Celentano, L.P.; et al. HPV vaccination in a context of public mistrust and uncertainty: A systematic literature review of determinants of HPV vaccine hesitancy in Europe. *Hum. Vaccin Immunother.* **2019**, *15*, 1615–1627. [CrossRef]
47. Trucchi, C.; Amicizia, D.; Tafuri, S.; Sticchi, L.; Durando, P.; Costantino, C.; Varlese, F.; Silverio, B.D.; Bagnasco, A.M.; Ansaldi, F.; et al. Assessment of Knowledge, Attitudes, and Propensity towards HPV Vaccine of Young Adult Students in Italy. *Vaccines* **2020**, *8*, 74. [CrossRef]
48. Harrington, N.; Chen, Y.; O'Reilly, A.M.; Fang, C.Y. The role of trust in HPV vaccine uptake among racial and ethnic minorities in the United States: A narrative review. *AIMS Public Health* **2021**, *8*, 352–368. [CrossRef] [PubMed]

49. Özdemir, S.; Akkaya, R.; Karaşahin, K.E. Analysis of community-based studies related with knowledge, awareness, attitude, and behaviors towards HPV and HPV vaccine published in Turkey: A systematic review. *J. Turk. Ger. Gynecol. Assoc.* **2020**, *21*, 111–123. [CrossRef] [PubMed]
50. Kim, H.W.; Lee, E.J.; Lee, Y.J.; Kim, S.Y.; Jin, Y.J.; Kim, Y.; Lee, J.L. Knowledge, attitudes, and perceptions associated with HPV vaccination among female Korean and Chinese university students. *BMC Women's Health* **2022**, *22*, 51. [CrossRef]
51. Mizumachi, K.; Aoki, H.; Kitano, T.; Onishi, T.; Takeyama, M.; Shima, M. How to recover lost vaccine acceptance? A multi-center survey on HPV vaccine acceptance in Japan. *J. Infect. Chemother. Off. J. Jpn. Soc. Chemother.* **2021**, *27*, 445–449. [CrossRef] [PubMed]
52. Lei, J.; Ploner, A.; Elfström, K.M.; Wang, J.; Roth, A.; Fang, F.; Sundström, K.; Dillner, J.; Sparén, P. HPV Vaccination and the Risk of Invasive Cervical Cancer. *N. Engl. J. Med.* **2020**, *383*, 1340–1348. [CrossRef] [PubMed]
53. Jentschke, M.; Kampers, J.; Becker, J.; Sibbertsen, P.; Hillemanns, P. Prophylactic HPV vaccination after conization: A systematic review and meta-analysis. *Vaccine* **2020**, *38*, 6402–6409. [CrossRef]
54. Valasoulis, G.; Pouliakis, A.; Michail, G.; Kottaridi, C.; Spathis, A.; Kyrgiou, M.; Paraskevaidis, E.; Daponte, A. Alterations of HPV-Related Biomarkers after Prophylactic HPV Vaccination. A Prospective Pilot Observational Study in Greek Women. *Cancers* **2020**, *12*, 1164. [CrossRef]
55. Tsakiroglou, M.; Bakalis, M.; Valasoulis, G.; Paschopoulos, M.; Koliopoulos, G.; Paraskevaidis, E. Women's knowledge and utilization of gynecological cancer prevention services in the Northwest of Greece. *Eur. J. Gynaecol. Oncol.* **2011**, *32*, 178–181.
56. Lutringer-Magnin, D.; Kalecinski, J.; Cropet, C.; Barone, G.; Ronin, V.; Régnier, V.; Leocmach, Y.; Jacquard, A.-C.; Vanhems, P.; Chauvin, F.; et al. Prevention of sexually transmitted infections among girls and young women in relation to their HPV vaccination status. *Eur. J. Public Health* **2013**, *23*, 1046–1053. [CrossRef]
57. Valasoulis, G.; Pouliakis, A.; Michail, G.; Daponte, A.-I.; Galazios, G.; Panayiotides, I.; Daponte, A. The Influence of Sexual Behavior and Demographic Characteristics in the Expression of HPV-Related Biomarkers in a Colposcopy Population of Reproductive Age Greek Women. *Biology* **2021**, *10*, 713. [CrossRef]
58. Ortiz, R.R.; Smith, A.; Coyne-Beasley, T. A systematic literature review to examine the potential for social media to impact HPV vaccine uptake and awareness, knowledge, and attitudes about HPV and HPV vaccination. *Hum. Vaccines Immunother.* **2019**, *15*, 1465–1475. [CrossRef] [PubMed]

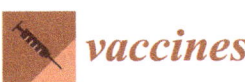

Article

Immunity after HPV Vaccination in Patients after Sexual Initiation

Dominik Pruski [1,2,*], Małgorzata Łagiedo-Żelazowska [3,4], Sonja Millert-Kalińska [1,4], Jan Sikora [3], Robert Jach [5] and Marcin Przybylski [1,2]

1. Department of Obstetrics and Gynecology, District Public Hospital in Poznan, 60-479 Poznań, Poland; millertsonja@gmail.com (S.M.-K.); nicramp@poczta.onet.pl (M.P.)
2. Gynecology Specialised Practise, 60-408 Poznań, Poland
3. Department of Immunology, Chair of Pathomorphology and Clinical Immunology, Poznan University of Medical Sciences, 60-806 Poznań, Poland; mlagiedo@ump.edu.pl (M.Ł.-Ż.); jan-sikora@wp.pl (J.S.)
4. Doctoral School, Poznan University of Medical Sciences, 61-701 Poznań, Poland
5. Department of Gynecological Endocrinology, Jagiellonian University Medical College, 31-008 Cracow, Poland; jach@cm-uj.krakow.pl
* Correspondence: dominik.pruski@icloud.com

Abstract: Vaccinations against human papillomavirus (HPV) are included in the primary prevention of precancerous intraepithelial lesions and HPV-related cancers. Despite the undeniable effectiveness of vaccination in the juvenile population, there is still little research on the effect in patients after sexual initiation. Our study aims to assess anti-HPV (L1 HPV) antibodies in healthy patients and diagnosed cervical pathology after 9-valent vaccination. We provide a prospective, ongoing 12-month, non-randomised pilot study in which 89 subjects were enrolled. We used an enzyme-linked immunosorbent assay to determine IgG class antibodies to HPV. We noted significantly higher levels of antibodies in vaccinated individuals than in the unvaccinated control group. The above work shows that vaccination against HPV might be beneficial in patients after sexual initiation as well as in those already diagnosed with HPV or SIL infection.

Keywords: HPV serum antibodies; L1 HPV; 9-valent vaccination; squamous intraepithelial neoplasia

1. Introduction

Squamous intraepithelial lesion (SIL) and cervical cancer are among the most common oncological diagnoses in women globally; therefore, they constitute a significant health problem. Cervical cancer remains the fourth most frequent cancer in women worldwide [1] unless it is theoretically preventable. The most critical risk factor for the development of cervical cancer is a persistent infection caused by highly oncogenic types of human papillomavirus (HPV). Neoplastic transformation begins with integrating HPV DNA into the genome of a typical epithelial cell. This situation may occur when the circular form of HPV DNA breaks, and then chromatin shifts within the chromosomal DNA of the host cells. Vaccination against HPV prevents infections with specific HPV types and, consequently, cervical cancer development due to infection with a given type [2–4]. Generally, during the human immune response to HPV, B cells detect the viral antigens and exhibit them to T helper type 2 cells, promoting the production of high-affinity antibodies (IgG, IgA, and IgM) against HPV antigens by B cells. It has already been demonstrated that anti-HPV IgG might be a reliable marker for past HPV exposure [5]. Studies have shown that the median seroconversion time was about 8.3–11.8 months. These data suggest that the development of IgG antibodies at a detectable level after a natural infection can be a slow process, and it does not necessarily occur in every woman. Following a human papillomavirus (HPV) vaccine, type 16 virus-like particles (VLPs), according to the authors, appear within 8.3 months and remain for approximately 36 months [6]. Antibodies could persist for a long period of time if the initial antibody levels were high or if there was continued antigenic exposure. At the same time, IgM may be detected in acute or current exposure, typically after one month following initial immunisation, as Harro et al. claim [7]. Vaccinations against HPV are included in the primary prevention of precancerous lesions—mainly SIL and cervical cancer. The other cancers associated with HPV infections affect the genital organs (vulva, vagina, and penis), anal canal, oral cavity, and upper respiratory tract [8,9]. Vaccination against HPV significantly reduced the incidence of HPV-related lesions in New Zealand and the United States [10,11]. In the European countries, and thus in Poland, vaccination against HPV has been introduced into the vaccination calendar. Local governments organise vaccination programmes in many provinces of our country. It is recommended that both girls and boys are vaccinated before sexual initiation. After identifying an HPV infection, many patients decide to vaccinate after sexual initiation due to the fear of developing intraepithelial neoplasia of the cervix, vagina, vulva, or HPV-dependent changes in the respiratory tract. After the treatment of HPV-related lesions, such as intraepithelial neoplasia of the cervix or genital warts, some patients decide to vaccinate to develop anti-HPV antibodies that can protect against re-infection and the formation of HPV-related lesions. However, there is still very little research into post-vaccination antibody levels (VLP), so it seems to us that this is a topic worth exploring [12–14].

The 9-valent vaccine contains the purified proteins of nine types of HPV, namely 6, 11, 16, 18, 31, 22, 45, 52, and 58. The vaccine is usually administered according to a three-dose schedule. Studies focusing on the presence of HPV genotypes in large populations may contribute to the development of further protective vaccinations [15].

Considering this, we aim to assess the level of anti-HPV (L1 HPV) antibodies in healthy patients and with diagnosed cervical pathology after vaccination. The introduction of tests for the detection of anti-HPV (L1 HPV) antibodies may, in the future, facilitate the assessment of the effectiveness of vaccine programmes. Moreover, it might be helpful in the identification of patients with immune disorders in whom infection with oncogenic types of HPV persisted, resulting in intraepithelial neoplasia. Analysing specific types of immune disorders will facilitate the identification of groups of women with the highest risk of developing high-grade squamous intraepithelial lesions and, consequently, malignancy.

The following meta-analysis compares the effectiveness of the vaccine administration in the population of patients before and after sexual initiation in either healthy individuals or those with diagnosed cervical pathology.

2. Materials and Methods

2.1. Study Design

We provide a prospective, ongoing 12-month, non-randomised pilot study to assess the level of anti-HPV (L1 HPV) antibodies in healthy patients and those with diagnosed cervix pathology after the 9-valent HPV vaccine. The Bioethical Committee of the Poznan University of Medical Sciences, Poland, approved the study protocol (597/19). We obtained written consent for the study from all patients. We included patients who met the following criteria: (i) only adult women, (ii) non-pregnant subjects, postpartum, (iii) patients not treated with immunosuppressive drugs, (iv) not previously vaccinated with other HPV vaccines, (v) expressing informed and written consent to participate in the study, (vi) agreeing to the proposed surgical diagnostics in the case of indications and possible surgical treatment, (vii) had taken three doses of the 9-valent vaccination against HPV according to the 0–2–6 months scheme, and (viii) provided blood samples after at least six months from the last dose of vaccination. The exclusion criteria were: (i) refusal of possible treatment of squamous intraepithelial lesions, and (ii) failure to complete the full vaccination schedule. A total of 61 women met the above criteria.

All subjects from the study group were undergoing a verification diagnostic of abnormal Pap-smear results by punch biopsy. We examined the status of HPV infection and looked for the presence of pre-neoplastic lesions, such as low-grade squamous intraepithelial lesions (LSIL) or high-grade squamous intraepithelial lesions (HSIL). All patients with histopathologically confirmed HSIL (CIN 2, CIN 3) were treated with the LEEP conization and curettage of the cervical canal.

The control group 1 covers 20 healthy, unvaccinated patients, in whom we excluded an infection with hrHPV or squamous intraepithelial lesions confirmed through punch biopsy. Control group 2 includes eight subjects both infected with highly oncogenic types of HPV and diagnosed with pre-neoplastic lesions who decided not to receive the HPV vaccine. Figure 1 presents the process of recruiting patients for the study, and Table 1 shows the basic division into study groups.

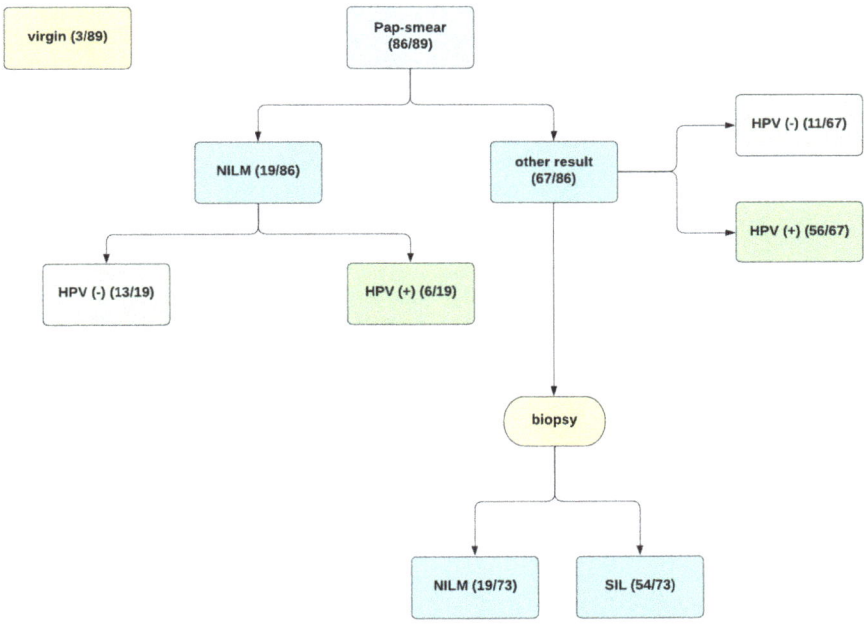

Figure 1. Flow chart. SIL—squamous intraepithelial lesion, NILM—negative for intraepithelial lesion or malignancy, HPV—human papillomavirus.

Table 1. Basic characteristics of study and control groups.

Group	n	HPV Status	Biopsy Result	Vaccination Status
Experimental	61	(+)/(−)	Normal/LSIL/HSIL	+
Control 1	20	(−)	Excluded LSIL and HSIL	−
Control 2	8	(+)/(−)	LSIL/HSIL	−

HPV—human papillomavirus, n—number.

All examination and follow-up groups are under regular oncogynaecological care. Patients diagnosed with HSIL (CIN 2, CIN 3) underwent proper treatment—the removal of the lesions according to the current recommendations of the Polish Colposcopic Society—and then subjected to close cytological and molecular control every six months.

2.2. Specimen Collection and Handling

Blood was drawn aseptically to the serum collection tubes (S-Monovette). The blood was collected at least six months after receiving the last vaccination dose. After that, the samples were centrifuged at 2000 rpm for 20 min. Supernatants (sera) were collected and frozen at −20 °C for further assays.

2.3. HPV Serological Measurements

We used an enzyme-linked immunosorbent assay to determine IgG class antibodies to human papillomavirus (Creative Diagnostics, New York, USA). The sera were diluted 1:101 into properly defined dilution tubes for the test. An ELISA microtiter plate was coated with recombinant VLP derived from HPV types 6, 11, 16, and 18. After incubation and washing, we added the diluted samples and quality control specimens to the microtiter plates along with a peroxidase-conjugated anti-human polyclonal antibody. Following incubation and washing, an enzyme substrate and chromogen were added to allow colour development. Reactions were stopped, and optical density (OD) was read at 450 and 620 nm, with the background measured at 620 nm and subtracted from the OD reading at 450 nm. A calculated formulation from the manufacturer determined the seropositive cut points. The cut points were set at 0.303 for HPV seronegative and >0.303 for HPV seropositive patients. We calculated the quantitative results of the assay as instructed in the kit insert (OD/CUT-OFF).

2.4. Statistical Analysis

We performed an analysis in SPSS, version 27. All tests were two-tailed, with $\alpha = 0.05$. The normality of the variables was validated based on the Shapiro–Wilk test. All three groups were characterised by reporting median with quartiles 1 and 3, or mean and standard deviation for quantitative variables, or n value and percentage for qualitative variables. The values of variables with normal distributions were compared between the experimental and control group 1 or 2 with the Student's t test. Variables without normal distributions were compared with the Mann–Whitney U test. Dependencies between the group and other variables were measured using Fisher's exact test. Odds ratios or median differences (experimental group–control group) with 95% confidence intervals were given when the results of the analyses were significant. Median differences were calculated using the Hodges–Lehmann estimator. The correlation was calculated with Pearson's r coefficient.

3. Results

As shown in Table 1, the experimental and control groups did not differ significantly in age or regarding pregnancies. Comorbidities were observed in 38% of women from the experimental group, 30% from control group 1, and 12.5% of women from control group 2. The dependency between the group and Pap-smear results was insignificant for the experimental vs. control group 2. The most common Pap-smear result in the experimental and control group 2 was LSIL, which accounted for 33% and 38%, respectively. A more significant proportion of women with positive HPV tests was found in the experimental group than in control group 1—nine times more. There was no considerable dependency between the groups and HPV test results in the case of the experimental group vs. control group 2. All women from control group 1 were histopathologically confirmed to have no pathology (NILM). An NILM result was observed in 19% of women in the experimental group, which is statistically significant. We did not find any dependency between the experimental/control group 2 and biopsy results. The most common histopathological result for women from the experimental group and control group 2 was HSIL (57% of women from both groups).

Figures 2 and 3 show the graphical arrangement of the levels of antibodies in individual research groups. Antibody levels were significantly higher in the experimental group than in both control group 1 and control group 2. The antibody level divided by the cut-off value (0.303) was also significantly higher in the experimental group than both of the control groups. There were significant dependences between group and sample being reactive ($p < 0.001$ for both analysis—experimental group vs. control group 1 and experimental group vs. control group 2). The sample was reactive for all women from the experimental group, 16% of women from control group 1, and one-fourth of women from control group 2, as presented in Table 2.

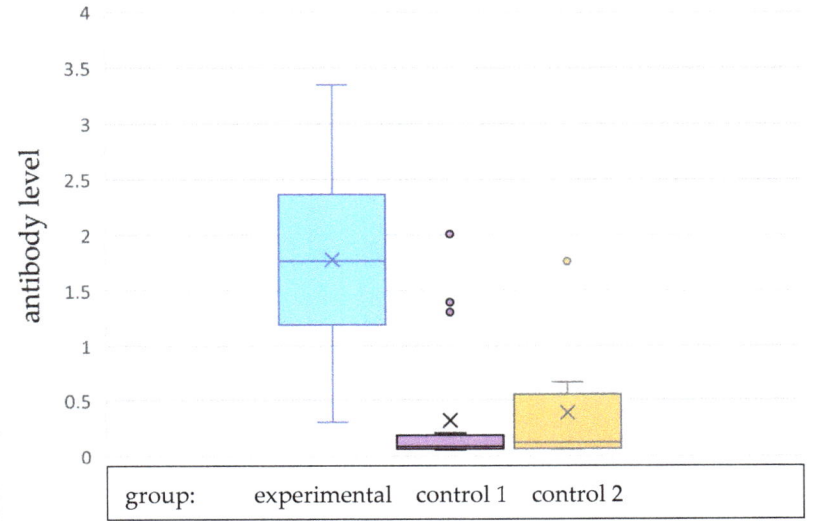

Figure 2. Antibody level.

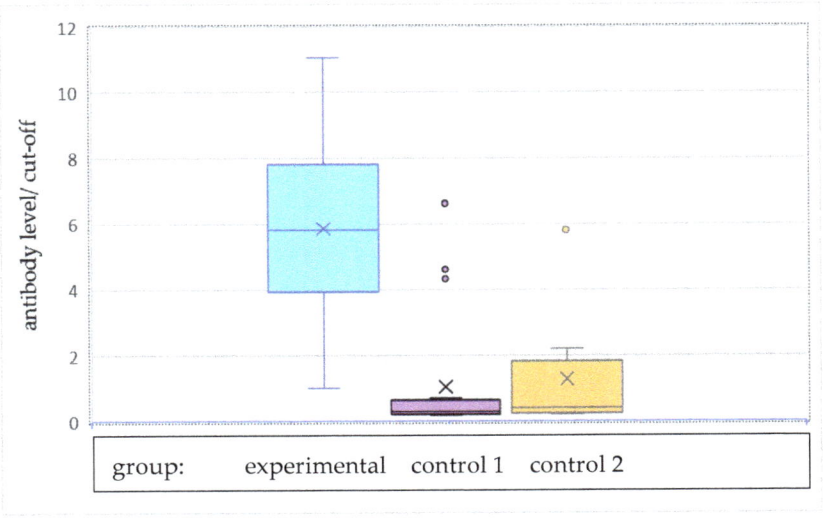

Figure 3. Antibody level divided by the cut-off value.

Table 2. Detailed group characteristics.

Characteristic	Experimental Group	Control Group 1	Control Group 2	p1	p2
n = 89	61	20	8		
Age, M ± SD	34.03 ± 7.32	36.40 ± 7.59	32.88 ± 7.77	0.217 [1]	0.667 [1]
Number of term pregnancies, n (%)					
0	26 (42.6)	7 (35.0)	5 (62.5)		
1	18 (29.5)	8 (40.0)	0 (0.0)	0.873	0.249
2	14 (23.0)	4 (20.0)	3 (37.5)		
3	3 (4.9)	1 (5.0)	0 (0.0)		
Number of pre-term pregnancies, n (%)					
0	60 (98.4)	20 (100.0)	8 (100.0)	>0.999	>0.999
1	1 (1.6)	0 (0.0)	0 (0.0)		
Number of miscarriages, n (%)					
0	55 (91.2)	18 (90.0)	8 (100.0)		
1	4 (6.6)	2 (10.0)	0 (0.0)	0.797	>0.999
2	2 (3.2)	0 (0.0)	0 (0.0)		
Number of pregnancies, Me (Q1; Q3)	1.00 (0.00; 2.00)	1.00 (0.00; 2.00)	0.00 (0.00; 2.00)	0.991 [2]	0.421 [2]
Comorbidities, n (%)	22 (37.7)	6 (30.0)	1 (12.5)	0.600	0.246
Cytology, n (%)	61	20	8		
NILM	7 (11.5)	12 (60.0)	0 (0.0)		
ASCUS	12 (19.7)	5 (25.0)	2 (25.0)		
ASC-H	10 (16.4)	1 (5.0)	1 (12.5)		
LSIL	20 (32.8)	1 (5.0)	3 (37.5)	0.001	0.903
HSIL	6 (9.8)	1 (5.0)	2 (25.0)		
AGC	2 (3.3)	0 (0.0)	0 (0.0)		
Virgin	3 (4.9)	0 (0.0)	0 (0.0)		
Cervical cancer	1 (1.6)	0 (0.0)	0 (0.0)		
HPV, n (%)	61	20	8		
Positive	52 (85.2)	2 (10.0)	8 (100.0)		
Negative	6 (9.9)	18 (90.0)	0 (0.0)	<0.001	>0.999
Virgin	3 (4.9)	0 (0.0)	0 (0.0)		
Biopsy, n (%)	n = 57	n = 8	n = 8		
NILM	11 (19.3)	8 (100.0)	0 (0.0)		
LSIL (CIN 1)	17 (29.8)	0 (0.0)	1 (12.5)	<0.001	0.285
HSIL (CIN2, CIN 3)	28 (49.1)	0 (0.0)	7 (87.5)		
Adenocarcinoma	1 (1.8)	0 (0.0)	0 (0.0)		
Antibody level, Me (Q1; Q3)	1.77 (1.22; 2.35)	0.09 (0.07; 0.19)	0.13 (0.07; 0.44)	<0.001 [2]	<0.001 [2]
Antibody level/cut-off, Me (Q1; Q3)	5.83 (4.01; 7.77)	0.29 (0.22; 0.62)	0.41 (0.23; 1.45)	<0.001 [2]	<0.001 [2]
Reactive, n (%)	61 (100.0)	3 (15.5)	2 (25.0)	<0.001	<0.001

NILM—negative for intraepithelial lesion or malignancy; ASCUS—atypical squamous cells of undetermined significance; ASC-H—atypical squamous cells cannot exclude HSIL; LSIL—low-grade squamous intraepithelial lesion; HSIL—high-grade squamous intraepithelial lesion; AGC—atypical glandular cells; Q1—first quartile; Q3—third quartile; n—number, p1—p-value for comparison between experimental group and control group 1; p2—p-value for comparison between the experimental group and control group 2. Comparisons were made with Student's t test [1] or Mann–Whitney U test [2] for quantitative variables and Fisher's exact test for qualitative variables.

Age was not significantly correlated with the antibody level, as seen in Table 3. The patients with LSIL diagnosis and those with HSIL or cancer diagnosis did not vary considerably in terms of antibody level and antibody level divided by cut-off value, as shown in Table 4.

Table 3. Correlation between age and antibody level.

Variable	Age	
	r	p
Antibody level	−0.11	0.137

r—Pearson's r correlation coefficient. p—p-value.

Table 4. Comparison of antibody level and antibody level/cut-off between groups with different diagnoses.

Variables	Diagnosis		p
	LSIL (CIN 1) n = 18	HSIL (CIN 2, CIN 3) and cancer n = 36	
Antibody level (M ± SD)	1.63 ± 0.88	1.53 ± 0.89	0.691
Antibody level/cut-off (M ± SD)	5.39 ± 2.90	5.04 ± 2.92	0.691

p—p-value; LSIL—low-grade squamous intraepithelial lesion; HSIL—high-grade squamous intraepithelial lesion; n—number.

Samples were reactive for 93% of women who received an LSIL diagnosis and 87% of women who received either an HSIL or cancer diagnosis.

Comparison made with Student's t test.

4. Discussion

Our study aimed to assess the level of anti-HPV antibodies in patients with diagnosed cervical pathology and in healthy patients after vaccination. Our work supports the practice of vaccinating HPV-infected patients after sexual initiation by showing the level of antibodies persisting after vaccination. Despite the proven and indisputable effectiveness of the 9-valent HPV vaccine as primary prevention in juveniles before sexual initiation, its efficacy has not yet been demonstrated in women with diagnosed cervical pathology.

As expected, in all patients vaccinated with the 9-valent vaccine, the samples turned out to be reactive. Additionally, the analysis confirmed a relationship between levels of antibodies and vaccination status. We noted significantly higher levels in vaccinated patients than in those of the unvaccinated control groups: 1.77 vs. 0.09 and 0.13, respectively. These results are consistent with the work published by Mirte Scherpenisse et al. Naturally induced HPV-specific antibodies from single-positive sera were genotype-specific and neutralising.

In contrast, the antibodies of multi-positive sera were less genotype-specific, cross-reactive, and tended to be non-neutralising. Post-vaccination antibody avidity was approximately three times higher than after HPV infection [16]. Post-vaccination antibody status assessment may help analyse the effectiveness of HPV preventative vaccination programmes. Vaccine efficacy against HPV16 and 18 infections were sustained over eight years post-vaccination [17]. HPV-specific IgG antibody levels and its neutralising activity remained well above the antibody levels induced by HPV infection [17,18]. Additionally, HPV vaccines offer cross-protection against several non-vaccine HPV types in patients without a previous HPV infection [19]. Antibodies that were also capable of neutralising non-vaccine HPV types were most frequently found to be directed against HPV31 and 45. Cross-neutralising antibody levels against HPV31, 33, 35, and 45 were significantly associated with their phylogenetically related vaccine-type antibody levels [20]. HPV genotypes frequently detected in cervical cancer are as follows: 31, 33, 45, and efficacious vaccines against these HPV types might further reduce malignancies. However, vaccine efficacy against non-vaccine HPV types decreased rapidly over time [19].

Interestingly, our results indicate that a current or persistent infection with human papillomavirus gives a lower antibody level percentage than in vaccinated patients, which is consistent with the reports presented by other researchers. In our study group, 18% of women infected with HPV had clinically significant levels of L1-HPV antibodies, and for comparison, we observed the antibodies in 100% of vaccinated women. Investigators argue that the rate of seroconversion associated with the vaccines is high, namely, >99% in women and men [21–24]. In contrast, the seroconversion results from natural infection are an estimated 50–70% in women [25] and men [26].

Although most of the patients in the control groups had antibody levels below the cut-off, we observed 3/20 reactive samples in control group 1 and 2/8 in control group 2. It is worth noting that only one woman with a reactive sample had no burden. In other cases, we observed the presence of infections with HR HPV and histopathologically confirmed HSIL or a history of Hashimoto's disease. This observation may provide new insight into the factors modulating the immune system. It is possible that comorbidities, dysfunctions of the immune system, or infection with HPV genotype 16 strongly stimulate the immune system to produce antibodies. Data provided by Aubin et al. suggest that autoimmune inflammatory diseases (AIID) and the drugs used to treat them are associated with an excess risk of genital HPV infection. Although this excess risk has not been specifically evaluated, the available data indicate a need for close monitoring of patients with AIID, regardless of their treatment, to ensure the prevention and treatment of benign and premalignant lesions [27].

Petter et al. [28] indicated that serological assays for HPV could help identify patients at risk of HPV-related cancers. In addition to strategies connected with antibody detection, DNA sequencing or the PCR method are also widely used to detect the viral DNA of HPV in tissue samples [29]. Therefore, antibody- and DNA- based assays can complement each other for the reliable identification of HPV-infected patients.

Researchers from Mexico presented somewhat similar work. Their study aimed to assess type-specific cervical HPV prevalence and their association with HPV-specific antibodies in a cohort of female university students. The observed study group was similar in terms of number. HPV genotyping was performed by amplifying and sequencing a fragment of the L1 protein. In addition to sexual behaviour, it was observed that the presence of serum-specific IgG antibodies against HPV can impact the prevalence of the virus. Alexander Pedroza-Gonzalez et al. suggest that seropositivity to HPV-16 and HPV-18 was associated with a lower prevalence of HPV-16, but not for other HPV types. Of note, there was a lower proportion of HPV-specific seropositivity in women who had the presence of the same HPV type in a cervical specimen, suggesting an immunoregulatory mechanism associated with the viral infection [30].

Efforts towards the detection of HPV antibodies as a tool to monitor and assess vaccine efficacy have increased significantly in recent years. In the study conducted by Bhatia et al., a standardised ELISA test developed for anti-HPV16L1 antibodies was validated against the WHO's international positive serum standard for HPV16. This assay was amenable to both venous blood and dried blood spots. The researchers also admit that the sample size used for the study was small; however, the presented technique has promise for widespread use in epidemiological and field studies of antibody prevalence and, coupled with the avidity measurement, may be of use in individual cases for monitoring vaccine responses such as failures [14].

A relatively small research group limited our methodological choices. However, in the future, we will be able to expand the group and test the level of antibodies over the next few years to assess the trend of changes. Fortunately, we observe an increasing awareness of patients and their partners and a growing number of vaccinations against HPV in both adults and those at the pre-contraceptive age.

5. Conclusions

The results of our study may indicate that high levels of antibodies are maintained after HPV vaccination. This further suggests that vaccinations are also effective in subjects after sexual initiation. These conclusions might help identify patients with immune disorders who have survived the infection with HR HPV, resulting in changes in the intraepithelial neoplasia. Analysing specific immune disorders might help identify groups of women with the highest risk of developing HSIL (CIN 2, CIN 3) lesions and, consequently, malignancies.

Author Contributions: Conceptualisation, D.P. and M.P.; methodology, D.P. and M.Ł.-Ż.; software, D.P. and S.M.-K.; validation, D.P. and M.Ł.-Ż.; formal analysis, D.P. and S.M.-K.; investigation, D.P. and M.P.; resources, D.P., M.Ł.-Ż. and J.S.; data curation, D.P. and M.P.; writing—original draft preparation, D.P., S.M.-K. and M.Ł.-Ż.; writing—review and editing, R.J., J.S. and D.P.; visualisation, D.P. and S.M.-K.; supervision, R.J. and J.S.; project administration, D.P. and M.P.; funding acquisition, D.P. and M.P. All authors have read and agreed to the published version of the manuscript.

Funding: This research received no external funding.

Institutional Review Board Statement: The study was conducted in accordance with the Declaration of Helsinki and approved by the Ethics Committee of the Poznan University of Medical Sciences, Poland (95/2021).

Informed Consent Statement: Informed consent was obtained from all subjects involved in the study.

Data Availability Statement: Not applicable.

Conflicts of Interest: The authors declare no conflict of interest.

References

1. Sung, H.; Ferlay, J.; Siegel, R.L.; Laversanne, M.; Soerjomataram, I.; Jemal, A.; Bray, F. Global Cancer Statistics 2020: GLOBOCAN Estimates of Incidence and Mortality Worldwide for 36 Cancers in 185 Countries. *CA Cancer J. Clin.* **2021**, *71*, 209–249. [CrossRef] [PubMed]
2. Bosch, F.X.; De Sanjosé, S. Chapter 1: Human Papillomavirus and Cervical Cancer–Burden and Assessment of Causality. *J. Natl. Cancer Inst. Monogr.* **2003**, *2003*, 3–13. [CrossRef] [PubMed]
3. Bosch, F.; Lorincz, A.; Muñoz, N.; Meijer, C.J.L.M.; Shah, K.V. The Causal Relation between Human Papillomavirus and Cervical Cancer. *J. Clin. Pathol.* **2002**, *55*, 244–265. [CrossRef] [PubMed]
4. Zur Hausen, H. Papillomaviruses Causing Cancer: Evasion from Host-Cell Control in Early Events in Carcinogenesis. *J. Natl. Cancer Inst.* **2000**, *92*, 690–698. [CrossRef] [PubMed]
5. Sitas, F.; Urban, M.; Stein, L.; Beral, V.; Ruff, P.; Hale, M.; Patel, M.; O'Connell, D.; Yu, X.Q.; Verzijden, A.; et al. The relationship between anti-HPV-16 IgG seropositivity and cancer of the cervix, anogenital organs, oral cavity and pharynx, oesophagus and prostate in a black South African population. *Infect. Agents Cancer* **2007**, *2*, 6. [CrossRef]
6. Ho, G.Y.F.; Studentsov, Y.Y.; Bierman, R.; Burk, R.D. Natural History of Human Papillomavirus Type 16 Virus-Like Particle Antibodies in Young Women. *Cancer Epidemiol. Biomark. Prev.* **2004**, *13*, 110–116. [CrossRef]
7. Harro, C.D.; Pang, Y.-Y.S.; Roden, R.B.S.; Hildesheim, A.; Wang, Z.; Reynolds, M.J.; Mast, T.C.; Robinson, R.; Murphy, B.R.; Karron, R.A.; et al. Safety and Immunogenicity Trial in Adult Volunteers of a Human Papillomavirus 16 L1 Virus-Like Particle Vaccine. *JNCI J. Natl. Cancer Inst.* **2001**, *93*, 284–292. [CrossRef]
8. Giuliano, A.R.; Tortolero-Luna, G.; Ferrer, E.; Burchell, A.N.; de Sanjose, S.; Kjaer, S.K.; Muñoz, N.; Schiffman, M.; Bosch, F.X. Epidemiology of human papillomavirus infection in men, cancers other than cervical and benign conditions. *Vaccine* **2008**, *26* (Suppl. 10), K17–K28. [CrossRef]
9. De Vuyst, H.; Clifford, G.M.; Nascimento, M.C.; Madeleine, M.M.; Franceschi, S. Prevalence and type distribution of human papillomavirus in carcinoma and intraepithelial neoplasia of the vulva, vagina and anus: A meta-analysis. *Int. J. Cancer* **2009**, *124*, 1626–1636. [CrossRef]
10. Oliphant, J.; Stewart, J.; Saxton, P.; Lo, M.; Perkins, N.; Ward, D. Trends in genital warts diagnoses in New Zealand five years following the quadrivalent human papillomavirus vaccine introduction. *N. Z. Med J.* **2017**, *130*, 9–16.
11. Markowitz, L.E.; Gee, J.; Chesson, H.; Stokley, S. Ten Years of Human Papillomavirus Vaccination in the United States. *Acad. Pediatr.* **2018**, *18*, S3–S10. [CrossRef] [PubMed]
12. Ramezani, A.; Aghakhani, A.; Soleymani, S.; Bavand, A.; Bolhassani, A. Significance of serum antibodies against HPV E7, Hsp27, Hsp20 and Hp91 in Iranian HPV-exposed women. *BMC Infect. Dis.* **2019**, *19*, 142. [CrossRef] [PubMed]
13. Bouassa, R.-S.M.; Péré, H.; Gubavu, C.; Prazuck, T.; Jenabian, M.-A.; Veyer, D.; Meye, J.-F.; Touzé, A.; Bélec, L. Serum and cervicovaginal IgG immune responses against α7 and α9 HPV in non-vaccinated women at risk for cervical cancer: Implication for catch-up prophylactic HPV vaccination. *PLoS ONE* **2020**, *15*, e0233084. [CrossRef]

14. Bhatia, R.; Stewart, J.; Moncur, S.; Cubie, H.; Kavanagh, K.; Pollock, K.G.; Busby-Earle, C.; Williams, A.R.; Howie, S.; Cuschieri, K. Development of an in-house ELISA to detect anti-HPV16-L1 antibodies in serum and dried blood spots. *J. Virol. Methods* 2018, *264*, 55–60. [CrossRef]
15. Przybylski, M.; Pruski, D.; Millert-Kalinska, S.; Madry, R.; Lagiedo-Zelazowska, M.; Sikora, J.; Zmaczynski, A.; Baran, R.; Twardowska, H.; Horbaczewska, A.; et al. Genotyping of human papillomavirus DNA in Wielkopolska region. *Ginekol. Polska* 2021. [CrossRef]
16. Scherpenisse, M.; Schepp, R.M.; Mollers, M.; Meijer, C.J.L.M.; Berbers, G.A.M.; Van Der Klis, F.R.M. Characteristics of HPV-Specific Antibody Responses Induced by Infection and Vaccination: Cross-Reactivity, Neutralizing Activity, Avidity and IgG Subclasses. *PLoS ONE* 2013, *8*, e74797. [CrossRef] [PubMed]
17. Roteli-Martins, C.M.; Naud, P.; de Borba, P.; Teixeira, J.C.; de Carvalho, N.S.; Zahaf, T.; Sanchez, N.; Geeraerts, B.; Descamps, D. Sustained Immunogenicity and Efficacy of the HPV-16/18 AS04-Adjuvanted Vaccine: Up to 8.4 Years of Follow-Up. *Hum. Vaccines Immunother.* 2012, *8*, 390–397. [CrossRef] [PubMed]
18. Kemp, T.J.; Safaeian, M.; Hildesheim, A.; Pan, Y.; Penrose, K.J.; Porras, C.; Schiller, J.T.; Lowy, D.R.; Herrero, R.; Pinto, L.A. Kinetic and HPV infection effects on cross-type neutralizing antibody and avidity responses induced by Cervarix®. *Vaccine* 2012, *31*, 165–170. [CrossRef]
19. Malagón, T.; Drolet, M.; Boily, M.-C.; Franco, E.L.; Jit, M.; Brisson, J.; Brisson, M. Cross-protective efficacy of two human papillomavirus vaccines: A systematic review and meta-analysis. *Lancet Infect. Dis.* 2012, *12*, 781–789. [CrossRef]
20. Draper, E.; Bissett, S.L.; Howell-Jones, R.; Edwards, D.; Munslow, G.; Soldan, K.; Beddows, S. Neutralization of non-vaccine human papillomavirus pseudoviruses from the A7 and A9 species groups by bivalent HPV vaccine sera. *Vaccine* 2011, *29*, 8585–8590. [CrossRef]
21. Paavonen, J.; Jenkins, D.; Bosch, F.X.; Naud, P.; Salmerón, J.; Wheeler, C.M.; Chow, S.-N.; Apter, D.; Kitchener, H.C.; Castellsagué, X.; et al. Efficacy of a prophylactic adjuvanted bivalent L1 virus-like-particle vaccine against infection with human papillomavirus types 16 and 18 in young women: An interim analysis of a phase III double-blind, randomised controlled trial. *Lancet* 2007, *369*, 2161–2170. [CrossRef]
22. Van Damme, P.; Olsson, S.E.; Block, S.; Castellsague, X.; Gray, G.E.; Herrera, T.; Huang, L.-M.; Kim, D.S.; Pitisuttithum, P.; Chen, J.; et al. Immunogenicity and Safety of a 9-Valent HPV Vaccine. *Pediatrics* 2015, *136*, e28–e39. [CrossRef] [PubMed]
23. Villa, L.L.; Costa, R.L.R.; Petta, C.A.; Andrade, R.P.; Paavonen, J.; Iversen, O.-E.; Olsson, S.-E.; Hoye, J.; Steinwall, M.; Riis-Johannessen, G.; et al. High sustained efficacy of a prophylactic quadrivalent human papillomavirus types 6/11/16/18 L1 virus-like particle vaccine through 5 years of follow-up. *Br. J. Cancer* 2006, *95*, 1459–1466. [CrossRef] [PubMed]
24. Viscidi, R.P.; Schiffman, M.; Hildesheim, A.; Herrero, R.; Castle, P.E.; Bratti, M.C.; Rodriguez, A.C.; Sherman, M.E.; Wang, S.; Clayman, B.; et al. Seroreactivity to Human Papillomavirus (HPV) Types 16, 18, or 31 and Risk of Subsequent HPV Infection. *Cancer Epidemiol. Biomark. Prev.* 2004, *13*, 324–327. [CrossRef] [PubMed]
25. Carter, J.J.; Koutsky, L.A.; Hughes, J.P.; Lee, S.K.; Kuypers, J.; Kiviat, N.; Galloway, D.A. Comparison of Human Papillomavirus Types 16, 18, and 6 Capsid Antibody Responses Following Incident Infection. *J. Infect. Dis.* 2000, *181*, 1911–1919. [CrossRef]
26. Edelstein, Z.R.; Carter, J.J.; Garg, R.; Winer, R.L.; Feng, Q.; Galloway, D.A.; Koutsky, L.A. Serum Antibody Response Following Genital 9 Human Papillomavirus Infection in Young Men. *J. Infect. Dis.* 2011, *204*, 209–216. [CrossRef]
27. Aubin, F.; Martin, M.; Puzenat, E.; Magy-Bertrand, N.; Segondy, M.; Riethmuller, D.; Wendling, D. Genital human Papillomavirus infection in patients with autoimmune inflammatory diseases. *Jt. Bone Spine* 2011, *78*, 460–465. [CrossRef]
28. Petter, A.; Christensen, N.; Nig, A.C.-K.; Zangerle, R.; Guger, M.; Pfister, H.; Heim, K.; Höpfl, R.; Wieland, U.; Sarcletti, M. Specific serum IgG, IgM and IgA antibodies to human papillomavirus types 6, 11, 16, 18 and 31 virus-like particles in human immunodeficiency virus-seropositive women. *J. Gen. Virol.* 2000, *81*, 701–708. [CrossRef]
29. Syrjänen, S.; Lodi, G.; von Bültzingslöwen, I.; Aliko, A.; Arduino, P.; Campisi, G.; Challacombe, S.; Ficarra, G.; Flaitz, C.; Zhou, H.; et al. Human papillomaviruses in oral carcinoma and oral potentially malignant disorders: A systematic review. *Oral Dis.* 2011, *17*, 58–72. [CrossRef]
30. Pedroza-Gonzalez, A.; Reyes-Reali, J.; Campos-Solorzano, M.; Blancas-Diaz, E.M.; Tomas-Morales, J.A.; Hernandez-Aparicio, A.A.; de Oca-Samperio, D.M.; Garrido, E.; Garcia-Romo, G.S.; Mendez-Catala, C.F.; et al. Human papillomavirus infection and seroprevalence among female university students in Mexico. *Hum. Vaccines Immunother.* 2022, *18*, 1–12. [CrossRef]

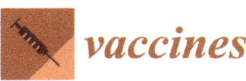

Article

Adherence to the Recommended HPV Vaccine Dosing Schedule among Adolescents Aged 13 to 17 Years: Findings from the National Immunization Survey-Teen, 2019–2020

Chinenye Lynette Ejezie [1,2,*,†], Ikponmwosa Osaghae [3,4,†], Sylvia Ayieko [1] and Paula Cuccaro [1]

[1] Department of Health Promotion and Behavioral Sciences, The University of Texas School of Public Health, 1200 Pressler St, Houston, TX 77030, USA; sylvia.a.ayieko@uth.tmc.edu (S.A.); paula.m.cuccaro@uth.tmc.edu (P.C.)
[2] Department of Investigational Cancer Therapeutics, The University of MD Anderson Cancer Center, Houston, TX 77030, USA
[3] Department of Biostatistics, The University of Texas MD Anderson Cancer Center, Houston, TX 77030, USA; ikponmwosa.osaghae@uth.tmc.edu
[4] Department of Epidemiology, Human Genetics & Environmental Sciences, The University of Texas School of Public Health, Houston, TX 77030, USA
* Correspondence: chinenye.l.ejezie@uth.tmc.edu; Tel.: +1-(832-513-3925)
† These authors contributed equally to this work.

Abstract: The 9-valent human papillomavirus (9-vHPV) vaccine uptake rate among adolescents has improved over the years; however, little is known about the adherence to the recommended dosing schedule. This study examines the prevalence and factors associated with adherence to the recommended 9vHPV vaccination dosing schedule among adolescents aged 13 to 17 years. The cross-sectional study was conducted using the 2019–2020 National Immunization Survey-Teen. The parents of 34,619 adolescents were included in our analyses. The overall up-to-date (UTD) prevalence was 57.1%. The UTD prevalence was 60.0% among females and 54.2% among males. Adolescents aged 16 years had the highest UTD prevalence of 63.0%. The UTD prevalence was 61.6% among Hispanics and 54.7% among non-Hispanic Whites. Overall, compared to females, males had 14% lower odds of UTD. The odds of UTD were 1.91 times, 2.08 times, and 1.98 times higher among adolescents aged 15–17 years, respectively, compared to those aged 13 years. Moreover, region, poverty, insurance status, mothers' educational level, and provider recommendation were associated with UTD. Our findings show that adherence to the recommended 9vHPV vaccine schedule is low in the US. Targeted public health efforts are needed to improve the rates of adherence to the recommended 9vHPV dose schedule.

Keywords: HPV vaccination; dosing schedule; dosing interval; 9-valent; low adherence

1. Introduction

In the United States, the Advisory Committee on Immunization Practices (ACIP) and the Centers for Disease Control and Prevention (CDC) recommend that adolescents prophylactically receive the 9-valent human papillomavirus (HPV) vaccine (9vHPV) [1–4]. Toward the end of 2016, the 9vHPV vaccine became the only HPV vaccine available in the US and the administration of other types of HPV vaccines were permanently discontinued [5]. Clinical trials have shown that 9vHPV is about 90% effective in preventing HPV-related cancers when administered on the recommended dosing schedule [6–9]. The dose schedule of 9vHPV differs across age categories: the ACIP and CDC recommends two doses administered at a schedule of 5 to 12 months for persons younger than 15 years [10,11]. The CDC recommends a third dose for people younger than 15 years who receive the second dose less than 5 months following the first dose [10,11]. Additionally, the CDC recommends three doses (second dose administered at a schedule of 1 to 2 months after the first dose;

and the third dose administered 6 months after the first dose) for persons who initiate the vaccine series on or after their 15th birthday, as well as those with a compromised immune system [11].

Despite the recommendation by the ACIP and CDC, the number of adolescents adhering to the recommended dosing schedule remains relatively low. Adherence to the recommended dosing schedule is crucial to optimize immune response to the HPV vaccine [12,13]. According to the CDC, only about half of adolescents aged 13 to 17 years adhere to the recommended HPV vaccine dosing schedule [1]. A possible contributing factor of low adherence to the recommended dosing schedule is little or no emphasis on the dosing schedule in reporting the vaccine series as complete [14–16]. Specifically, the vaccine is often categorized as complete based on the uptake of the required number of doses (two or three doses depending on age category) without considering the interval between doses [14–16]. For example, in Munn et al.'s study conducted to examine the uptake and completion of HPV vaccine series among adolescent users and nonusers of school-based health centers, completion was defined as the uptake of the required number of doses per age category, with no information about the interval between doses [15]. Similarly, another study conducted by Simons et al. to estimate and examine predictors of HPV vaccine series completion defined completion based on the receipt of three doses of HPV vaccine within one year without considering adherence to the recommended dosing schedule [14]. Given that adherence to the recommended number of doses and interval between doses is necessary for efficacy [17,18], considerations should be made to note both requirements when categorizing HPV vaccination as complete.

Observational studies have identified several factors that influence the uptake of the HPV vaccine among adolescents [13–15]; however, the factors that influence adherence to the recommended dosing schedule remain unexplored. It is plausible that the factors associated with HPV vaccine uptake are also associated with adherence to the recommended HPV dosing schedule. For example, sociodemographic characteristics, including age, race/ethnicity, income level, insurance status, census region, and sex; and factors such as provider recommendation, parental hesitancy, structural barriers, and knowledge influence HPV vaccine uptake [13–16,19] and, therefore, may affect adherence to the recommended dosing schedule.

Receiving two or three doses of 9vHPV is not enough to offer the expected protection from HPV-related diseases [10,18]. Complying with the recommended interval between doses is also essential to ensure HPV vaccine efficacy [10,17,18]. Since adherence to the recommended dosing schedule seems necessary for protection from HPV-related infections [10,17,18], the efficacy of the 9vHPV vaccine may be reduced when the intervals between doses are not according to the recommended schedule. Adverse effects associated with not receiving the HPV vaccine, such as risk of HPV-related cancers [10], may be associated with non-adherence to the recommended HPV vaccine dosing schedule. Although previous research has shown that HPV vaccine uptake among adolescents aged 13 to 17 years has improved over the years, limited research on HPV vaccine completion has examined the adherence to the recommended dosing schedule. Thus, the goal of this research is to examine the prevalence and factors associated with adherence to the recommended HPV vaccination dosing schedule among adolescents aged 13 to 17 years. Findings could help researchers and policy makers to improve adherence to the recommended dosing schedule by highlighting the importance of dosing intervals when creating programs aimed at improving HPV vaccination.

2. Materials and Methods

Study Design, Setting, and Participants

In this secondary analysis, we utilized the 2019–2020 National Immunization Survey Teen (NIS-Teen) conducted by the CDC [20]. The NIS-Teen is conducted annually with samples of parents or caregivers of adolescents who are aged 13 to 17 years and reside in the US. The sampling frame includes a representative sample of eligible parents with landlines or cell phones. The survey consists of provider-verified data on vaccines from adolescents aged 13 to 17 years in the 50 states, the District of Columbia, and territories.

The survey occurs in two phases: in phase 1, parents or caregivers are contacted via telephone to provide information pertaining to their adolescents' sociodemographic characteristics, contact information, and vaccination history. Additionally, parents or caregivers are asked to provide consent for the adolescents' healthcare provider to be contacted. In phase 2, healthcare providers are contacted through a mailed survey to verify the accuracy of the information obtained from parents or caregivers. Detailed information about the methods for the NIS-Teen study are available elsewhere [20].

3. Measures

3.1. Dependent Variable

HPV Vaccine Uptake

The dependent variable assessed whether an adolescent adhered to the required dosing schedule when completing the HPV vaccine series. Specifically, the variable assessed whether adolescents were HPV vaccine up-to-date (UTD) in line with the required dosing and interval between HPV vaccine shots. This variable was first included in the NIS-teen survey in 2016. UTD was defined as 3+ human papillomavirus shots (9V, 4 V, UV, CV, or HP) or 2+ human papillomavirus shots, with the first shot received before age 15 and an interval between first and second shots of at least 5 months (minus 4 days), excluding any vaccinations after the random digit dialing interview date [20]. This variable was binary, i.e., "UTD" versus "Not UTD".

3.2. Independent Variables

Provider Recommendation

To assess provider recommendation, respondents were asked, "Had or has a doctor or other health care professional ever recommended that teen receive HPV shots?" Responses were either "Yes", "No", "Don't Know", or "Refused". This variable was operationalized as binary, with only responses "Yes" or "No" retained for our analysis.

3.3. Sociodemographic Characteristics

Sociodemographic characteristics assessed based on previous literature were adolescent's age (categorical variable 13–17 years), gender (male or female), race/ethnicity (non-Hispanic White, non-Hispanic Black, Hispanic, and non-Hispanic Other), region (West, Midwest, Northeast, and South), and insurance status (any Medicaid, private insurance only, other insurance, and uninsured). Other sociodemographic characteristics assessed were poverty status, defined as percentage of poverty line (categorized as above poverty ≤USD 75 k, above poverty >USD 75 k, and below poverty), and mother's education status (categorized as college graduate, some college, high school only, and less than high school).

3.4. Statistical Analysis

All analyses were conducted using Stata/IC V.15.1. The analyses accounted for the complex study design and survey sampling weights used in the NIS-Teens survey. The inclusion criterion was the presence of adequate provider data for UTD and not UTD adolescents. We excluded all "Don't Know" and "Refused" responses for provider recommendation, and "Unknown" responses for poverty status. A complete case analysis was conducted; as such, respondents with missing data for provider recommendation (1.79%) and region (0.84%) were excluded from the analysis. Weighted percentages were reported and are, therefore, representative of the general population. Descriptive statistics were presented in the overall population and in populations stratified by gender using simple proportions and chi-square test. Furthermore, we presented the weighted prevalence of UTD by sociodemographic characteristics and provider recommendations in the overall population and stratified by gender. Bivariable and multivariable logistic regression analyses were used to estimate the association between sociodemographic characteristics and provider recommendation with HPV UTD among adolescents aged 13–17 years in our overall study sample and separately among females and males. Each model was adjusted for sociodemographic characteristics, provider recommendation, and survey year. Statistical significance was defined as a two-sided p-value < 0.05 for all comparisons.

4. Results

4.1. Overall Population

A total of 34,619 adolescents were included in our final analyses. Among those who were UTD in the overall population, most were females (51.8%), 16 years old (22.0%), non-Hispanic White (50.7%), resided in the southern region (36.5%), had private insurance only (55.0%), had income above poverty >USD 75 k (51.0%), had mothers who were college graduates (45.8%), and had received a provider recommendation (88.9%) (Table 1).

The overall UTD prevalence among all adolescents was 57.1% (95% CI: 56.0–58.1%). In the overall population, the UTD prevalence was 60.0% among females and 54.2% among males. Adolescents aged 16 years had the highest UTD prevalence of 63.0%. The UTD prevalence was also highest (61.6%) among Hispanics and highest (63.9%) among adolescents residing in the Northeast region. Moreover, adolescents who had any Medicaid had the highest (60.7%) UTD prevalence, while adolescents below the poverty line had the highest (60.8%) UTD prevalence. The UTD prevalence was highest (61.7%) among adolescents with mothers having less than high school education and highest (62.8%) among adolescents who received a provider recommendation. Additionally, the UTD prevalence was 54.6% in 2019 and 59.5% in 2020 (Table 2).

In the overall population, results of multivariable regression analysis showed that, compared to uninsured adolescents, adolescents who had any Medicaid had over twofold higher adjusted odds of UTD (AOR: 2.13; 95% CI: 1.64–2.76). Moreover, compared to adolescents below the poverty line, those living above poverty <= USD 75 k had 22% lower adjusted odds of UTD (AOR: 0.78; 95% CI: 0.66–0.92). Adolescents residing in the Midwest and Northeast regions had 1.19- and 1.49-times higher odds of UTD, respectively, compared to those residing in the Southern region (AOR: 1.19; 95% CI: 1.08–1.31, AOR: 1.49; 95% CI:1.33–1.66, respectively). Additionally, adolescents who received a provider recommendation had about twofold higher adjusted odds of UTD compared to those who did not (AOR: 1.85; 95% CI: 1.74–1.97). We also found 22% higher odds of UTD in 2020 compared to 2019 (Table 2).

Table 1. Descriptive statistics of teens aged 13–17 years, stratified by gender, National Immunization Survey—Teen (2019–2020).

Characteristics	Overall Sample (n = 34,619)			Female (n = 16,623)			Male (n = 17,996)		
	Not UTD (n = 14,322) (n (w%))	UTD (n = 20,297) (n (w%))	p-Value	Not UTD (n = 6554) (n (w%))	UTD (n = 10,069) (n (w%))	p-Value	Not UTD (n = 7768) (n (w%))	UTD (n = 10,228) (n (w%))	p-Value
Sex			<0.001						
Female	6554 (45.8)	10069 (51.8)							
Male	7768 (54.2)	10228 (48.2)							
Age, years			<0.001			<0.001			<0.001
13	3799 (24.7)	3450 (15.3)		1826 (26.3)	1693 (16.3)		1973 (23.3)	1757 (14.2)	
14	3111 (21.8)	4168 (20.1)		1427 (22.4)	2031 (19.2)		1684 (21.3)	2137 (21.1)	
15	2631 (18.7)	4257 (21.7)		1186 (18.1)	2094 (22.3)		1445 (19.2)	2163 (21.1)	
16	2477 (17.2)	4432 (22.0)		1093 (16.3)	2238 (21.6)		1384 (17.9)	2194 (22.4)	
17	2304 (17.7)	3990 (20.9)		1022 (16.9)	2013 (20.7)		1282 (18.3)	1977 (21.2)	
Race/ethnicity			<0.001			<0.001			0.054
Non-Hispanic White	9589 (56.5)	12750 (50.7)		4395 (57.1)	6257 (50.1)		5194 (56.0)	6493 (51.4)	
Non-Hispanic Black	1035 (13.4)	1608 (13.7)		471 (13.8)	804 (13.2)		564 (13.1)	804 (14.2)	
Hispanic	2154 (20.8)	3579 (25.2)		966 (19.4)	1767 (25.4)		1188 (22.1)	1812 (25.0)	
Non-Hispanic Other	1544 (9.2)	2360 (10.4)		722 (9.7)	1241 (11.3)		822 (8.8)	1119 (9.5)	
Region			<0.001			0.002			<0.001
West	3365 (23.4)	4295 (24.5)		1546 (21.8)	2157 (25.2)		1819 (24.7)	2138 (23.7)	
Midwest	2986 (21.2)	4583 (21.4)		1315 (21.8)	2206 (21.0)		1671 (20.6)	2377 (22.0)	
Northeast	2255 (13.2)	4458 (17.6)		1068 (14.0)	2167 (16.7)		1187 (12.6)	2291 (18.5)	
South	5716 (42.3)	6961 (36.5)		2625 (42.5)	3539 (37.1)		3091 (42.1)	3422 (35.9)	
Insurance status			<0.001			<0.001			<0.001
Any Medicaid	3800 (30.9)	5803 (35.9)		1713 (30.3)	2857 (34.7)		2087 (31.4)	2946 (37.2)	
Private insurance only	8625 (56.3)	12558 (55.0)		3991 (57.5)	6240 (56.4)		4634 (55.3)	6318 (53.5)	
Other insurance	1252 (7.6)	1470 (6.3)		552 (7.1)	740 (6.2)		700 (8.0)	730 (6.4)	
Uninsured	645 (5.2)	466 (2.9)		298 (5.2)	232 (2.8)		347 (5.3)	234 (2.9)	
Poverty status, % of poverty line			<0.001			0.009			0.016
Above poverty ≤USD 75 k	4454 (33.3)	5444 (29.5)		2041 (33.6)	2639 (29.0)		2413 (33.1)	2805 (30.1)	
Above poverty >USD 75 k	7999 (50.1)	11867 (51.0)		3671 (49.5)	5910 (51.9)		4328 (50.6)	5957 (50.2)	
Below poverty	1869 (16.6)	2986 (19.4)		842 (16.9)	1520 (19.1)		1027 (16.4)	1466 (19.8)	

Table 1. Cont.

Characteristics	Overall Sample (n = 34,619)			Female (n = 16,623)			Male (n = 17,996)		
	Not UTD (n = 14,322) (n (w%))	UTD (n = 20,297) (n (w%))	p-Value	Not UTD (n = 6554) (n (w%))	UTD (n = 10,069) (n (w%))	p-Value	Not UTD (n = 7768) (n (w%))	UTD (n = 10,228) (n (w%))	p-Value
Mother's education status			<0.001			0.001			0.058
College graduate	7004 (42.3)	10974 (45.8)		3205 (42.5)	5404 (46.7)		3799 (42.2)	5570 (44.8)	
Some college	4206 (26.4)	4982 (23.9)		1945 (26.9)	2464 (22.9)		2261 (26.0)	2518 (25.0)	
High school only	2140 (22.4)	2744 (19.6)		965 (22.2)	1390 (19.6)		1175 (22.6)	1354 (19.6)	
Less than high school	972 (8.9)	1597 (10.8)		439 (8.4)	811 (10.8)		533 (9.3)	786 (10.7)	
Provider recommendation			<0.001			<0.001			<0.001
No	4200 (30.2)	1932 (11.1)		1588 (25.7)	789 (8.9)		2612 (33.9)	1143 (13.5)	
Yes	10122 (69.8)	18365 (88.9)		4966 (74.3)	9280 (91.1)		5156 (66.1)	9085 (86.5)	
Survey year			<0.001			<0.001			0.009
2019	7294 (53.2)	9382 (48.2)		3325 (53.9)	4667 (47.9)		3969 (52.5)	4715 (48.4)	
2020	7028 (46.8)	10915 (51.9)		3229 (46.1)	5402 (52.1)		3799 (47.5)	5513 (51.6)	

n = unweighted number of participants; w% = weighted percentages. UTD = up-to-date was defined as 3+ human papillomavirus shots (9 V, 4 V, UV, CV, or HP) or 2+ human papillomavirus shots, with first shot received before age 15 and interval between first and second shots of at least 5 months (minus 4 days), excluding any vaccinations after the random digit dialing interview date.

Table 2. Prevalence and association between sociodemographic characteristics and provider recommendation among teens aged 13–17 years and UTD in the overall sample, National Immunization Survey—Teen (2019–2020).

Characteristics		Overall Sample (n = 34,619)	
	w% (95% CI)	Crude OR (95% CI)	Adjusted OR (95% CI) [a]
Overall	57.1% (56.0–58.1%)		
Sex			
Female	60.0 (58.5–61.5)	Ref	Ref
Male	54.2 (52.7–55.7)	0.79 (0.72–0.86)	0.83 (0.76–0.91)
Age, years			
13	45.1 (42.9–47.3)	Ref	Ref
14	55.1 (52.6–57.6)	1.49 (1.30–1.71)	1.52 (1.32–1.75)
15	60.7 (58.4–62.9)	1.88 (1.64–2.14)	1.91 (1.67–2.19)
16	63.0 (60.7–65.2)	2.09 (1.84–2.37)	2.09 (1.82–2.40)
17	61.2 (58.5–63.7)	1.99 (1.73–2.27)	1.93 (1.66–2.23)
Race/ethnicity			
Non-Hispanic White	54.4 (53.2–55.6)	Ref	Ref
Non-Hispanic Black	57.5 (54.2–60.7)	1.13 (1.18–1.54)	1.22 (1.04–1.43)
Hispanic	61.6 (58.7–64.5)	1.35 (0.99–1.31)	1.51 (1.31–1.74)
Non-Hispanic Other	60.0 (57.0–63.0)	1.26 (1.10–1.44)	1.27 (1.11–1.46)
Region			
South	53.4 (51.9–55.0)	Ref	Ref
West	58.2 (55.1–61.3)	1.22 (1.05–1.40)	1.12 (0.97–1.31)
Midwest	57.4 (55.7–59.0)	1.17 (1.07–1.29)	1.19 (1.08–1.31)
Northeast	63.9 (61.8–65.8)	1.54 (1.39–1.71)	1.49 (1.33–1.66)
Insurance status			
Uninsured	42.1 (36.4–47.9)	Ref	Ref
Any Medicaid	60.7 (58.6–62.7)	2.13 (1.65–2.73)	2.13 (1.64–2.76)
Private insurance only	56.5 (55.1–57.8)	1.79 (1.40–2.28)	1.61 (1.23–2.09)
Other insurance	52.3 (48.4–56.2)	1.51 (1.14–2.01)	1.49 (1.10–2.01)
Poverty status, % of poverty line			
Below poverty	60.8 (58.0–63.6)	Ref	Ref
Above poverty ≤USD 75 k	54.1 (52.1–56.1)	0.76 (0.66–0.88)	0.78 (0.66–0.92)
Above poverty >USD 75 k	57.5 (56.1–58.9)	0.87 (0.77–1.00)	0.89 (0.73–1.08)
Mother's education status			
College graduate	59.0 (57.6–60.4)	Ref	Ref
Some college	54.6 (52.5–56.7)	0.84 (0.75–0.93)	0.80 (0.71–0.89)
High school only	53.7 (50.9–56.4)	0.81 (0.71–0.91)	0.76 (0.65–0.88)
Less than high school	61.7 (57.7–65.4)	1.12 (0.94–1.33)	1.02 (0.82–1.28)

Table 2. *Cont.*

Characteristics	Overall Sample (n = 34,619)		
	w% (95% CI)	Crude OR (95% CI)	Adjusted OR (95% CI) [a]
Provider recommendation			
No	32.8 (30.5–35.3)	Ref	Ref
Yes	62.8 (61.7–64.0)	1.86 (1.75–1.97)	1.85 (1.74–1.97)
Survey year			
2019	54.6 (53.0–56.2)	Ref	Ref
2020	59.5 (58.2–60.9)	1.22 (1.12–1.34)	1.22 (1.11–1.33)

w% = weighted percentages; OR = odds ratio; CI = confidence interval; Ref = reference category. UTD = up-to-date was defined as 3+ human papillomavirus shots (9 V, 4 V, UV, CV, or HP) or 2+ human papillomavirus shots, with first shot received before age 15 and interval between first and second shots of at least 5 months (minus 4 days), excluding any vaccinations after the random digit dialing interview date. [a] Model adjusted for sociodemographic characteristics, provider recommendation, and survey year.

4.2. Female Adolescents

Following stratification by gender, among females, the UTD prevalence was 60.0% (95% CI: 58.5–61.5%). Moreover, UTD prevalence was 63.2% among female adolescents on any Medicaid and 44.8% among uninsured females. Female adolescents below the poverty line had a UTD prevalence of 62.9%, while those above the poverty line ≤USD 75 k had a UTD prevalence of 56.4%. Female adolescents who received a recommendation from a provider had a UTD prevalence of 64.8%, while those who received no provider recommendation had a UTD prevalence of 34.2% (Table 3).

Among females, results of multivariable regression analysis showed that, compared to female adolescents that are uninsured, those with any Medicaid, private insurance only, and other insurance had 124%, 68%, and 62% higher adjusted odds of UTD, respectively. Moreover, females who had received a provider recommendation had 92% (AOR: 1.92; 95% CI: 1.75–2.11) higher adjusted odds of UTD compared to those who received no recommendation (Table 3).

4.3. Male Adolescents

Following stratification by gender, among males, the UTD prevalence was 54.2% (95% CI: 52.7–55.7%). Male adolescents who had any Medicaid insurance had the highest (58.3%) UTD prevalence, while those who were uninsured had the lowest (39.6%) UTD prevalence. Male adolescents below the poverty line had a UTD prevalence of 58.8%, while those above the poverty line >USD 75 k had a UTD prevalence of 54.0%. Male adolescents who received a recommendation from a provider had a UTD prevalence of 60.8%, while those who received no provider recommendation had a UTD prevalence of 31.9% (Table 3).

Furthermore, among male adolescents, results of multivariable logistic regression analysis were mostly similar but slightly attenuated compared to what was seen among female adolescents. Male adolescents with any Medicaid had 102% higher adjusted odds of being UTD compared to those who were uninsured. In terms of poverty status, compared to male adolescents below the poverty line, those living above poverty ≤USD 75 k had 27% lower adjusted odds of UTD (AOR: 0.73; 95% CI: 0.58–0.92) (Table 3).

Table 3. Prevalence and association between sociodemographic characteristics and provider recommendation among teens aged 13–17 years and UTD, stratified by gender, National Immunization Survey—Teen (2019–2020).

Characteristics	Female (n = 16,623)			Male (n = 17,996)		
	w% (95% CI)	Crude OR (95% CI)	Adjusted OR (95% CI) [a]	w% (95% CI)	Crude OR (95% CI)	Adjusted OR (95% CI) [a]
Overall	60.0 (58.5–61.5)			54.2 (52.7–55.7)		
Age, years						
13	48.1 (44.8–51.4)	Ref	Ref	41.8 (38.9–44.7)	Ref	Ref
14	56.3 (52.7–59.8)	1.39 (1.14–1.69)	1.40 (1.14–1.71)	53.9 (50.4–57.5)	1.63 (1.35–1.97)	1.65 (1.36–1.99)
15	64.8 (61.8–67.8)	1.99 (1.65–2.40)	2.06 (1.70–2.50)	56.5 (53.2–59.8)	1.81 (1.51–2.17)	1.80 (1.49–2.18)
16	66.5 (63.2–69.7)	2.14 (1.76–2.60)	2.14 (1.74–2.64)	59.7 (56.6–62.8)	2.06 (1.73–2.46)	2.05 (1.72–2.45)
17	64.8 (61.1–68.4)	1.98 (1.61–2.44)	2.00 (1.64–2.44)	57.7 (54.0–61.4)	1.90 (1.57–2.30)	1.87 (1.52–2.30)
Race/ethnicity						
Non-Hispanic White	56.8 (55.1–58.6)	Ref	Ref	52.0 (50.4–53.7)	Ref	Ref
Non-Hispanic Black	59.1 (54.4–63.6)	1.10 (0.89–1.34)	1.21 (0.97–1.52)	56.0 (51.4–60.5)	1.17 (0.96–1.43)	1.22 (0.98–1.51)
Hispanic	66.3 (62.3–70.0)	1.49 (1.24–1.80)	1.67 (1.36–2.05)	57.2 (53.0–61.4)	1.23 (1.03–1.48)	1.39 (1.13–1.70)
Non-Hispanic Other	63.6 (59.5–67.6)	1.33 (1.10–1.60)	1.33 (1.10–1.60)	56.0 (51.7–60.3)	1.17 (0.97–1.42)	1.22 (1.00–1.48)
Region						
South	56.7 (54.5–58.8)	Ref	Ref	50.2 (48.0–52.4)	Ref	Ref
West	63.5 (59.0–67.8)	1.33 (1.08–1.64)	1.19 (0.96–1.48)	53.2 (48.8–57.5)	1.13 (0.93–1.37)	1.06 (0.86–1.30)
Midwest	59.1 (56.6–61.5)	1.10 (0.97–1.26)	1.13 (0.98–1.29)	55.7 (53.4–58.0)	1.25 (1.10–1.42)	1.25 (1.10–1.43)
Northeast	64.3 (61.4–67.1)	1.37 (1.18–1.60)	1.30 (1.11–1.52)	63.4 (60.6–66.2)	1.72 (1.48–2.00)	1.68 (1.44–1.96)
Insurance status						
Uninsured	44.8 (37.0–52.9)	Ref	Ref	39.6 (31.7–48.0)	Ref	Ref
Any Medicaid	63.2 (60.3–66.1)	2.12 (1.50–3.00)	2.24 (1.55–3.24)	58.3 (55.4–61.1)	2.14 (1.49–3.07)	2.02 (1.40–2.90)
Private insurance only	59.6 (57.6–61.4)	1.81 (1.30–2.53)	1.68 (1.16–2.42)	53.4 (51.5–55.2)	1.75 (1.23–2.48)	1.53 (1.05–2.22)
Other insurance	56.6 (51.4–61.8)	1.61 (1.09–2.37)	1.62 (1.09–2.42)	48.5 (43.0–54.1)	1.44 (0.95–2.17)	1.35 (0.87–2.11)
Poverty status, % of poverty line						
Below poverty	62.9 (58.9–66.7)	Ref	Ref	58.8 (54.7–62.8)	Ref	Ref
Above poverty ≤USD 75 k	56.4 (53.5–59.3)	0.76 (0.62–0.94)	0.84 (0.67–1.07)	51.8 (49.0–54.6)	0.75 (0.62–0.92)	0.73 (0.58–0.92)
Above poverty >USD 75 k	61.2 (59.2–63.1)	0.93 (0.77–1.12)	1.00 (0.75–1.33)	54.0 (52.0–55.9)	0.82 (0.68–0.99)	0.80 (0.62–1.04)

Table 3. Cont.

Characteristics	Female (n = 16,623)			Male (n = 17,996)		
	w% (95% CI)	Crude OR (95% CI)	Adjusted OR (95% CI) [a]	w% (95% CI)	Crude OR (95% CI)	Adjusted OR (95% CI) [a]
Mother's education status						
College graduate	62.3 (60.3–64.2)	Ref	Ref	55.7 (53.7–57.6)	Ref	Ref
Some college	56.1 (53.2–59.0)	0.78 (0.67–0.90)	0.75 (0.64–0.88)	53.2 (50.2–56.2)	0.90 (0.78–1.04)	0.85 (0.72–1.00)
High school only	56.9 (53.0–60.8)	0.80 (0.67–0.96)	0.78 (0.63–0.97)	50.6 (46.7–54.5)	0.82 (0.68–0.97)	0.74 (0.60–0.90)
Less than high school	65.9 (60.2–71.2)	1.17 (0.90–1.52)	1.11 (0.80–1.55)	57.6 (52.2–62.9)	1.08 (0.86–1.37)	0.94 (0.70–1.27)
Provider recommendation						
No	34.2 (30.6–38.0)	Ref	Ref	31.9 (28.8–35.2)	Ref	Ref
Yes	64.8 (63.2–66.4)	1.88 (1.72–2.06)	1.92 (1.75–2.11)	60.8 (59.1–62.4)	1.82 (1.67–1.97)	1.81 (1.67–1.97)
Survey year						
2019	57.1 (54.8–59.5)	Ref	Ref	52.1 (49.9–54.4)	Ref	Ref
2020	62.9 (61.1–64.8)	1.27 (1.12–1.44)	1.28 (1.12–1.45)	56.2 (54.3–58.2)	1.18 (1.04–1.33)	1.17 (1.03–1.33)

w% = weighted percentages; OR = odds ratio; CI = confidence interval; Ref = reference category. UTD = up-to-date was defined as 3+ human papillomavirus shots (9 V, 4 V, UV, CV, or HP) or 2+ human papillomavirus shots, with first shot received before age 15 and interval between first and second shots of at least 5 months (minus 4 days), excluding any vaccinations after the random digit dialing interview date. [a] Model adjusted for sociodemographic characteristics, provider recommendation, and survey year.

5. Discussion

To our knowledge, our study is among the first to employ the 2019–2020 NIS-Teen dataset to examine the prevalence and factors associated with the adherence to the ACIP recommended 9vHPV vaccine schedule among teenagers aged 13 to 17 years. Nationally, only about half of females and males completed the vaccine series with adherence to the recommended schedule. Our finding is consistent with previous research, which shows that only 58.6% of teenagers adhered to the recommended dosing schedule [1]. Without adherence to the recommended dosing schedule, immune response imparting expected protection from the HPV vaccine is uncertain [18]. It is possible that expected immune protection might be reduced or absent outside of the recommended vaccination schedule [9].

Our low adherence finding could be related to a number of possible reasons, including providers not scheduling follow-up doses at the time of the initial dose, or few or no reminders for follow-up dose scheduling. Since lack of knowledge is a factor associated with low HPV vaccine uptake [21–23], it could also be a reason for low adherence to the recommended vaccination schedule. Based on previous studies, knowledge is an important predictor of HPV vaccine uptake, and improvement in knowledge results in improvements in HPV vaccine behaviors [21–23]. Providing parents with information about the importance of adhering to the appropriate dosing interval may encourage parents to pay attention to the time points when vaccinating their adolescents. Moreover, creating intervention programs aimed at increasing knowledge on adherence to the recommended dosing may improve adherence to the recommended vaccination schedule.

In our provider recommendation analysis, we found that provider recommendation was consistently associated with HPV vaccine completion with adherence to the recommended dosing schedule. Our results are in agreement with other studies that have shown that parents are more likely to vaccinate their adolescents when they receive a recommendation from a healthcare provider [24]. How providers introduce and recommend vaccines is robustly associated with vaccine behaviors [25,26]. Specifically, "strong" provider recommendation (which encompasses the recommendation of same-day vaccination, emphasizing the completion of the vaccine series, and specifying the recommended dosing schedule) is associated with nine times the odds of HPV vaccine uptake compared to a weak recommendation [26]. Moreover, providing parents with information regarding the differences in dosing schedules and requirements by age provides an incentive for on-time vaccination [27]. Our provider-recommendation-related finding is possibly because parents who are rule followers adhere to the recommended schedule, or because parents who go to their primary care provider for vaccination are more likely to have a follow-up appointment scheduled and get a reminder call/postcard/text about their upcoming appointment. Although parental hesitancy discourages providers from having HPV-vaccine-related conversations with parents [25], it is important that providers understand that even hesitant parents are willing to change with provider encouragement. These findings offer early evidence for the need for provider education to improve the quality of provider recommendations, which could increase adherence to the recommended dosing schedule.

In our income analysis, we found that the odds of complying with the dosing schedule were higher among those below the poverty line. We found that adolescents who had any Medicaid had higher odds of adhering to the recommended HPV vaccine dosing schedule. According to Hoff et al. [28], Medicaid expansion resulted in a significant increase in HPV vaccine uptake among people living below the poverty level. Under the Vaccines for Children program (VFC), adolescents enrolled in Medicaid are eligible to receive all vaccines recommended by the ACIP at no cost to them or their families [29–31]. These factors may contribute to greater compliance with the vaccination schedule. Because VFC also covers uninsured adolescents, it is surprising that adherence to the recommended dosing schedule is lower in uninsured adolescents than in adolescents with only Medicaid. Therefore, the lower rates of adherence to the dosing schedule among uninsured adolescents should be investigated further.

In our census region analysis, we found that, in the South (where HPV vaccine completion is the lowest in the nation: Mississippi 28.8% and Wyoming 30.9%) [32], parents had lower odds of adhering to the recommended dosing schedule compared to other regions. This finding has important public health implications. If lower adherence to the recommended dosing schedule in the South census region persists, this region could face a disproportionately higher burden of HPV-related infections in future decades compared to regions with higher adherence to the recommended dosing schedule. Further research is needed to explore possible factors impacting adherence to the recommended HPV vaccine dosing schedule in the South census region and to determine how best to design interventions aimed at improving the adherence to the recommended HPV vaccine dosing schedule in the South census region.

While we found that the odds of vaccine completion with adherence to the recommended dosing schedule was higher in 2020 than in 2019, rates remain relatively low. Structural barriers, such as transportation difficulties, could make complying with the recommended vaccination schedule difficult for adolescents and their parents [33]. Thus, there is a need for improving vaccine accessibility for adolescents with parental consent by making the vaccine available in alternative settings, such as schools without the need for parents to be present. Increasing access to vaccination through systems-level interventions, such as school-based vaccination, can improve vaccination uptake with adherence to the vaccine schedule.

A limitation of this study is that the respondent is one parent/guardian of the adolescent and may not be the most knowledgeable about the adolescent's health status and vaccinations. However, we addressed this limitation by including only respondents with adequate provider data. Another limitation is that our dependent variable was designed to account for adolescents who received the 9vHPV vaccine as well as those who may have received other types of HPV vaccines (4 V, UV, CV, or HP) prior to the discontinuation in 2017. While this limitation did not affect the goal of our study, which is to examine the adherence to the recommended dose schedule, there is a need for the NIS-Teen researchers to include a variable that focuses on the adherence to the dosing schedule of the 9vHPV vaccine. This strategy will allow HPV-vaccine researchers to better examine adherence to the recommended dosing schedule of the only HPV vaccine currently administered in the US. Our study may be prone to residual confounding from father's educational status, as this variable is unavailable in the NIS-Teens dataset and was not accounted for in all our analyses. Other limitations, such as social desirability bias and recall bias, were also addressed by using respondents with adequate provider data. Strengths of the study include its large sample size and nationally representative data, and use of provider verified data.

Our study contributes to previous research by examining the sociodemographic factors associated with adherence to the HPV vaccine dosing schedule. Our findings suggest that adherence to the recommended dosing schedule remains relatively low. Adherence to the recommended dosing schedule is important for adequate immune response and expected protection from HPV infection. Therefore, findings from this research are important for the improvement in adherence to the HPV vaccine schedule.

6. Conclusions

It is important to investigate nonadherence to the recommended dosing schedule for HPV vaccination. Our cross-sectional analysis depicts salient factors, including provider recommendation, that can be targeted through interventions to improve adherence to the 9vHPV dosing schedule to offer better protection from HPV-related cancers. More research is needed to examine correlates of adherence to the recommended schedule for 9vHPV. Multilevel interventions to increase knowledge of the 9vHPV dosing schedule, improve the quality of provider recommendation, and remove access barriers to vaccination are warranted to improve the overall rates of adherence to the recommended 9vHPV dose schedule across races, age categories, and census regions.

Author Contributions: C.L.E. and I.O. are co-first authors, had full access to all of the data in the study, and take responsibility for the integrity of the data and the accuracy of the data analysis. *Study concept and design*: C.L.E., P.C., I.O. *Acquisition, analysis, and interpretation of data*: C.L.E., I.O., P.C. *Drafting of the manuscript*: C.L.E., I.O., S.A. *Critical revision of the manuscript for important intellectual content*: P.C., C.L.E. *Statistical analysis*: I.O., C.L.E. *Obtained funding*: NA. *Administrative, technical, or material support*: S.A., C.L.E. *Study supervision*: P.C. All authors have read and agreed to the published version of the manuscript.

Funding: This study was supported in part by: the authors did not receive any funding support for this study.

Financial Disclosure: None reported.

All Financial Interests (Including Pharmaceutical and Device Product(s)): The authors declare no financial interest.

Institutional Review Board Statement: Ethical review and approval for this study was waived because the NIS-Teen data is de-identified and publicly available.

Informed Consent Statement: All participants in the NIS-Teen survey provided informed consent to participate in the survey.

Data Availability Statement: Data supporting reported results can be found at https://www.cdc.gov/vaccines/imz-managers/nis/datasets-teen.html, accessed on 5 April 2022.

Conflicts of Interest: The authors declare no conflict of interest.

References

1. Pingali, C.; Yankey, D.; Elam-Evans, L.D.; Markowitz, L.E.; Williams, C.L.; Fredua, B.; McNamara, L.A.; Stokley, S.; Singleton, J.A. National, regional, state, and selected local area vaccination coverage among adolescents aged 13–17 years—United States, 2020. *Morb. Mortal. Wkly. Rep.* **2021**, *70*, 1183. [CrossRef] [PubMed]
2. Walker, T.Y.; Elam-Evans, L.D.; Yankey, D.; Markowitz, L.E.; Williams, C.L.; Fredua, B.; Singleton, J.A.; Stokley, S. National, regional, state, and selected local area vaccination coverage among adolescents aged 13–17 years—United States, 2018. *Morb. Mortal. Wkly. Rep.* **2019**, *68*, 718. [CrossRef] [PubMed]
3. Yusupov, A.; Popovsky, D.; Mahmood, L.; Kim, A.S.; Akman, A.E.; Yuan, H. The nonavalent vaccine: A review of high-risk HPVs and a plea to the CDC. *Am. J. Stem Cells* **2019**, *8*, 52. [PubMed]
4. Laprise, J.F.; Markowitz, L.E.; Chesson, H.W.; Drolet, M.; Brisson, M. Comparison of 2-dose and 3-dose 9-valent human papillomavirus vaccine schedules in the United States: A cost-effectiveness analysis. *J. Infect. Dis.* **2016**, *214*, 685–688. [CrossRef] [PubMed]
5. Meites, E.; Kempe, A.; Markowitz, L.E. Use of a 2-dose schedule for human papillomavirus vaccination—Updated recommendations of the Advisory Committee on Immunization Practices. *Morb. Mortal. Wkly. Rep.* **2016**, *65*, 1405–1408. [CrossRef]
6. Gilca, V.; Sauvageau, C.; Panicker, G.; De Serres, G.; Ouakki, M.; Unger, E.R. Immunogenicity and safety of a mixed vaccination schedule with one dose of nonavalent and one dose of bivalent HPV vaccine versus two doses of nonavalent vaccine—A randomized clinical trial. *Vaccine* **2018**, *36*, 7017–7024. [CrossRef]
7. Pinto, L.A.; Dillner, J.; Beddows, S.; Unger, E.R. Immunogenicity of HPV prophylactic vaccines: Serology assays and their use in HPV vaccine evaluation and development. *Vaccine* **2018**, *36*, 4792–4799. [CrossRef]
8. Bergman, H.; Buckley, B.S.; Villanueva, G.; Petkovic, J.; Garritty, C.; Lutje, V.; Riveros-Balta, A.X.; Low, N.; Henschke, N. Comparison of different human papillomavirus (HPV) vaccine types and dose schedules for prevention of HPV-related disease in females and males. *Cochrane Database Syst. Rev.* **2019**, *11*, CD013479. [CrossRef]
9. Hoes, J.; Pasmans, H.; Schurink-van't Klooster, T.M.; van der Klis, F.R.; Donken, R.; Berkhof, J.; de Melker, H.E. Review of long-term immunogenicity following HPV vaccination: Gaps in current knowledge. *Hum. Vaccines Immunother.* **2021**, *18*, 1–11. [CrossRef]
10. Meites, E.; Szilagyi, P.G.; Chesson, H.W.; Unger, E.R.; Romero, J.R.; Markowitz, L.E. Human papillomavirus vaccination for adults: Updated recommendations of the Advisory Committee on Immunization Practices. *Am. J. Transplant.* **2019**, *19*, 3202–3206. [CrossRef]
11. Centers for Disease Control and Prevention. Human papillomavirus (HPV): Vaccine Schedule and Dosing. Available online: https://www.cdc.gov/hpv/hcp/schedules-recommendations.html (accessed on 1 November 2021).
12. Markowitz, L.E.; Dunne, E.F.; Saraiya, M.; Chesson, H.W.; Curtis, C.R.; Gee, J.; Bocchini, J.A., Jr.; Unger, E.R. Human papillomavirus vaccination: Recommendations of the Advisory Committee on Immunization Practices (ACIP). *Morb. Mortal. Wkly. Rep. Recomm. Rep.* **2014**, *63*, 1–30.

13. Sauver, J.L.; Rutten, L.J.; Ebbert, J.O.; Jacobson, D.J.; McGree, M.E.; Jacobson, R.M. Younger age at initiation of the human papillomavirus (HPV) vaccination series is associated with higher rates of on-time completion. *Prev. Med.* **2016**, *89*, 327–333. [CrossRef] [PubMed]
14. Simons, H.R.; Unger, Z.D.; Lopez, P.M.; Kohn, J.E. Predictors of human papillomavirus vaccine completion among female and male vaccine initiators in family planning centers. *Am. J. Public Health* **2015**, *105*, 2541–2548. [CrossRef] [PubMed]
15. Munn, M.S.; Kay, M.; Page, L.C.; Duchin, J.S. Completion of the human papillomavirus vaccination series among adolescent users and nonusers of school-based health centers. *Public Health Rep.* **2019**, *134*, 559–566. [CrossRef] [PubMed]
16. Rand, C.M.; Tyrrell, H.; Wallace-Brodeur, R.; Goldstein, N.P.; Darden, P.M.; Humiston, S.G.; Albertin, C.S.; Stratbucker, W.; Schaffer, S.J.; Davis, W.; et al. A learning collaborative model to improve human papillomavirus vaccination rates in primary care. *Acad. Pediatr.* **2018**, *18*, S46–S52. [CrossRef]
17. Gertig, D.M.; Brotherton, J.M.; Budd, A.C.; Drennan, K.; Chappell, G.; Saville, A.M. Impact of a population-based HPV vaccination program on cervical abnormalities: A data linkage study. *BMC Med.* **2013**, *11*, 227. [CrossRef]
18. Blomberg, M.; Dehlendorff, C.; Sand, C.; Kjaer, S.K. Dose-related differences in effectiveness of human papillomavirus vaccination against genital warts: A nationwide study of 550,000 young girls. *Clin. Infect. Dis.* **2015**, *61*, 676–682. [CrossRef]
19. Mansfield, L.N.; Silva, S.G.; Merwin, E.I.; Chung, R.J.; Gonzalez-Guarda, R.M. Factors Associated with Human Papillomavirus Vaccine Series Completion Among Adolescents. *Am. J. Prev. Med.* **2021**, *61*, 701–708. [CrossRef]
20. Centers for Disease Control and Prevention, National Opinion Research Center at the University of Chicago. *National Immunization Survey-Teen: A user's Guide for the 2020 Public-Use Data File*; National Opinion Research Center: Chicago, IL, USA, 2020.
21. Mohammed, K.A.; Subramaniam, D.S.; Geneus, C.J.; Henderson, E.R.; Dean, C.A.; Subramaniam, D.P.; Burroughs, T.E. Rural-urban differences in human papillomavirus knowledge and awareness among US adults. *Prev. Med.* **2018**, *109*, 39–43. [CrossRef]
22. Hirth, J.M.; Fuchs, E.L.; Chang, M.; Fernandez, M.E.; Berenson, A.B. Variations in reason for intention not to vaccinate across time, region, and by race/ethnicity, NIS-Teen (2008–2016). *Vaccine* **2019**, *37*, 595–601. [CrossRef]
23. Boyd, E.D.; Phillips, J.M.; Schoenberger, Y.M.; Simpson, T. Barriers and facilitators to HPV vaccination among rural Alabama adolescents and their caregivers. *Vaccine* **2018**, *36*, 4126–4133. [CrossRef] [PubMed]
24. Burdette, A.M.; Webb, N.S.; Hill, T.D.; Jokinen-Gordon, H. Race-specific trends in HPV vaccinations and provider recommendations: Persistent disparities or social progress? *Public Health* **2017**, *142*, 167–176. [CrossRef] [PubMed]
25. Shay, L.A.; Baldwin, A.S.; Betts, A.C.; Marks, E.G.; Higashi, R.T.; Street, R.L.; Persaud, D.; Tiro, J.A. Parent-provider communication of HPV vaccine hesitancy. *Pediatrics* **2018**, *141*, e20172312. [CrossRef] [PubMed]
26. Gilkey, M.B.; Calo, W.A.; Moss, J.L.; Shah, P.D.; Marciniak, M.W.; Brewer, N.T. Provider communication and HPV vaccination: The impact of recommendation quality. *Vaccine* **2016**, *34*, 1187–1192. [CrossRef] [PubMed]
27. Margolis, M.A.; Brewer, N.T.; Shah, P.D.; Calo, W.A.; Alton Dailey, S.; Gilkey, M.B. Talking about recommended age or fewer doses: What motivates HPV vaccination timeliness? *Hum. Vaccines Immunother.* **2021**, *17*, 3077–3080. [CrossRef] [PubMed]
28. Hoff, B.M.; Livingston, M.D., III; Thompson, E.L. The association between state Medicaid expansion and human papillomavirus vaccination. *Vaccine* **2020**, *38*, 5963–5965. [CrossRef] [PubMed]
29. Keim-Malpass, J.; Mitchell, E.M.; DeGuzman, P.B.; Stoler, M.H.; Kennedy, C. Legislative activity related to the human papillomavirus (HPV) vaccine in the United States (2006–2015): A need for evidence-based policy. *Risk Manag. Healthc. Policy* **2017**, *10*, 29. [CrossRef] [PubMed]
30. Levinson, D.R.; General, I. *Vaccines for Children Program: Vulnerabilities in Vaccine Management*; Department of Health and Human Services, Office of Inspector General: Washington, DC, USA, 2012.
31. Conis, E. Clinton's vaccines for children program. In *Vaccine Nation*; University of Chicago Press: Chicago, IL, USA, 2021; pp. 161–178.
32. Hirth, J. Disparities in HPV vaccination rates and HPV prevalence in the United States: A review of the literature. *Hum. Vaccines Immunother.* **2019**, *15*, 146–155. [CrossRef]
33. Vamos, C.A.; Kline, N.; Vázquez-Otero, C.; Lockhart, E.A.; Lake, P.W.; Wells, K.J.; Proctor, S.; Meade, C.D.; Daley, E.M. Stakeholders' perspectives on system-level barriers to and facilitators of HPV vaccination among Hispanic migrant farmworkers. *Ethn. Health* **2021**, 1–23. [CrossRef]

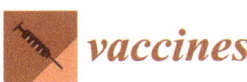

Article

Real-Life Safety Profile of the 9-Valent HPV Vaccine Based on Data from the Puglia Region of Southern Italy

Antonio Di Lorenzo, Paola Berardi, Andrea Martinelli, Francesco Paolo Bianchi, Silvio Tafuri * and Pasquale Stefanizzi

Department of Biomedical Science and Human Oncology, Aldo Moro University of Bari, 70124 Bari, Italy; antoniodilorenzo95@gmail.com (A.D.L.); paola.berardi28@libero.it (P.B.); dott.a.martinelli@gmail.com (A.M.); frapabi@gmail.com (F.P.B.); pasquale.stefanizzi@uniba.it (P.S.)
* Correspondence: silvio.tafuri@uniba.it

Abstract: Human Papillomavirus (HPV) is responsible for epithelial lesions and cancers in both males and females. The latest licensed HPV vaccine is Gardasil-9®, a 9-valent HPV vaccine which is effective not only against the high-risk HPV types, but also against the ones responsible for non-cancerous lesions. This report describes adverse events following Gardasil-9® administration reported in Puglia, southern Italy, from January 2018 to November 2021. This is a retrospective observational study. Data about the adverse events following immunization (AEFIs) with Gardasil-9® were collected from the Italian Drug Authority database. AEFIs were classified as serious or non-serious accordingly to World Health Organization guidelines, and serious ones underwent causality assessment. During the study period, 266,647 doses of 9vHPVv were administered in Puglia and 22 AEFIs were reported, with a reporting rate (RR) of 8.25 per 100,000 doses. The most reported symptoms were neurological ones (7/22). A total of 5 (22.7%) AEFIs were classified as serious, and 2 of these led to the patient's hospitalization. In one case, permanent impairment occurred. Following causality assessment, only 2 out of 5 serious AEFIs were deemed to be consistently associated with the vaccination (RR: 0.750 per 100,000 doses). The data gathered in our study are similar to the pre-licensure evidence as far as the nature of the AEFIs is concerned. The reporting rate, though, is far lower than the ones described in clinical trials, likely due to the different approach to data collection: in our study, data were gathered via passive surveillance, while pre-marketing studies generally employ active calls for this purpose. Gardasil-9®'s safety profile appears to be favorable, with a low rate of serious adverse events and a risk/benefits ratio pending for the latter.

Keywords: HPV; vaccines; AEFIs; causality assessment

Citation: Di Lorenzo, A.; Berardi, P.; Martinelli, A.; Bianchi, F.P.; Tafuri, S.; Stefanizzi, P. Real-Life Safety Profile of the 9-Valent HPV Vaccine Based on Data from the Puglia Region of Southern Italy. *Vaccines* **2022**, *10*, 419. https://doi.org/10.3390/vaccines10030419

Academic Editor: Gloria Calagna

Received: 11 February 2022
Accepted: 7 March 2022
Published: 10 March 2022

Publisher's Note: MDPI stays neutral with regard to jurisdictional claims in published maps and institutional affiliations.

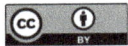

Copyright: © 2022 by the authors. Licensee MDPI, Basel, Switzerland. This article is an open access article distributed under the terms and conditions of the Creative Commons Attribution (CC BY) license (https://creativecommons.org/licenses/by/4.0/).

1. Introduction

Human Papillomaviruses (HPVs) are responsible for multiple epithelial lesions and cancers in both males and females. They are the etiological agent of cutaneous and anogenital warts which may progress to carcinoma depending on the virus' subtype. Subtypes 16 and 18 are the ones most commonly associated with pre-cancerous and cancerous lesions of the cervix in females and of the anogenital and oropharyngeal areas in both sexes [1].

In Italy, the prevalence of high-risk HPV subtypes has been estimated at around 8% of the female population, with no significant geographical differences, while the incidence of cervical cancer is lower in the south of Italy. This uneven distribution of the incidence of HPV-related cancers has been explained by an increase in high-risk HPV prevalence in younger generations, thus predicting an increase in the burden of cervical cancer in the south of Italy in the coming decades [2].

The HPV vaccine is effective in reducing the risk of HPV infection, pre-cancerous lesions and cancer. Without HPV-vaccination, 7 out of 10 women and men will be infected with HPV, 1 in 10 women and men will get genital warts, 1 in 10 women will get pre-cancerous lesions, 1 in 100 women will develop cervical cancer and 1 in 500 women will die of cervical cancer. In men, HPV is the cause of cancer of the penis, anus, oral cavity and throat, and it has been estimated that about 1 in 200 men will get cancer caused by HPV [3–5]. Anti-HPV vaccination is therefore an essential means of prevention both in HPV-naïve subjects and in subjects with high-risk-HPV-related pre-cancerous lesions.

Nowadays, three vaccines against HPV are available. Gardasil® (Sanofi Pasteur MSD)/Silgard® (Merck Sharp & Dohme, Kenilworth, NJ, USA), a quadrivalent recombinant vaccine against the HPV types 6, 11, 16 and 18 (qHPVv), was licensed by the Food and Drug Administration (FDA) in 2006, whereas Cervarix® (GlaxoSmithKline Biologicals, Brentford, Middlesex, UK), a bivalent recombinant vaccine for immunization against HPV types 16 and 18 (bHPVv), was licensed in 2007. Both vaccines contain non-infectious inactivated subunits, and protect against the high-risk HPV types 16 and 18, responsible for more than 70% of cervical cancer cases. The qHPVv also protects against subtypes 6 and 11, which cause most cases of genital warts [6,7].

The latest licensed HPV vaccine is Gardasil-9®, a 9-valent HPV vaccine (9vHPVv) which is effective against all of the HPV types covered by the qHPVv (6, 11, 16, and 18), as well as five additional oncogenic types (31, 33, 45, 52, and 58), showing strong protection against cervical infections caused by these HPV types as well as condylomas and some HPV-related cancers, including oropharyngeal, vaginal, vulvar, penile, and anal cancers [8].

The 9vHPVv was approved by the FDA on 10 December 2014, for use in females aged 9 to 26 years and males aged 9 to 15 years. For these recommendations, the Advisory Committee on Immunization Practices (ACIP) reviewed additional data on 9vHPVv in males aged 16 to 26 years. 9vHPVv and 4vHPVv are currently licensed for use in both females and males. 2vHPVv, on the other hand, is licensed for use in females only [9].

Immunization strategies in Italy are designed by the Ministry of Health and described in the National Immunization Plan (NIP). Each of the 20 Italian regions must follow the guidelines stated by the NIP, but may also offer other vaccines to target populations not covered by the National Plan itself. Furthermore, since 2012 the Ministry of Health has promoted the "Vaccination schedule for life", an immunization schedule that follows every phase of an individual's life with the objective of protecting them for the whole duration of their life [10].

The Italian Vaccination schedule for life, contained within the National Vaccine Prevention Plan 2017–2019, provides for two or three doses of HPV vaccine, according to the vaccine and to the patient's age. Two doses are recommended for subjects aged from 9 to 14 years (both males and females), with a 6- to 12-month interval between the doses, while three doses are recommended for patients aged from 15 to 26 years, with administration at 0, 1 to 2, and 6 months (only for women) [10].

Puglia is a region in the south of Italy (around 4 million inhabitants); the 2018 Apulian edition of the Vaccination schedule for life follows the same immunization schedule as the national one, while also offering the HPV vaccination to adult women considered at higher risk for cervical cancer due to high-risk sexual behaviors; in this case, the HPV vaccine may be requested by the patient herself via co-payment, or offered during periodic screening for cervical pre-cancerous lesions [11].

Three years after the implementation of the universal mass-vaccination program using 9vHPVv, it is useful, from a public health perspective, to assess the real-life safety profile of this vaccine. The World Health Organization (WHO, Geneva, Switzerland) recommends surveillance of Adverse Events Following Immunization (AEFIs) during the post-marketing life of new vaccines as a mean to better understand the safety profile and effectiveness of new drugs [12]. Thanks to the revision of AEFIs' reporting rates, post-marketing surveillance is indeed capable of detecting rare adverse events which pre-licensure studies could not observe, as well as studying the vaccine's safety profile in subgroups that were not represented in pre-marketing trials [13,14]. The WHO has recommended the application of a standardized causality assessment methodology in order to grant a more ordinate approach to the surveillance of AEFIs, as well as to surpass the "emotional" approach, which may increase vaccine hesitancy while decreasing the quality of the surveillance data [15].

This report describes the adverse events following Gardasil-9® administration reported in Puglia from 2018 to 2021, focusing on serious AEFIs and taking into consideration the causality assessment. We aim to design the product's safety profile in a real-life scenario and compare it with the safety profile highlighted in phase-three clinical studies.

2. Materials and Methods

This is a retrospective observational study. Data were collected from the list of AEFIs recorded following 9vHPVv (Gardasil-9®) administration from January 2018 to November 2021, which was obtained from the Italian Drug Authority (AIFA, Rome, Italy) database. Reporting AEFIs is indeed mandatory for all healthcare workers in Italy, and reports must be submitted to the National Pharmacovigilance Network (RNF), an online platform managed by AIFA itself. AEFIs may also be reported by the person experiencing them or by their legal representative. The overall number of Gardasil-9® doses administered during the study period in Puglia was extrapolated from the regional online immunization database (GIAVA).

For every subject who suffered from one or more AEFIs, a form was completed which included information about date of birth, gender, date of vaccine administration, and other vaccines administered at the same time. AEFIs were described by providing the following data: date of onset and date of computing in RNF, clinical characteristics, duration, treatment, final outcome, hospitalization or emergency room access, and a description of the case.

An Excel spreadsheet was used to build the database and perform the required analyses. The total reporting rate was calculated as the total number of reported AEFIs divided by the number of Gardasil-9® administrations during the study period, while the annual reporting rate was calculated as the number of AEFIs that occurred in a year divided by the number of doses administered in the same year.

AEFIs were classified as "serious" or "non-serious" following WHO guidelines, that define an AEFI as serious if it results in death, is life threatening, requires in-patient hospitalization or prolongation of existing hospitalization, results in persistent or significant disability/incapacity, results in a congenital anomaly/birth defect, or requires intervention to prevent permanent damage or impairment. Additionally, in 2016, AIFA published a list of particular health conditions that must be considered as serious AEFIs when occurring after vaccination. This list is the Italian version of the European Medicines Agency's important medical events list [16,17].

For serious AEFIs, the WHO's causality assessment algorithm was applied in order to classify AEFIs as having a "consistent causal association", having an "inconsistent causal association", "indeterminate", or "non-classifiable". In particular, for AEFIs requiring hospitalization, the patient's medical records were examined for a better understanding of the event's characteristics [18]. Causality assessment was carried out by two different physicians with expertise in vaccinology and results were compared; in cases of divergent results, the literature was reviewed and a third physician was consulted in order to decide how to classify the adverse event.

3. Results

A total of 266,647 doses of 9vHPVv (Gardasil-9®) were administered in Puglia from January 2018 to November 2021. During the same period, 22 adverse events following Gardasil-9® administration were reported in Puglia (reporting rate (RR): 8.25 per 100,000 doses). Reporting rates were higher during the first two years after the vaccine's authorization, significantly decreasing over the following years (Table 1).

Table 1. AEFIs reporting rates during 2018–2021.

Year	Total Number of Administered Doses	AEFIs	RR (/100,000 Doses)
2018	68,756	5	7.27
2019	78,895	10	12.7
2020	56,411	3	5.32
2021	62,585	4	6.39

The overall male/female ratio of AEFIs was 0.833 (10 males vs. 12 females). The majority of AEFIs were reported in subjects aged from 10 to 18, with 15 reports out of 22 (68.2%) for subjects between 11 and 12 years of age. In detail, 17 AEFIs (77.3%) were reported in subjects aged from 10 to 14, an AEFI (4.50%) was reported for a 17-year-old subject and the remaining 4 AEFIs (18.2%) were observed in subjects over 25 years of age.

Table 2 describes the prevalence of specific signs and symptoms reported in the AEFI data. Neurological symptoms were the most common, followed by local events of pain, tenderness, oedema and/or swelling and allergic reactions.

Table 2. Prevalence of specific signs and symptoms described in the AEFI reports, and reporting rates (RR) per 100,000 doses.

Signs/Symptoms	N°	% out of 22 AEFIs	RR per 100,000 Doses
Neurological symptoms	7	31.8	2.62
Local pain/tenderness/oedema/swelling	6	27.3	2.25
Allergic reactions	6	27.3	2.25
Gastro-intestinal symptoms	3	13.6	1.12
Fever/hyperpyrexia/chills	2	9.09	0.750
Other symptoms	14	63.6	5.25

Out of 22 AEFIs, 5 (22.7%) were classified as serious and 17 (77.3%) as non-serious, according to the latest WHO guidelines. A total of 2 out of 5 (40.0%) serious AEFIs led to the patients' hospitalization, and one of them (20.0%) caused impairment. The RR for serious AEFIs was 1.87 per 100,000 doses.

Out of the five serious AEFIs, two (40.0%) were deemed to be consistently associated with the vaccine's administration, while for another two of them (40.0%), no consistent causal association was found between the adverse event and the vaccination. For the fifth adverse event, the causality assessment outcome was undetermined.

The results show that 1 of the 2 AEFIs with consistent causal association caused the patient's hospitalization, but in both cases the subjects had fully healed by the time the report was completed. The RR for vaccine-related serious AEFIs was 0.750 per 100,000 doses.

The final outcome for 15 out of 22 AEFIs (68.2%) was the patient's complete recovery, while for three of them (13.6%) only partial improvement occurred. In total, 2 out of 22 patients (9.10%) had still not healed from the reported adverse events, while for another 2 (9.10%) the AEFI's outcome was not known.

We will now focus on the five serious AEFIs. We will describe these adverse events based on the data provided by the reporting subjects, and causality assessment will be taken into consideration in order to better understand the outcomes of the AEFIs' evaluations.

3.1. AEFI 1

The first case was reported in a female subject, aged 33 at the time of onset of the adverse event. The subject was already known to have had mild allergic reactions to food allergens. About six hours after Gardasil-9® administration, the patient manifested a skin rash localized to the chest and abdomen, followed by glottis oedema on the next day. The subject was therefore hospitalized, and the adverse event was treated by intravenous corticosteroid infusion and intramuscular injection of an antihistaminic (active ingredients were not reported), which were gradually discontinued over the following days. The adverse event healed completely. The reaction was deemed to be consistently associated with the vaccine's administration, as anaphylaxis has been observed as a rare serious adverse event following vaccination with Gardasil-9®.

3.2. AEFI 2

The second case was reported in a female subject, aged 11 at the time of onset of the adverse event. The subject was administered with Gardasil-9®, injected in the left deltoid, and anti-meningococcal serotype $ACW_{135}Y$ conjugated vaccine Menveo®, injected in the right deltoid. On the following day, the patient reported a syncopal episode with mild hypotension and significant oedema and hematoma were observed on the right arm. The subject required neither hospitalization nor pharmacological therapy, and the AEFI healed completely. The reaction was deemed to be non-associated with the vaccine's administration, as it happened more than 12 h after the vaccine's administration.

3.3. AEFI 3

The third case was reported in a male subject, aged 11 years at the time of onset of the adverse event. About one hour after Gardasil-9® administration, the subject lost consciousness for approximately one minute, falling and reporting mild cranial trauma. Witnesses reported that the patient appeared pale and sweating shortly before the event. The subject was put in the Trendelenburg position and an ice-bag was placed on his head, leading to complete recovery. Hospitalization was not needed, as the symptoms resolved in a few hours. The reaction was deemed to be consistently associated with the vaccine's administration.

3.4. AEFI 4

The fourth case was reported in a female subject, aged 25 at the time of onset of the adverse event. Ten days after Gardasil-9® administration, the subject reported prolonged asthenia of the lower limbs, muscle stiffness, fatigue and persistent paresthesia, with such intensity that ordinary activities were impeded. Myorelaxants were administered, followed by duloxetine, and the patient was diagnosed with fibromyalgia. It is interesting to note that this AEFI was reported only three years after its occurrence, mainly due to the symptoms' persistence and their significant impact on the patient's quality of life. The reaction was deemed to be non-associated with the vaccine's administration.

3.5. AEFI 5

The fifth case was reported in a female subject, aged 11 at the time of onset of the adverse event. The subject was administered with both Gardasil-9® and anti-meningococcal serotype B recombinant absorbed vaccine Trumenba® during the same immunization session. Following vaccination, the patient manifested headache, vertigo and extrasystoles with bigeminal rhythm (time of onset after vaccination was not noted in the report), and was therefore hospitalized. In hospital, laboratory analysis showed that their troponin level was 3 pg/mL, while the creatinine-kinase level was 106 U/L. No further action was taken, and the subject's health condition improved. The adverse event was defined as undetermined following causality assessment, due to the co-administration of two different vaccines and the lack of more specific information.

4. Discussion

Our study describes data referring to the safety profile of Gardasil-9®, which is currently the most used anti-HPV vaccine. Gardasil-9® is offered in Puglia to subjects aged

9 and older as part of the region's routine vaccination schedule. The vaccine was offered actively and free-of-charge, and 266,647 vaccine doses were administered in Puglia from 2018 to 2021.

Data from the passive surveillance of AEFIs showed that more than 8 subjects out of 100,000 receiving Gardasil-9® suffered from one or more adverse events. Serious AEFIs were reported in five patients, or less than 2 cases out of 100,000 administered doses, and the most common adverse events were neurological symptoms, reported in seven patients, local events of pain, tenderness, oedema or swelling, reported in six patients, and allergic reactions, reported in six patients.

Following causality assessment, a significant causal association between the adverse event and the vaccination was found for 2 out of 5 serious AEFIs. One of them was a case of loss of consciousness which occurred one hour after the vaccine's administration, and which spontaneously resolved in a few seconds; other symptoms, such as pallor and sweating, disappeared in less than a day. The episode did not determine any permanent damage to the patient. The second AEFI which was deemed related to the vaccine was an allergic reaction with mild glottis oedema and erythema located on the chest and abdomen, which occurred in a subject with a previous history of anaphylaxis, and which was successfully treated with corticosteroid and antihistaminic drugs after hospitalization.

Permanent impairment was reported in one case, but causality assessment ruled out the hypothesis of a causal correlation between the disability and the vaccine's administration; in this case, the patient reported asthenia, muscular stiffness, fatigue to the lower limbs and the formication of both hands and feet ten days after the vaccination, and was later diagnosed with fibromyalgia. While muscular symptoms are a common side effect of Gardasil-9® [19], no data exist regarding a plausible biological association between this vaccine and fibromyalgia, which was therefore defined as a non-vaccine-related AEFI. No cases of death were reported.

Comparing these data with pre-licensure evidence, reporting rates in our study are significantly lower. The United States Food and Drug Administration (FDA), for instance, reported local events of pain, swelling and erythema, and headache in more than 10% of patients treated with Gardasil-9® [19]. This discrepancy is likely due to the different surveillance methods employed in these studies: whereas pre-licensure evidence is gathered via active call, our data were collected through a passive surveillance network. Passive surveillance is in fact undermined by the risk of under-reporting, as Italian patients and healthcare professionals tend not to report adverse events, especially when mild and self-limiting. This phenomenon has already been documented by other studies of our research group [18].

On the other hand, our data are similar to pre-licensure evidence as far the symptoms distribution is concerned. In fact, neurological symptoms and local reactions were the most reported symptoms both in FDA authorization studies and in ours [19].

A 2018 review on HPV vaccines' safety profile highlighted that injection-site reactions are fairly common with 9vHPVv, likely due to the greater amount of adjuvant contained in this product. Headache too was reported commonly, thus confirming the trend that emerged in our study. The higher reporting rates in this review are likely related to the active surveillance protocol employed in many of the considered studies. The review also focused on various adverse events of special interest, such as allergic reactions and anaphylaxis; the latter's reporting rate was 0.17 per 100,000 doses in the United States, about 0.30 per 100,000 doses in Australia and Canada and 1 per 100,000 doses in the United Kingdom. These data are slightly lower than the ones regarding allergic reactions we extrapolated from the RNF, which indicate an RR of 2.25 per 100,000 doses. Therefore, despite being flawed by under-reporting, Italian data may be considered a good estimate of the real incidence rate of AEFIs as far as serious reactions are concerned [20].

A 2017 review of clinical trials and case series regarding AEFIs after HPV vaccination included a clinical trial in which systemic adverse events were reported by 59.7% of patients who were administered with 9vHPVv. However, the difference between this group and the control one was not significant. Another study included in this review mentioned significant differences between 9vHPVv and 4vHPVv, with the 9-valent vaccine causing severe injection-site reactions and systemic adverse events more frequently than the 4-valent product. Systemic AEFIs were especially frequent, having been reported in nearly 30% of patients [21].

Our study's main strength is the high numerosity of the reference population: The Apulian population is over 4 million, and 266,647 doses of Gardasil-9® were administered over the course of four years. This is a significantly larger population than the ones examined in pre-licensure clinical trials. Moreover, Gardasil-9® has been licensed for use in Italy since 2018. During the immediate post-licensure period, the attention on new vaccines is higher from both the physicians' and the patients' perspectives. Studies that focus on the first stage of a drug's post-marketing life are fundamental not only to identify rare AEFIs and to better understand these new products' safety profile, but also to discern adverse events which are related to the vaccine from those that are not, building the public's trust towards vaccinations. In addition to this, our study focuses on causality assessment for serious AEFIs, an aspect that is often overlooked by post-marketing studies [15].

On the other hand, as already stated, our study is affected by our data collection method: passive surveillance carries a high risk of under-reporting and tends to alter the serious/non-serious AEFIs ratio. One of the reported adverse events, moreover, had not undergone causality assessment, thus reducing the available information regarding serious AEFIs.

The safety profile of vaccines is currently one of the main points of argument with anti-vaccination groups. This is also one of the most important reasons for vaccination skepticism among the general public, thus representing an essential building block of effective medical information [22]. As already demonstrated by the recent withdrawal of the AstraZeneca ChAdOx-1S anti-SARS-CoV-2 vaccine from the market, failures in communication between the scientific community and the public can cause a significant distrust of the general population towards vaccination practices [23].

As far as HPV vaccines are concerned, gaining optimal vaccination coverage is especially important. According to a 2020 modelling study, the recent crisis of HPV vaccinations in Japan is expected to result in 24,600–27,300 cases of cervical cancer in 1994–2007 birth cohorts, predicting at least 5000 deaths in the next few years; a further increase in HPV-related cancers might occur if vaccination coverages are not restored in the immediate future [24].

5. Conclusions

The risk of AEFIs is conclusively very low in subjects both under and over 18 years of age (<0.1‰ of administered doses), reinforcing the available evidence about the favorable risks/benefits ratio for Gardasil-9® [25]. Since the beginning of Gardasil-9®'s marketing, only one of the reported AEFIs led to permanent impairment, and it was not deemed to be consistently associated with the vaccine's administration. Furthermore, the outcomes of all the remaining serious AEFIs were at least a partial recovery.

Effective communication between the scientific world and the public is therefore imperative in order to ensure that people keep trusting vaccination practices and understand their importance.

Author Contributions: A.D.L. and P.B. conceived the study, collected data and drafted the manuscript. A.M. and F.P.B. contributed to the analysis of data. S.T. and P.S. reviewed the paper and carried out the causality assessment of serious AEFIs detected. All authors have read and agreed to the published version of the manuscript.

Funding: This research received no external funding.

Institutional Review Board Statement: Not applicable.

Informed Consent Statement: Not applicable.

Data Availability Statement: Data regarding the total number of Gardasil-9® doses administered in Puglia during the study period were extrapolated from the regional online immunization database (GIAVA). Data regarding adverse events following immunization with Gardasil-9® were gathered from the Italian Drug Authority (AIFA) database.

Conflicts of Interest: The authors declare no conflict of interest.

References

1. Luria, L.; Cardoza-Favarato, G. *Human Papillomavirus*; StatPearls: Treasure Island, FL, USA, 2021. [PubMed]
2. Rossi, P.G.; Chini, F.; Borgia, P.; Guasticchi, G.; Carozzi, F.M.; Confortini, M.; Angeloni, C.; Buzzoni, C.; Buonaguro, F.M. Gruppo di lavoro HPV Prevalenza. Epidemiologia del Papilloma virus umano (HPV), incidenza del cancro della cervice uterina e diffusione dello screening: Differenze fra macroaree in Italia. *Epidemiol. Prev.* **2012**, *36*, 1–12.
3. Orumaa, M.; Kjaer, S.K.; Dehlendorff, C.; Munk, C.; Olsen, A.O.; Hansen, B.T.; Campbell, S.; Nygård, M. The impact of HPV multi-cohort vaccination: Real-world evidence of faster control of HPV-related morbidity. *Vaccine* **2020**, *38*, 1345–1351. [CrossRef] [PubMed]
4. Drolet, M.; Bénard, É.; Pérez, N.; Brisson, M.; HPV Vaccination Impact Study Group. Population-level impact and herd effects following the introduction of human papillomavirus vaccination programmes: Updated systematic review and meta-analysis. *Lancet* **2019**, *394*, 497–509. [CrossRef]
5. Kjaer, S.K.; Tran, T.N.; Sparen, P.; Tryggvadottir, L.; Munk, C.; Dasbach, E.; Liaw, K.; Nygård, J.; Nygård, M. The Burden of Genital Warts: A Study of Nearly 70,000 Women from the General Female Population in the 4 Nordic Countries. *J. Infect. Dis.* **2007**, *195*, 1447–1454. [CrossRef] [PubMed]
6. Stillo, M.; Santisteve, P.C.; Lopalco, P.L. Safety of human papillomavirus vaccines: A review. *Expert Opin. Drug Saf.* **2015**, *14*, 697–712. [CrossRef] [PubMed]
7. Schmiedeskamp, M.R.; Kockler, D.R. Human Papillomavirus Vaccines. *Ann. Pharmacother.* **2006**, *40*, 1344–1352. [CrossRef] [PubMed]
8. Cheng, L.; Wang, Y.; Du, J. Human Papillomavirus Vaccines: An Updated Review. *Vaccines* **2020**, *8*, 391. [CrossRef] [PubMed]
9. Petrosky, E.; Bocchini, J.A., Jr.; Hariri, S.; Chesson, H.; Curtis, C.R.; Saraiya, M.; Unger, E.R.; Markowitz, L.E. Use of 9-valent human papillomavirus (HPV) vaccine: Updated HPV vaccination recommendations of the advisory committee on immunization practices. *MMWR Morb. Mortal. Wkly. Rep.* **2015**, *64*, 300–304. [PubMed]
10. Conferenza Permanente per i Rapporti tra lo Stato le Regioni e le Province Autonome di Trento e Bolzano. Intesa, ai Sensi Dell'articolo 8, Comma 6, Della Legge 5 Giugno 2003, n. 131, tra il Governo, le Regioni e le Province Autonome di Trento e Bol-zano sul Documento Recante "Piano Nazionale Prevenzione Vaccinale 2017–2019" (Rep. Atti n. 10/CSR) (17°01195). Available online: https://www.trovanorme.salute.gov.it/norme/dettaglioAtto?id=58185&completo=true (accessed on 11 October 2021).
11. Regione Puglia. Calendario Vaccinale Per La Vita 2018—Regione Puglia. 2019. Available online: https://www.sanita.puglia.it/documents/20182/26673928/Calendario+vaccinale+per+la+vita+2018/f36429b9-5f76-44c2-b495-d5b9228959ef?version=1.0&t=1549553827908 (accessed on 11 October 2021).
12. World Health Organization (WHO). *Causality Assessment of an Adverse Event Following Immunization (AEFI): User Manual for the Revised WHO Classification*, 2nd ed.; 2019 Update; WHO: Geneva, Switzerland, 2019. Available online: https://www.who.int/publications/i/item/causality-assessment-aefi-user-manual-2019 (accessed on 11 October 2021).
13. Stefanizzi, P.; De Nitto, S.; Spinelli, G.; Lattanzio, S.; Stella, P.; Ancona, D.; Dell'Aera, M.; Padovano, M.; Soldano, S.; Tafuri, S.; et al. Post-Marketing Active Surveillance of Adverse Reactions Following Influenza Cell-Based Quadrivalent Vaccine: An Italian Prospective Observational Study. *Vaccines* **2021**, *9*, 456. [CrossRef] [PubMed]
14. Tafuri, S.; Fortunato, F.; Gallone, M.S.; Stefanizzi, P.; Calabrese, G.; Boccalini, S.; Martinelli, D.; Prato, R. Systematic causality assessment of adverse events following HPV vaccines: Analysis of current data from Apulia region (Italy). *Vaccine* **2018**, *36*, 1072–1077. [CrossRef] [PubMed]
15. Tafuri, S.; Gallone, M.S.; Calabrese, G.; Germinario, C. Adverse events following immunization: Is this time for the use of WHO causality assessment? *Expert Rev. Vaccines* **2015**, *14*, 625–627. [CrossRef] [PubMed]
16. AIFA—Gruppo di Lavoro Sull'analisi dei Segnali dei Vaccini. Guida alla Valutazione delle Reazioni Avverse Osservabili Dopo Vaccinazione. 2016. Available online: http://www.aifa.gov.it/sites/default/files/Guida_valutazione_reazioni_avverse_osservabili_dopo_vaccinazione_2.pdf (accessed on 7 December 2021).
17. European Medical Agency. Important Medical Event Terms List Version (MedDRA)—Version 24.0. Available online: https://www.ema.europa.eu/en/human-regulatory/research-development/pharmacovigilance/eudravigilance/eudravigilance-system-overview (accessed on 7 December 2021).
18. Stefanizzi, P.; Stella, P.; Ancona, D.; Malcangi, K.N.; Bianchi, F.P.; De Nitto, S.; Ferorelli, D.; Germinario, C.A.; Tafuri, S. Adverse Events Following Measles-Mumps-Rubella-Varicella Vaccination and the Case of Seizures: A Post Marketing Active Surveillance in Puglia Italian Region, 2017–2018. *Vaccines* **2019**, *7*, 140. [CrossRef] [PubMed]
19. U.S. Food and Drug Administration. Gardasil 9. Package Insert. 2020. Available online: https://www.fda.gov/media/90064/download (accessed on 15 December 2021).

20. Phillips, A.; Patel, C.; Pillsbury, A.; Brotherton, J.; Macartney, K. Safety of Human Papillomavirus Vaccines: An Updated Review. *Drug Saf.* **2018**, *41*, 329–346. [CrossRef] [PubMed]
21. Martínez-Lavín, M.; Amezcua-Guerra, L. Serious adverse events after HPV vaccination: A critical review of randomized trials and post-marketing case series. *Clin. Rheumatol.* **2017**, *36*, 2169–2178. [CrossRef] [PubMed]
22. Tafuri, S.; Gallone, M.S.; Cappelli, M.G.; Martinelli, D.; Prato, R.; Germinario, C. Addressing the anti-vaccination movement and the role of HCWs. *Vaccine* **2014**, *32*, 4860–4865. [CrossRef] [PubMed]
23. Faranda, D.; Alberti, T.; Arutkin, M.; Lembo, V.; Lucarini, V. Interrupting vaccination policies can greatly spread SARS-CoV-2 and enhance mortality from COVID-19 disease: The AstraZeneca case for France and Italy. *Chaos Interdiscip. J. Nonlinear Sci.* **2021**, *31*, 41105. [CrossRef] [PubMed]
24. Simms, K.T.; Hanley, S.J.B.; Smith, M.; Keane, A.; Canfell, K. Impact of HPV vaccine hesitancy on cervical cancer in Japan: A modelling study. *Lancet Public Health* **2020**, *5*, e223–e234. [CrossRef]
25. Moreira, E.D.; Block, S.L.; Ferris, D.; Giuliano, A.R.; Iversen, O.-E.; Joura, E.A.; Kosalaraksa, P.; Schilling, A.; Van Damme, P.; Bornstein, J.; et al. Safety Profile of the 9-Valent HPV Vaccine: A Combined Analysis of 7 Phase III Clinical Trials. *Pediatrics* **2016**, *138*, e20154387. [CrossRef] [PubMed]

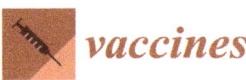

Article

Availability of the HPV Vaccine in Regional Pharmacies and Provider Perceptions Regarding HPV Vaccination in the Pharmacy Setting

Jill M. Maples [1,*], Nikki B. Zite [1], Oluwafemifola Oyedeji [2], Shauntá M. Chamberlin [3], Alicia M. Mastronardi [1], Samantha Gregory [1], Justin D. Gatwood [4], Kenneth C. Hohmeier [4], Mary E. Booker [1], Jamie D. Perry [1], Heather K. Moss [1] and Larry C. Kilgore [1]

[1] Department of Obstetrics and Gynecology, Graduate School of Medicine, University of Tennessee, Knoxville, TN 37920, USA; nzite@utmck.edu (N.B.Z.); ammastronardi@utmck.edu (A.M.M.); sgregory1@utmck.edu (S.G.); mbooker@utmck.edu (M.E.B.); jperry@utmck.edu (J.D.P.); hmoss@utmck.edu (H.K.M.); lkilgore@utmck.edu (L.C.K.)
[2] Department of Public Health, University of Tennessee, Knoxville, TN 37996, USA; oonaade@vols.utk.edu
[3] Department of Family Medicine, Graduate School of Medicine, University of Tennessee, Knoxville, TN 37920, USA; schamberlin@utmck.edu
[4] Department of Clinical Pharmacy and Translational Science, College of Pharmacy, University of Tennessee Health Science Center, Nashville, TN 37211, USA; jgatwood@uthsc.edu (J.D.G.); khohmeier@uthsc.edu (K.C.H.)
* Correspondence: jmaple13@uthsc.edu

Citation: Maples, J.M.; Zite, N.B.; Oyedeji, O.; Chamberlin, S.M.; Mastronardi, A.M.; Gregory, S.; Gatwood, J.D.; Hohmeier, K.C.; Booker, M.E.; Perry, J.D.; et al. Availability of the HPV Vaccine in Regional Pharmacies and Provider Perceptions Regarding HPV Vaccination in the Pharmacy Setting. *Vaccines* **2022**, *10*, 351. https://doi.org/10.3390/vaccines10030351

Academic Editor: Gloria Calagna

Received: 29 January 2022
Accepted: 22 February 2022
Published: 24 February 2022

Publisher's Note: MDPI stays neutral with regard to jurisdictional claims in published maps and institutional affiliations.

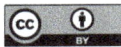

Copyright: © 2022 by the authors. Licensee MDPI, Basel, Switzerland. This article is an open access article distributed under the terms and conditions of the Creative Commons Attribution (CC BY) license (https://creativecommons.org/licenses/by/4.0/).

Abstract: There is increasing support for HPV vaccination in the pharmacy setting, but the availability of the HPV vaccine is not well known. Additionally, little is known about perceptions of medical providers regarding referring patients to community pharmacies for HPV vaccination. The purpose of this study was to determine HPV vaccine availability in community pharmacies and to understand, among family medicine and obstetrics–gynecology providers, the willingness of and perceived barriers to referring patients for HPV vaccination in a pharmacy setting. HPV vaccine availability data were collected from pharmacies in a southern region of the United States. Family medicine and obstetrics–gynecology providers were surveyed regarding vaccine referral practices and perceived barriers to HPV vaccination in a community pharmacy. Results indicated the HPV vaccine was available in most pharmacies. Providers were willing to refer patients to a community pharmacy for HPV vaccination, despite this not being a common practice, likely due to numerous barriers reported. Pharmacist-administered HPV vaccination continues to be a commonly reported strategy for increasing HPV vaccination coverage. However, coordinated efforts to increase collaboration among vaccinators in different settings and to overcome systematic and legislative barriers to increasing HPV vaccination rates are still needed.

Keywords: HPV; HPV vaccine; pharmacy; vaccine referral; family medicine; obstetrics and gynecology; HPV vaccine barriers; provider perspectives

1. Introduction

Human papillomavirus (HPV) is the leading cause of most anogenital (i.e., anal, vulvar, vaginal, cervical, penile) and oropharyngeal cancers in both men and women, and the number of cancer cases linked to HPV has increased significantly over the past 15 years [1–3]. HPV-related cancers are the only cancers that can be prevented by a highly effective and safe vaccine [1,3]. In 2020, 75.1% of adolescents received at least one dose of an HPV vaccine, and 58.6% of adolescents were up to date with the entire series [4]. However, recent evidence suggests the COVID-19 pandemic resulted in fewer adolescents initiating the HPV vaccine series [4]. Among adults, the rates of HPV vaccination have increased moderately among certain populations over the past decade. For example, HPV vaccination coverage among males aged 19–26 years and Hispanic females aged 19–26 years increased, but approximately 50% of females aged 19–26 years and 70% of males aged 19–26 years remained unvaccinated [5]. Disparities in HPV vaccination coverage and HPV-cancer incidence exist in geographic locations in the United States [6–8]. Specifically, those living in rural areas [8] and in the Southern United States [6,7] have lower HPV vaccination rates and higher HPV-related cancer incidence rates.

To address vaccination shortfalls, the President's Cancer Panel (2018) [9] and National Vaccine Advisory Committee (2016) [10] released statements supporting HPV vaccination utilizing community pharmacies. Pharmacists are ideally positioned to overcome some of the barriers to HPV vaccination initiation and series completion [11]. HPV vaccine administered in a pharmacy is a frequently mentioned strategy for increasing HPV vaccination coverage. Pharmacies are conveniently located for many families with easier access, especially in rural communities. In fact, most U.S. residents (91%) live within five miles of a community pharmacy [12]. Additionally, compared to doctors' offices, pharmacies are open for longer hours and on weekends, which potentially facilitates improved access to vaccines [13]. Pharmacists in most states are authorized to administer vaccines and provide a convenient option for patients [14]. The extent to which pharmacies stock and administer the HPV vaccine, particularly in rural settings, is unknown.

While pharmacies could potentially serve a powerful role in providing HPV vaccine access, administration, and series completion, relatively little is known about the willingness of physicians to refer patients to a pharmacy setting for HPV vaccination. Campos-Outcalt et al. (2010) reported that 34.2% of family physicians referred adult patients to a pharmacy for routinely recommended vaccines, but the authors did not report if they would refer adolescents and/or adult patients to a pharmacy setting for HPV vaccination specifically [15]. A recent study by O'Leary et al. (2020) reported that among obstetrician–gynecologists that routinely assess for patient vaccination status, 92% screened for HPV vaccination status [16]. However, not all of these providers stocked and/or administered the HPV vaccine [16]. For obstetrician–gynecologists that are unable to stock and administer vaccinations onsite, the American College of Obstetrics and Gynecology (ACOG) has created guidance to develop immunization referral systems [17]. This guidance was developed with the goal of future pharmacy–physician practice collaboration. However, to our knowledge, there are no studies reporting the willingness of and perceived barriers to referring patients for HPV vaccination in a pharmacy setting among family medicine and obstetrics–gynecology providers.

The purpose of this study was to determine HPV vaccine availability in community pharmacy settings in a southern region of the United States. Additionally, this study aimed to understand, among family medicine and obstetrics–gynecology providers, the willingness of and perceived barriers to referring patients for HPV vaccination in a community pharmacy setting. This was accomplished by surveying family medicine and obstetrics–gynecology providers at a single academic medical center in the same geographic region.

2. Materials and Methods

2.1. Pharmacy Data Collection

The availability of the HPV vaccine in the pharmacy setting was determined by the percentage of pharmacies that administer and stock the HPV vaccine. To accomplish this, a list of all pharmacies in a southern region of the United States (consisting of 17 counties in Eastern Tennessee) was generated. First, a list of zip codes for the target counties was generated and then an online search for pharmacies located in those zip codes was performed. Each pharmacy was called by a research team member acting as a "secret shopper", where the team member acted as a customer inquiring about pharmacy services from October 2020 through April 2021. A standardized script for data collection was developed primarily based on study outcomes, including HPV vaccine availability and other measures of accessibility (if the pharmacy stocked the HPV vaccine, how soon one could get the HPV vaccine, and if an appointment was needed to get the HPV vaccine).

The script was discussed and confirmed by consensus among coauthors (J.M.M., O.O., S.G., J.D.G., K.C.H.). Using this standardized script, data regarding HPV vaccine availability were collected. The pharmacy staff member was first asked if the pharmacy administered the HPV vaccine. If the pharmacy stocked the HPV vaccine, they were then asked how soon one could get the HPV vaccine at their location, and if an appointment was required. Pharmacies were deemed "successfully contacted" if a research team member was able to call the pharmacy and get a definitive answer to any of the HPV vaccine-related questions. All pharmacies were considered in analyses. Up to three attempts were made to contact each pharmacy.

To better understand the impact of pharmacy type on HPV vaccine availability, pharmacies were categorized into the following groups: single independent, multiple independent, regional chain, grocery store chain (e.g., Kroger, Publix), national chain (e.g., Walgreens, CVS), and mass merchandiser (e.g., Wal-Mart, Target). To interpret the impact of pharmacy geographic location, categorizations of rural versus nonrural were created for each pharmacy location's zip code based on Health Resources and Services Administration's Federal Office of Rural Health Policy (HRSA FORHP) designations [18].

2.2. Family Medicine and Obstetrics–Gynecology Provider Surveys

An electronic survey was adapted from a previously published survey on adult immunization and preventative care practices by Hurley et al. [19]. The survey asked providers if their practice administered and stocked the HPV vaccine. Questions about Advisory Committee on Immunization Practices (ACIP)-recommended vaccine referral practices and then specifically about referral and prescription practices for the HPV vaccine across three different age categories for patients (age 11–18 years, age 19–26 years, and age 27–49 years) were included. Additionally, the survey asked about perceived barriers to HPV vaccination in a community pharmacy setting. The survey was emailed, via REDCap, to family medicine and obstetrics–gynecology providers (including physicians and midwives) at a single academic medical center. Research Electronic Data Capture (REDCap) is a secure, HIPAA-compliant, web application hosted by the University of Tennessee Graduate School of Medicine for building and managing online surveys and databases.

2.3. Statistical Analysis

Data analysis was primarily descriptive, using categorical data, means, and frequencies to determine vaccine availability and accessibility. Chi-squared analyses determined if HPV vaccine availability differed by pharmacy type and geographic location and if pharmacy type differed by geographic location. To determine HPV vaccine availability in the family medicine and obstetrics–gynecology providers' practices and to understand HPV vaccine referral practices, survey data analysis was primarily descriptive, using categorical data, means, and frequencies. Data were analyzed using Microsoft Excel (Office 365) and SPSS (Released 2019. IBM SPSS Statistics for Windows, Version 26.0. IBM Corp, Armonk, NY, USA).

3. Results

3.1. Pharmacy Data Collection

A total of 233 out of 240 (97.1%) pharmacies were successfully contacted. Characteristics of the pharmacies contacted are presented in Table 1 along with measures of HPV vaccine accessibility and availability. Among the pharmacies contacted, the majority were national chain pharmacies (35.2%), followed by single independent pharmacies (27.5%). More than half of the pharmacies administered the HPV vaccine (60.1%), and among those that administered it, over two-thirds (67.1%) reported having it "in stock". Ninety percent of the locations did not require an appointment to receive the vaccine, and 76.4% reported that the vaccine could be received the same day as the call of inquiry.

Table 1. Pharmacy characteristics.

All Pharmacies (n = 233)	
Pharmacy Type	
Single independent	64 (27.5%)
Multiple independent	24 (10.3%)
Grocery store chain	32 (13.7%)
Mass merchandiser	25 (10.7%)
National chain	82 (35.2%)
Regional chain	6 (2.6%)
Geographic location	
Nonrural	171 (73.4%)
Rural	62 (26.6%)
HPV Vaccine Availability	
No	93 (39.9%)
Yes	140 (60.1%)
Pharmacies with HPV Vaccine Availability (n = 140)	
Stock HPV Vaccine	
No	46 (32.9%)
Yes	94 (67.1%)
Appointment Needed	N = 140
No	126 (90.0%)
Yes	14 (10.0%)
Length of Time Needed for Desired HPV Vaccination	
Same Day	107 (76.4%)
Within 24 h	9 (6.4%)
24–48 h	6 (4.3%)
More than 48 h	11 (7.9%)
Other	7 (5.0%)

HPV vaccine availability differed significantly ($p < 0.01$) across pharmacy type (Figure 1). A larger percentage of mass merchandisers (24 out of 25, 96.0%), national chain pharmacies (76 out of 82, 92.7%), and grocery store pharmacies (23 out of 32, 71.9%) provide the HPV vaccine compared to single independent pharmacies (13 out of 64, 20.3%), multiple independent pharmacies (2 out of 24, 8.3%), and regional chain pharmacies (2 out of 6, 33.3%). HPV vaccine availability in pharmacies stratified by geographic location (rural vs. nonrural) was not significantly different ($p = 0.704$). Additionally, there were no significant differences in pharmacy type when stratified by geographic location ($p = 0.704$).

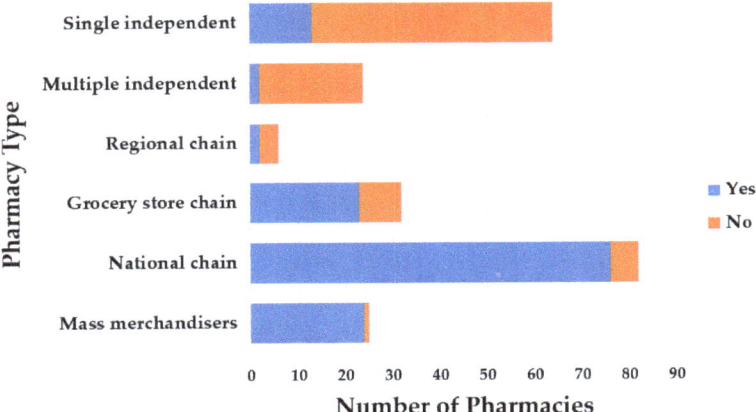

Figure 1. Reported HPV vaccine availability by pharmacy type. The total number of pharmacies, stratified by type, is indicated by each bar. Each bar is stacked to display the proportion of pharmacies, within that pharmacy type, that have the HPV vaccine available and those that do not have the HPV vaccine available. Chi-squared analysis revealed a significant difference in HPV vaccine availability across pharmacy type ($p < 0.001$).

3.2. Family Medicine and Obstetrics–Gynecology Providers

3.2.1. Provider Characteristics

The survey was distributed to 70 family medicine and Ob/Gyn providers; 60 providers completed the survey (85.7% response rate). Among the respondents, 34 (56.7%) were affiliated with the Department of Family Medicine at the University of Tennessee Graduate School of Medicine and 26 (43.3%) were affiliated with the Department of Obstetrics and Gynecology at the same institution. The majority identified as female ($n = 38$, 63.3%), and the age of the respondents ranged from 26 to 69 years of age (mean = 35.9 ± 10.6 years). In terms of role, 55.0% ($n = 33$) were resident physicians, 41.7% ($n = 25$) were attending physicians, and 3.3% ($n = 2$) were midwife practitioners.

3.2.2. HPV Vaccination Availability and Referral Practices

Most respondents indicated their practice administered and stocked the HPV vaccine. Nearly all (98.3%, $n = 59$) respondents reported their practice administers the HPV vaccine, and 95.0% stock the vaccine. When asked if they had ever referred a patient to receive an ACIP-recommended vaccine outside of their practice, 81.7% ($n = 49$) reported they had referred a patient for vaccination. When asked specifically if they have ever referred a patient for HPV vaccination outside of their practice, 20.0% ($n = 12$) had referred a patient age 11–18 years, 21.7% ($n = 13$) had referred a patient age 19–26 years, and 20.0% ($n = 12$) had referred a patient age 27–49 years. Among those that had ever referred a patient for HPV vaccination outside of their practice, over 90.0% referred patients to a local health department for HPV vaccination and did so across all patient age groups. Regarding referrals to a community pharmacy for HPV vaccination, 50% of those ever referring a patient for HPV vaccination referred a patient age 27–49 years, 53.8% referred a patient age 19–26 years, and 33.3% referred a patient age 11–18 years.

When asked if they had ever prescribed the HPV vaccine for a patient to be received at a community pharmacy location, 6.7% ($n = 4$) reported they had prescribed the HPV vaccine for patients age 19–26 years, followed by 5.0% ($n = 3$) and 3.3% ($n = 2$) for patients age 27–49 and 11–18 years respectively. Most providers (>90%) were willing or very willing to refer an eligible patient to receive an HPV vaccination at a community pharmacy across all age groups (Table 2).

Table 2. Willingness of provider to refer an eligible patient for HPV vaccination in a community pharmacy, stratified by patient age group.

	Not Willing at All	Not Really Willing	Somewhat Willing	Willing	Very Willing
Patient Age Group	% (n)	% (n)	% (n)	% (n)	% (n)
11–18 years	0 (0)	0 (0)	5.2 (3)	25.9 (15)	68.9 (40)
19–26 years	0 (0)	0 (0)	8.3 (5)	25.0 (15)	66.7 (40)
27–49 years	0 (0)	0 (0)	10.0 (6)	23.3 (14)	66.7 (40)

Perceived barriers to referring a patient for HPV vaccination in a pharmacy setting are shown in Figure 2. The most-reported barrier (61.7% of respondents) indicated that providers felt it made the most sense that their patients receive the HPV vaccine in their office (Figure 2).

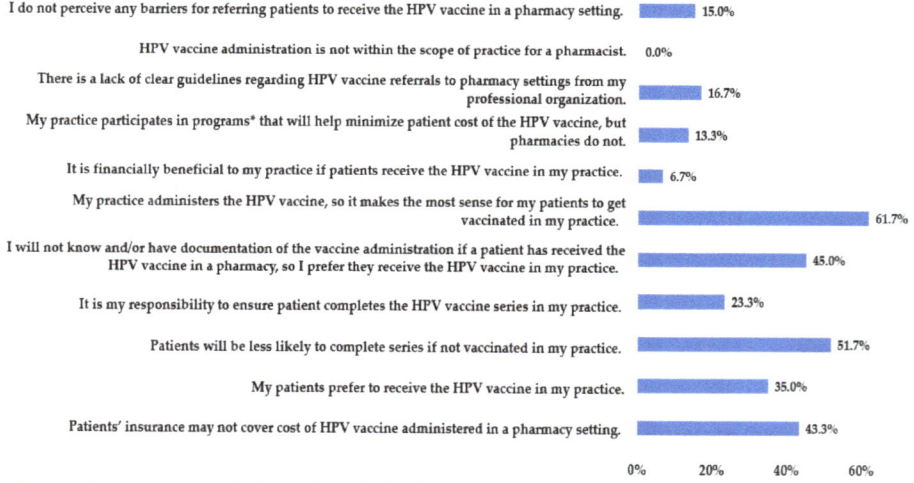

Figure 2. Perceived barriers to providers referring patients for HPV vaccination at community pharmacies. Each bar presents the percentage of respondents that indicated the barrier listed was a barrier for referring patients for HPV vaccination at a community pharmacy. The total percentage summed from all bars exceeds 100% because this survey question was a "mark all that apply" format question.

When asked what percentage of pharmacies in their region administer and stock the HPV vaccine, 88.3% (n = 53) of providers answered, "I do not know". Among the few respondents (11.7%, n = 7) that provided a numeric answer to the question regarding the percentage of pharmacies that administer the HPV vaccine, answers ranged from 25% to 85%, which was similar to the answers provided in response to the question of percentage of pharmacies that stock the HPV vaccine (ranging from 10% to 90%).

4. Discussion

The purpose of this study was to determine HPV vaccine accessibility in pharmacy settings in a southern region of the United States and to understand, among family medicine and obstetrics–gynecology providers, the willingness of and perceived barriers to referring patients to community pharmacies for HPV vaccination. The primary findings indicated that the majority of pharmacies in Eastern Tennessee (a state in the Southern United States) administer and stock the HPV vaccine. Family medicine and obstetrics–gynecology providers surveyed in this study were willing to refer patients to a community pharmacy for HPV vaccination, despite this not being a common practice. Most providers did not know the extent to which community pharmacies in their region administered and/or stocked the HPV vaccine. Providers also reported several perceived barriers to referring patients for HPV vaccination in a pharmacy setting. The most common barriers expressed included their desire for patients to be vaccinated in their office; concern that patients would not complete the HPV vaccine series if referred outside their practice for vaccination; providers not knowing or having documentation of vaccination if performed in a pharmacy setting; and potential financial burdens for patients, associated with lack of insurance coverage, for the HPV vaccine in a pharmacy setting.

In the current study, a larger proportion of pharmacies (60.1%) reported administering the HPV vaccine (Table 1) compared to previous reports [13,20]. A study by Hastings et al. (2017) reported that only 11.7% of community pharmacies in the state of Alabama, which is another state located in the Southern United States, had the HPV vaccine in their inventory [20]. A study by Westrick et al. (2018) reported that, among a nationally representative sample of pharmacies in the United States, 38.9% of pharmacies offered the HPV vaccine [13]. However, 44.2% of the sample consisted of independently owned pharmacies, and the percentage of pharmacies offering the HPV vaccine was not stratified by pharmacy type [13]. In the current study, mass merchandisers (96.0%), national chain pharmacies (92.7%), and grocery store pharmacies (71.9%) reported administering the HPV vaccine, while fewer single independent pharmacies (20.3%), multiple independent pharmacies (8.3%), and regional chain pharmacies (33.3%) offered the HPV vaccine (Figure 1). This is consistent with previous reports that describe barriers to HPV vaccination among independent pharmacies [21,22]. These include organizational barriers to HPV vaccine administration including lack of space and staff.

Reports indicate HPV vaccination coverage is lower in rural areas, despite these areas having higher rates of HPV-associated cancers [4,8]. In the current study, we surveyed pharmacies in a region where approximately 38% of the population lives in a rural area [23]. We found that HPV vaccine availability in pharmacy settings was not different between those in rural and nonrural locations. Additionally, there were no significant differences in pharmacy type when stratified by geographic location, which suggests that, in the region surveyed, the HPV vaccine is likely available in a chain, mass merchandiser, and/or grocery pharmacy setting even in rural locations. This is consistent with the concept that pharmacies in rural locations could potentially serve a powerful role in providing HPV vaccine administration [12,22]. However, the benefit of the HPV vaccine in the rural pharmacy setting alone is clearly not enough to increase HPV vaccination coverage as HPV vaccination uptake and accessibility is impacted by legislative, social, and environmental factors unique to HPV vaccination, nor would availability overcome other obstacles for vaccination including medical literacy, socioeconomics, and personal choice [11].

In the current study, family medicine and obstetrics–gynecology providers were willing to refer patients to a community pharmacy for HPV vaccination, despite this not being a common practice. A study by Hurley et al. (2014) reported on vaccination referral practices by alternate vaccinators, including general internists and family medicine providers, where financial barriers made them less likely to stock and administer vaccines [19]. Although the report was not specific to the HPV vaccine, the providers surveyed indicated they "always, often or sometimes" referred patients to a pharmacy for vaccination [19]. Additionally, the study reported that most providers agreed it was helpful to have pharmacists share a role in patient vaccination. However, one-third of providers had reservations about pharmacists as vaccinators. Some of these reservations were related to communication, or lack thereof, between physicians and pharmacists and concerns about inadequate documentation of patient vaccines. They disagreed that it was more convenient for their patients to get vaccines at a pharmacy compared to their office, and the majority reported their patients preferred to receive vaccines at their office, rather than a pharmacy. The results of the current study suggest similar themes presented in the Hurley et al. study. Providers support the idea of pharmacists as vaccinators (Table 2) but would prefer to vaccinate their patients in their offices (Figure 2). Perhaps this is tied to concern about fragmented care and the importance of patients receiving care in their medical home.

It is worthwhile to mention that among the providers surveyed in the current study, none of them perceived HPV vaccination as outside the scope of a pharmacist. This suggests the training and knowledge of a pharmacist surrounding the HPV vaccine may not be problematic for many family medicine and obstetrics–gynecology providers. Overall, these findings are in contrast to a study by Welch et al. (2003) that found most family medicine physicians were neither very knowledgeable about nor supportive of pharmacists as vaccinators [24]. It is possible the providers surveyed in the current study are inherently different compared to the providers surveyed in the Welch et al. study. For example, the providers included in the current study were from a single academic institution where the majority work in clinics that administer and stock the HPV vaccine. Similarly, it is possible that providers in clinical settings that are unable to or that chose not to administer or stock the HPV vaccine may have different HPV vaccine referral practices and/or attitudes towards referring patients to a pharmacy setting for HPV vaccination. In terms of generalizing the findings of the current study more broadly, several of the providers surveyed indicated they treat primarily adult patients, which could have influenced their willingness and comfort to refer patients to a pharmacy setting for HPV vaccination.

While the majority of pharmacies in the current study had the HPV vaccine available, the majority of providers in the current study were not actively referring patients to a pharmacy setting for HPV vaccination. Providers reported concerns their patients may not complete the HPV vaccine series if referred outside of their office for vaccination and expressed concern they would not be informed whether their patients received vaccines in a pharmacy setting (Figure 2). The lack of coordinated up-to-date immunization registries has been cited as a barrier in previous studies [21]. Promoting the wider use of immunization registries could be a strategy to overcome some provider concerns related to referring patients outside the office setting for vaccination.

In the current study, we did not specifically ask providers to distinguish their opinions and/or practices regarding HPV vaccine series initiation versus booster. For example, it is possible some providers prefer to administer the first HPV vaccine dose that a patient receives in their clinic, but would be willing to refer patients to a pharmacy setting for HPV vaccine series completion. Additional studies are needed to determine if providers might be more willing to refer patients to a pharmacy for HPV vaccine series completion and to determine the rate of follow-up for HPV vaccination among patients that are referred to a community pharmacy for HPV vaccination series completion. A recent study by Douchette et al. (2019) described a coordinated delivery of an HPV vaccine program using a clinic–pharmacy partnership. In their study, less than 50% of patients referred to a pharmacy received an HPV vaccine [25]. However, 100% of the patients that received the HPV vaccine in the pharmacy setting, after referral to the pharmacy for vaccination, completed the series. Further evidence of successful vaccine series completion in a community pharmacy setting is described in a recent report by Frederick et al. (2020). In this study, they describe the use of "nudge"-based clinical decision support embedded within a community pharmacy's software system to improve vaccine series completion in a community pharmacy setting [26].

This study has limitations. These results may not be generalizable beyond this specific region in the Southern United States, as HPV vaccination uptake and accessibility are impacted by several factors that are state- and region-specific. These may include legislation and policies regarding HPV vaccination, social and environmental factors, religiosity, political ideology, and vaccine hesitancy. However, these data suggest that more research is needed to better understand perceived barriers and opportunities for HPV vaccination among providers in a variety of clinical settings. The providers included in the current study were from a single academic institution, working in clinics that administer and stock the HPV vaccine. It is possible that providers working in different settings would not be as willing to refer patients to a pharmacy setting for the HPV vaccine. Future work should include providers that are not affiliated with an academic medical center and those that do not work in practices that administer and stock the HPV vaccine. Finally, this study did not attempt to evaluate pharmacists as facilitators of HPV vaccines or their comfort in counseling patients about HPV vaccination. Nor did this study attempt to evaluate perceptions of facilitators to HPV vaccination in the pharmacy setting among family medicine and obstetrics–gynecology providers. Additional studies are needed to understand barriers and overcome obstacles to HPV vaccination, particularly in the community pharmacy setting.

5. Conclusions

Findings suggest that the HPV vaccine is commonly available in nonindependent pharmacies in Eastern Tennessee. Family medicine and obstetrics–gynecology providers report they are willing to refer patients for HPV vaccination in a pharmacy setting; however, several barriers were reported that might limit this practice. While pharmacist-administered HPV vaccination continues to be a commonly reported strategy for increasing HPV vaccination coverage and the availability of the HPV vaccine in the pharmacy setting is common, coordinated efforts to increase collaboration among vaccinators in different settings and overcome systematic and legislative barriers to increasing HPV vaccination rates are still needed.

Author Contributions: Conceptualization, L.C.K., N.B.Z., J.M.M., O.O., S.G., J.D.G. and K.C.H.; Methodology, L.C.K., N.B.Z., J.M.M., O.O., S.G., A.M.M., J.D.G., K.C.H., S.M.C., J.D.P. and H.K.M.; Validation, J.M.M., O.O., S.G. and A.M.M.; Formal Analysis, J.M.M., M.E.B. and A.M.M.; Investigation, L.C.K., N.B.Z., J.M.M., O.O., S.G., A.M.M., M.E.B., J.D.G., K.C.H. and S.M.C.; Writing—Original Draft Preparation, J.M.M.; Writing—Review and Editing, L.C.K., N.B.Z., J.M.M., O.O., S.G., A.M.M., J.D.G., K.C.H., S.M.C., J.D.P., M.E.B. and H.K.M.; Visualization, J.M.M. and A.M.M.; Supervision, L.C.K. and J.M.M.; Project Administration, J.M.M., O.O., S.G. and S.M.C.; Funding Acquisition, L.C.K., N.B.Z. and J.M.M. All authors have read and agreed to the published version of the manuscript.

Funding: This work was funded by a University of Tennessee Medical Center Cancer Institute Research Grant awarded to L.C.K., N.B.Z. and J.M.M.

Institutional Review Board Statement: This study was conducted according to the guidelines of the Declaration of Helsinki and approved by the Institutional Review Board of the University of Tennessee Graduate School of Medicine (IRB# 4691 approved 26 October 2020; IRB# 4884 approved 2 December 2021).

Informed Consent Statement: For the pharmacy data collection portion of this study, respondent consent was waived due to the "secret shopper" nature of the study design. No identifiable information was collected from those contacted in the pharmacy setting and all pharmacy-related data were presented in aggregate. For the provider survey, informed consent was obtained from all respondents involved in the study.

Data Availability Statement: These data are not publicly available, but the data presented in this study are available upon reasonable request from the corresponding author.

Acknowledgments: The study team would like to acknowledge Mara Walters, Zachary Shelton, Emma Mitchell, Allison Zisko, and Cara Rubin for their assistance in collecting pharmacy data.

Conflicts of Interest: Kenneth C. Hohmeier reports vaccine-related funding from Genentech, Merck & Co., Kenilworth, NJ, USA and GlaxoSmithKline, Philadelphia, PA, USA. Justin D. Gatwood reports vaccine-related funding from Merck & Co., Kenilworth, NJ, USA and GlaxoSmithKline, Philadelphia, PA, USA. The funders, the University of Tennessee Medical Center Cancer Institute, had no role in the design of the study; in the collection, analyses, or interpretation of data; in the writing of the manuscript; or in the decision to publish the results.

References

1. Senkomago, V.; Henley, S.J.; Thomas, C.C.; Mix, J.M.; Markowitz, L.E.; Saraiya, M. Human papillomavirus-attributable cancers-united states, 2012–2016. *MMWR Morb. Mortal. Wkly. Rep.* **2019**, *68*, 724–728. [CrossRef] [PubMed]
2. Van Dyne, E.A.; Henley, S.J.; Saraiya, M.; Thomas, C.C.; Markowitz, L.E.; Benard, V.B. Trends in human papillomavirus-associated cancers-united states, 1999–2015. *MMWR Morb. Mortal. Wkly. Rep.* **2018**, *67*, 918–924. [CrossRef] [PubMed]
3. Viens, L.J.; Henley, S.J.; Watson, M.; Markowitz, L.E.; Thomas, C.C.; Thompson, T.D.; Razzaghi, H.; Saraiya, M. Human papillomavirus-associated cancers-united states, 2008–2012. *MMWR Morb. Mortal. Wkly. Rep.* **2016**, *65*, 661–666. [CrossRef] [PubMed]
4. Pingali, C.; Yankey, D.; Elam-Evans, L.D.; Markowitz, L.E.; Williams, C.L.; Fredua, B.; McNamara, L.A.; Stokley, S.; Singleton, J.A. National, regional, state, and selected local area vaccination coverage among adolescents aged 13–17 years-united states, 2020. *MMWR Morb. Mortal. Wkly. Rep.* **2021**, *70*, 1183–1190. [CrossRef] [PubMed]
5. Lu, P.J.; Hung, M.C.; Srivastav, A.; Grohskopf, L.A.; Kobayashi, M.; Harris, A.M.; Dooling, K.L.; Markowitz, L.E.; Rodriguez-Lainz, A.; Williams, W.W. Surveillance of vaccination coverage among adult populations -united states, 2018. *MMWR Surveill. Summ.* **2021**, *70*, 1–26. [CrossRef]
6. Damgacioglu, H.; Sonawane, K.; Zhu, Y.; Li, R.; Balasubramanian, B.A.; Lairson, D.R.; Giuliano, A.R.; Deshmukh, A.A. Oropharyngeal cancer incidence and mortality trends in all 50 states in the US, 2001–2017. *JAMA Otolaryngol. Head Neck Surg.* **2021**, *148*, 155–165. [CrossRef] [PubMed]
7. Rahman, M.; McGrath, C.J.; Berenson, A.B. Geographic variation in human papillomavirus vaccination uptake among 13–17 year old adolescent girls in the united states. *Vaccine* **2014**, *32*, 2394–2398. [CrossRef] [PubMed]
8. Zahnd, W.E.; Rodriguez, C.; Jenkins, W.D. Rural-urban differences in human papillomavirus-associated cancer trends and rates. *J. Rural Health* **2019**, *35*, 208–215. [CrossRef] [PubMed]
9. Hpv Vaccination for Cancer Prevention: Progress, Opportunities, and a Renewed Call to Action. Available online: https://prescancerpanel.cancer.gov/report/hpvupdate/pdf/PresCancerPanel_HPVUpdate_Nov2018.pdf (accessed on 1 December 2021).
10. National Vaccine Advisory Committee. Overcoming barriers to low hpv vaccine uptake in the united states: Recommendations from the national vaccine advisory committee: Approved by the national vaccine advisory committee on 9 June 2015. *Public Health Rep.* **2016**, *131*, 17–25. [CrossRef] [PubMed]
11. Cartmell, K.B.; Young-Pierce, J.; McGue, S.; Alberg, A.J.; Luque, J.S.; Zubizarreta, M.; Brandt, H.M. Barriers, facilitators, and potential strategies for increasing hpv vaccination: A statewide assessment to inform action. *Papillomavirus Res.* **2018**, *5*, 21–31. [CrossRef] [PubMed]
12. Face-to-Face with Community Pharmacies. Available online: https://www.nacds.org/pdfs/about/rximpact-leavebehind.pdf (accessed on 1 December 2021).
13. Westrick, S.C.; Patterson, B.J.; Kader, M.S.; Rashid, S.; Buck, P.O.; Rothholz, M.C. National survey of pharmacy-based immunization services. *Vaccine* **2018**, *36*, 5657–5664. [CrossRef] [PubMed]
14. Pharmacist Administered Vaccines, Updated July 2021, Based on Apha/Naspa Survey of State Iz Laws/Rules. Available online: https://aphanet.pharmacist.com/sites/default/files/practice/07-2020/pharmacist-administered-vaccines-june-2020.pdf (accessed on 15 September 2021).
15. Campos-Outcalt, D.; Jeffcott-Pera, M.; Carter-Smith, P.; Schoof, B.K.; Young, H.F. Vaccines provided by family physicians. *Ann. Fam. Med.* **2010**, *8*, 507–510. [CrossRef] [PubMed]
16. O'Leary, S.T.; Riley, L.E.; Lindley, M.C.; Allison, M.A.; Crane, L.A.; Hurley, L.P.; Beaty, B.L.; Brtnikova, M.; Collins, M.; Albert, A.P.; et al. Vaccination practices among obstetrician/gynecologists for non-pregnant patients. *Am. J. Prev. Med.* **2019**, *56*, 429–436. [CrossRef] [PubMed]
17. Developing an Immunization Referral System. Available online: https://www.nacds.org/ceo/2018/0628/2018-Immun-Referral-TipSheet.pdf (accessed on 1 December 2021).
18. Federal Office of Rural Health Policy (Forhp) Data Files. Available online: https://www.hrsa.gov/rural-health/about-us/definition/datafiles.html (accessed on 1 September 2021).
19. Hurley, L.P.; Bridges, C.B.; Harpaz, R.; Allison, M.A.; O'Leary, S.T.; Crane, L.A.; Brtnikova, M.; Stokley, S.; Beaty, B.L.; Jimenez-Zambrano, A.; et al. U.S. Physicians' perspective of adult vaccine delivery. *Ann. Intern. Med.* **2014**, *160*, 161. [CrossRef] [PubMed]
20. Hastings, T.J.; Hohmann, L.A.; McFarland, S.J.; Teeter, B.S.; Westrick, S.C. Pharmacists' attitudes and perceived barriers to human papillomavirus (hpv) vaccination services. *Pharmacy* **2017**, *5*, 45. [CrossRef] [PubMed]

21. Oyedeji, O.; Maples, J.M.; Gregory, S.; Chamberlin, S.M.; Gatwood, J.D.; Wilson, A.Q.; Zite, N.B.; Kilgore, L.C. Pharmacists' perceived barriers to human papillomavirus (hpv) vaccination: A systematic literature review. *Vaccines* **2021**, *9*, 1360. [CrossRef] [PubMed]
22. Ryan, G.; Daly, E.; Askelson, N.; Pieper, F.; Seegmiller, L.; Allred, T. Exploring opportunities to leverage pharmacists in rural areas to promote administration of human papillomavirus vaccine. *Prev. Chronic. Dis.* **2020**, *17*, E23. [CrossRef] [PubMed]
23. Just How Rural or Urban are Tennessee's 95 Counties? Finding a Measure for Policy Makers. Tennessee Advisory Commission on Intergovernmental Relations Staff Report. Available online: https://www.tn.gov/content/dam/tn/tacir/documents/2016JustHowRuralOrUrban.pdf (accessed on 16 February 2022).
24. Welch, A.C.; Ferreri, S.P.; Blalock, S.J.; Caiola, S.M. North carolina family practice physicians' perceptions of pharmacists as vaccinators. *J. Am. Pharm. Assoc.* **2005**, *45*, 486–491. [CrossRef] [PubMed]
25. Doucette, W.R.; Kent, K.; Seegmiller, L.; McDonough, R.P.; Evans, W. Feasibility of a coordinated human papillomavirus (hpv) vaccination program between a medical clinic and a community pharmacy. *Pharmacy* **2019**, *7*, 91. [CrossRef] [PubMed]
26. Frederick, K.D.; Gatwood, J.D.; Atchley, D.R.; Rein, L.J.; Ali, S.G.; Brookhart, A.L.; Crain, J.; Hagemann, T.M.; Ramachandran, S.; Chiu, C.Y.; et al. Exploring the early phase of implementation of a vaccine-based clinical decision support system in the community pharmacy. *J. Am. Pharm. Assoc.* **2020**, *60*, e292–e300. [CrossRef] [PubMed]

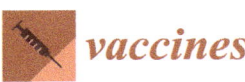

Article

Parents' Knowledge and Attitude towards HPV and HPV Vaccination in Poland

Katarzyna Smolarczyk [1,*], Anna Duszewska [2], Slawomir Drozd [3] and Slawomir Majewski [1]

[1] Department of Dermatology Immunodermatology and Venereology, Medical University of Warsaw, 02-008 Warsaw, Poland; slawomir.majewski@wum.edu.pl
[2] Division of Histology and Embryology, Department of Morphological Sciences, Faculty of Veterinary Medicine, Warsaw University of Life Sciences, 02-776 Warsaw, Poland; duszewskaanna@hotmail.com
[3] Institute of Physical Culture Studies, College of Medical Sciences, University of Rzeszow, 35-959 Rzeszów, Poland; slawek.drozd@op.pl
* Correspondence: ksmolarczyk@gmail.com; Tel.: +48-607-243-963

Abstract: HPV is one of the diseases of civilization that causes cervical cancer, among other diseases. For this reason, a vaccination program has been introduced worldwide for preadolescent, sexually inactive seronegative girls. However, the decision to vaccinate young girls must be made by the parents. In Poland, vaccinations are recommended but not financed by the government, which affects their choices, and there is insufficient knowledge of the diseases caused by genital HPV types. In addition, there are cultural, social, and even religious factors to be considered. Therefore, the aim of the study was to analyze the state of knowledge about HPV and HPV vaccines among parents. Two hundred and eighty-eight parents participated in the study, but only 180 of them declared that they had ever heard of HPV (62.5%). Therefore, only these parents completed the entire questionnaire consisting of 34 questions. The parents' answers were analyzed with the Fisher's and chi-squared tests. The study showed that parents' knowledge of HPV and HPV vaccination in Poland is low (49.4% of correct answers). Parents' attitudes were only influenced by knowledge and education and not by other parameters such as age, gender, place of residence, and the number of children. This study indicates that parents need to be educated about the threats of HPV and the possibilities of prophylactic vaccination.

Keywords: HPV; HPV vaccine; human papillomavirus

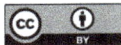

1. Introduction

Human papillomaviruses (HPVs) belong to the family *Papillomaviridae* and are non-enveloped icosahedral, circular, dsDNA viruses [1]. HPVs infect the cutaneous and mucosal epithelia, hence its wide spectrum of occurrence (skin, oral cavity, oropharynx, larynx, anogenital tract) [2]. There are more than 207 types of HPV [3], most of which do not cause any symptoms, lesions, or warts and are referred to as low-oncogenic (types). However, some types of HPVs are highly oncogenic and can induce intraepithelial neoplasia or cancers [2,4]. Among other diseases, cervical cancer is associated with types 16, 18, 31, 33, 35, 39, 45, 51, 52, 56, 58, 68, 73, 82, and especially 26, 53, and 66 [2]. In the European population, eight types are of particular importance (16, 18, 31, 33, 35, 45, 56, and 58), with 16 and 18 being responsible for 70 percent of all cases of cervical cancer [5].

In 2012, there were 530,000 cases of cervical cancer related to HPV, of which 370,000 were caused by HVP16/18 (71%) [6]. In addition, more than two-thirds of the cases are diagnosed in less developed countries [7,8]. Interestingly, the highest number of cases of HPV cervical cancer occurs in Asia (India 120,000) and Sub-Saharan Africa (93,000), and one of the lowest in Australia/New Zealand (940) [6]. The age-standardized mortality rate for cervical cancer is lower in developed nations at 2.2 per 100,000 compared with 4.3 per 100,000 in the developing nations [4].

In the European Union, about 34,000 new cases of cervical cancer related to HPV are diagnosed every year. The highest prevalence of cervical cancer associated with HPV infection are observed in Latvia (25.0/100,000 women), Bosnia and Herzegovina (23.9/100,000), and Estonia (22.5/100,000). On the other hand, the lowest prevalence is found in Malta (3.5/100,000), Switzerland (3.8/100,000), and Finland (4.7/100,000). In Poland, the prevalence is 9.4/100,000 women [9].

Currently, three vaccines are used in the world: 1. Cervarix (GlaxoSmithKline), a bivalent (2-V) vaccine targeting HPV16 and HPV18, the two most carcinogenic types; 2. Gardasil (Merck Inc., Meguro City, Tokyo), a quadrivalent (4-V) vaccine targeting HPV16/18 and the low risk types, HPV6 and HPV11, that cause genital warts; and 3. Gardasil 9 (Merck Inc.), a nonavalent (9-valent, 9-V) vaccine targeting HPV6/11/16/18 and the next five most carcinogenic types (HPV31/33/45/52/58).

Most recommendations, including from the WHO, recommend routine HPV vaccination in girls aged 9–14 years before becoming sexually active. The secondary target group is girls over the age of 15 years and young women. HPV vaccination of males is currently not recommended as a priority [10,11]. However, the CDC recommends HPV vaccination at the age of 11 or 12 years (but it can start from the age of 9 years) and for men up to the age of 26 years, if not vaccinated already [12].

HPV vaccination was first introduced in 2007 in Australia and, since then, many countries have joined the vaccination program. In 2020, HPV vaccination has been introduced in 107 (55%) of the 194 WHO Member States. In the Americas and Europe, 85% and 77% of the countries have already introduced HPV vaccination. A lower number of countries with a HPV vaccination programme was observed in Oceania (56%), Asia (40%), and Africa (31%) [13].

The implementation of an HPV vaccine programme has created many controversies. The two most frequently cited sources of negative knowledge about HPV vaccination are the Canadian article "Guinea pigs" and the Danish paradocumentary "De Vaccinerede Piger" (The Vaccinated Girls—Sick and Abandoned). The article describes the vaccination programme as "the biggest Canadian science experiment in decades". The paradocumentary tells the story of some girls who allegedly had a reaction to a HPV vaccination and suffered from POTS—postural orthostatic tachycardia syndrome. The paradocumentary presents the HPV vaccine in a very negative light, although no studies confirmed the described symptoms.

The vaccination coverage level depends on at what age the first dose of vaccination is being administered (higher coverage level in younger groups). However, in general, a high level of vaccination coverage was observed in Australia (78.6%) and in the United Kingdom (81%), in contrast with countries with low vaccination coverage level such as Georgia (36.2%), Lithuania (29%) [13], and Poland (7.5–10%) [14].

Until now, Poland was one of the EU countries where vaccination against HPV was recommended but not government-funded [14]. There are no restrictions to access of any type of HPV vaccine in Poland, but they are expensive. Difficulties limiting or even preventing the implementation of HPV vaccination in Poland include:

1. Lack of knowledge about HPV infections and vaccines.
2. Motivational obstacles for vaccination, including:
   a. lack of recommendations from the National Health Fund (NHF) and doctors,
   b. "bad attitude" towards vaccination in anti-vaccine environments,
   c. lack of support and conversations with parents about sexuality.
3. Logistical barriers, including:
   a. availability of vaccination,
   b. the price of the vaccine,
   c. the need to repeat vaccination (compliance).
4. Myths about the vaccine—mistaken beliefs, including:
   a. sexual promiscuity,

b. negative information about the vaccine in the media (ineffective, not very well studied, dangerous).

Of these many barriers, the lack of support and conversations with parents about sexuality deserves special attention. This issue is critical because prophylactic vaccination of girls against HPV should be carried out in the period preceding sexual initiation. Therefore, the decision to vaccinate girls is the responsibility of parents who, by giving their consent, give them the chance to avoid a disease that is dangerous to their health and even their life when they become adults.

The attitudes of parents and adolescents, using many research models [15–17], have already been the subject of many studies globally, including those conducted in Europe, and a review in this field was undertaken by Lopez et al. [18]. However, the situation in Poland was not considered in that review, so it is well-justified to present the results of studies that aim to assess: 1. The state of knowledge of parents about HPV infections and HPV vaccines; and 2. Parents' attitude to vaccination, including HPV vaccines.

Cervical cancer remains high in incidence and mortality rankings in Poland. Despite this, HPV vaccines are not covered by the government. Many local governments in Poland organize free HPV vaccination programs, but HPV immunization remains low.

This study, the first of its kind to be undertaken in Poland, undertook an analysis to determine the barriers to vaccination acceptance.

This study aimed to assess parents' knowledge about HPV infections, assess parents' knowledge about HPV vaccines, and assess the impact of parents' knowledge about HPV infection and HPV vaccines on their attitude to primary prevention, i.e., vaccinations.

2. Materials and Methods

2.1. Design of the Study

An observational cross-sectional descriptive study was undertaken.

All subjects gave their informed consent for inclusion before they participated in the study. The study was conducted in accordance with the Declaration of Helsinki, and the protocol was approved by the Ethics Committee of the Medical University of Warsaw (AKBE/123/16).

2.2. Data Collection

The survey was conducted in 2018 in Warsaw, Poland, and included parents of the children admitted to the Department of Pediatric Dermatology at a multidisciplinary regional hospital.

Data was collected using questionnaires presented on electronic devices (such as tablets, laptops, mobile phones) during the admission of the patients to the Department of Pediatric Dermatology. A researcher who monitored the study and helped with technical problems was present to ensure that only one parent was involved in the study.

Four parents refused to fill in the questionnaire, answering "no time" as the reason. The study was completed when questionnaires from a minimum of 200 parents were obtained. None of the children of the surveyed parents were diagnosed with HPV-related lesions as a reason for admission to the department.

2.3. Sample Size

A goal of the study was to include as many participants as possible. At the initial stage, no formal calculation of sample size was carried out. The final number of 288 parents ensured precision (measured at half the length of the 95% confidence interval) of 4 percentage points for assessing a trait whose true prevalence was 50% (for which 50% is needed in the most significant sample to reach a particular precision value).

2.4. Statistical Analysis

The analysis was conducted mainly with the use of descriptive statistics. The results are presented in the form of frequency tables and cross tables. Statistical inference was performed using the chi-squared test or, in the case of low frequencies of the analyzed features, Fisher's exact test.

Fisher's exact test is used in the case of samples that are too small—when the observed values calculated with the chi-squared test are below 5. The calculations were performed using the statistics program R 3.5.1. All tests were performed at a significance level $p = 0.05$.

The parents' responses regarding their knowledge about HPV were presented depending on their age, sex, their place of residence, and education. The parents' knowledge about vaccination was also analyzed. The parents' responses to the questions regarding their knowledge about vaccinations were classified as correct or incorrect. Total test result and results regarding the parents' knowledge about HPV and HPV vaccine was expressed as a percentage of available points.

2.5. Questionnaire

The questionnaire survey (Appendix A) for parents consisted of 34 questions and was designed by the authors. It was preceded by preliminary information, which consisted of explaining the purpose of the study, details on how to contact the author, and information about the voluntary and anonymous nature of the survey.

The survey consisted of both single-choice and multiple-choice questions. The age question was an open-ended question. The rest of the questions were closed questions. Seven questions related to their knowledge about the HPV virus, and seven questions related to their knowledge about the HPV vaccine. The rest of the questions were about the parents' attitudes to vaccination and demographic data. One hundred and eighty of the surveyed parents declared that they had heard about the HPV virus and filled in the entire questionnaire. The rest of the respondents answered "no" or "I do not know" and were asked to provide their age, gender, place of residence, and education.

3. Results

3.1. Group Characteristics

The study included the parents of the children admitted to the Department of Pediatric Dermatology in Warsaw, Poland. Two hundred and eighty-eight parents participated in the study. Most of the respondents were women (78.8%). Parents between the ages of 30 and 40 years accounted for 61% (n = 155) of the respondents, parents between the ages of 20 and 30 years accounted for 24% (n = 61), and parents between the ages of 40 and 70 years accounted for 15% (n = 38).

Furthermore, 38 parents (13.2%) lived in the countryside, 26 (9%) lived in a city with up to 20,000 inhabitants, 33 (11.5%) lived in a city with 20,000–100,000 inhabitants, 36 (12.5%) lived in a city with 100,000–500,000 inhabitants, and 155 (53.8%) lived in a city with more than 500,000 inhabitants.

Most of the respondents had higher education (71.2%, n = 205). Sixty-eight people had secondary education (23.6%), 13 people had basic vocational education (4.5%), and 2 people had primary education (0.7%). A summary of these data is presented in Table 1.

Table 1. Characteristic of the group.

Characteristic	Group Size	Options	N (%)
Sex	288	Women	227 (78.8%)
		Men	61 (21.2%)
Age	254	(20–30)	61 (24%)
		(31–40)	155 (61%)
		(41–70)	38 (15%)
Education	288	primary	2 (0.7%)
		vocational	13 (4.5%)
		secondary	68 (23.6%)
		higher	205 (71.2%)

Table 1. Cont.

Characteristic	Group Size	Options	N (%)
Residence	288	countryside	38 (13.2%)
		city up to 20,000 inhabitants	26 (9.0%)
		city from 20,000 to 100,000 inhabitants	33 (11.5%)
		city from 100,000 to 500,000 inhabitants	36 (12.5%)
		city > 500,000 inhabitants	155 (53.8%)

Among those surveyed, 180 declared that they had heard of the HPV virus and filled in the entire questionnaire. The characteristics differentiating these two groups are presented in Table 2. Most people declaring knowledge about HPV were women. The numbers of men who declared that they had heard about the virus (n = 33) and had not heard about the virus (n = 28) were similar.

Table 2. Characteristics of the group of parents divided into two groups, declaring knowledge about HPV and HPV vaccination and declaring the lack of knowledge.

			No Knowledge	Declaring Knowledge	p
Age	<30	N	23	38	0.073
		%	37.7	62.3	
	(30–35)	N	31	79	
		%	28.2	71.8	
	(36–40)	N	19	26	
		%	42.2	57.8	
	(41–65)	N	19	19	
		%	50	50	
Sex	Women	N	70	157	<0.001
		%	30.8	69.2	
	Men	N	33	28	
		%	54.1	45.9	
Education	Rest	N	54	29	<0.001
		%	65.1	34.9	
	Higher	N	49	156	
		%	23.9	76.1	
Place of residence	countryside	N	29	9	<0.001
		%	76.3	23.7	
	city up to 20,000 inhabitants	N	11	15	
		%	42.3	57.7	
	city from 20,000 to 100,000 inhabitants	N	18	15	
		%	54.5	45.5	
	city from 100,000 to 500,000 inhabitants	N	11	25	
		%	30.6	69.4	
	city > 500,000 inhabitants	N	34	121	
		%	21.9	78.1	

3.2. Test Results

Table 3 provides a summary of the total test scores and the number and percentage of parents with a particular test score. The first division presents all the scores together with the frequency and percentage of parents who achieved them. The highest score was 86.5% of correct answers, and the lowest score was 21.6% of correct answers.

From an analysis of the second part of the table, 2.8% of the parents achieved a score of up to 30% of correct answers, 47.8% scored in the range of 31–60 (n = 86), and 49.4% scored in the range of 61–100 (n = 89). Therefore, as many as 50.6% of parents would not pass the test if the pass mark for this test was a score above 61% of correct answers.

Table 4 provides summary statements for the percentage of the parental test for HPV vaccination knowledge. The first division presents the test scores together with the frequency and percentage of parents who achieved them. The highest score was 92.3% of correct answers, and the lowest score was 23.1% of correct answers.

From an analysis of the second part of the table, 2.2% of parents achieved a score of up to 30% of correct answers, 32.8% scored in the range of 31–60, and 65.0% scored in the range 61–100. Therefore, 35% of parents would not pass the test if the pass mark for this test was a score above 61% of correct answers.

Table 5 contains the summary result of the parents' test of knowledge about HPV infections. The first division presents the test scores together with the frequency and percentage of parents who achieved them. The highest test score was 84% of correct answers, and the lowest score was 16% of correct answers.

From an analysis of the second division, 6.7% of parents achieved a score of up to 30% of correct answers, 56.7% scored in the range of 31–60 (n = 102), and 36.7% scored in the range 61–100 (n = 66). Therefore, 63.4% of parents would not pass the test if the pass mark for this test was a score above 61% of correct answers.

Table 3. Summary test results.

Total Test Result (% of Correct Answers)	N	%
21.6	4	2.2%
29.7	1	0.6%
32.4	4	2.2%
35.1	5	2.8%
37.8	6	3.3%
40.5	6	3.3%
43.2	1	0.6%
45.9	10	5.6%
48.6	7	3.9%
51.4	14	7.8%
54.1	14	7.8%
56.8	5	2.8%
59.5	14	7.8%
62.2	13	7.2%
64.9	13	7.2%
67.6	13	7.2%
70.3	17	9.4%
73.0	10	5.6%
75.7	10	5.6%
78.4	5	2.8%
81.1	3	1.7%
83.8	3	1.7%
86.5	2	1.1%
(% points)		
(0–30)	5	2.8%
(31–60)	86	47.8%
(61–100)	89	49.4%

Total test result = overall knowledge points scored in test by parents. N = number of parents who achieved this test score; % = percentage of parents who achieved this test score.

Table 4. Summary test results—knowledge about HPV vaccine.

Knowledge about HPV Vaccine (% of Correct Answers)	N	%
23.1	4	2.2%
30.8	6	3.3%
38.5	8	4.4%
46.2	21	11.7%
53.8	24	13.3%
61.5	36	20.0%
69.2	37	20.6%
76.9	24	13.3%
84.6	13	7.2%
92.3	7	3.9%
(% points)		
(0–30)	4	2.2%
(31–60)	59	32.8%
(61–100)	117	65.0%

Total test result = overall knowledge points scored in test by parents; N = number of parents who achieved this test score; % = percentage of parents who achieved this test score.

Table 5. Summary test results—knowledge about HPV.

Knowledge about HPV (% of Correct Answers)	N	%
16.0	2	1.1%
20.0	4	2.2%
24.0	2	1.1%
28.0	4	2.2%
32.0	10	5.6%
36.0	1	0.6%
40.0	15	8.3%
44.0	20	11.1%
48.0	11	6.1%
52.0	7	3.9%
56.0	16	8.9%
60.0	22	12.2%
64.0	15	8.3%
68.0	21	11.7%
72.0	16	8.9%
76.0	8	4.4%
80.0	4	2.2%
84.0	2	1.1%
(% points)		
(0–30)	12	6.7%
(31–60)	102	56.7%
(61–100)	66	36.7%

Total test result = overall knowledge points scored in test by parents; N = number of parents who achieved this test score; % = percentage of parents who achieved this test score.

3.3. Parents' Knowledge—Correct Answers

Table 6 contains a summary list of answers to questions concerning parents' knowledge about the HPV virus and HPV vaccinations. In this comparison, only 39.4% correctly indicated the association of HPV with cancers of the genitourinary organs, and 42.8% correctly indicated an association of HPV with papillary lesions of the genital organs. In addition, only 8.9% of parents indicated the answer "children" as a group exposed to HPV infection.

Table 6. Knowledge about the HPV virus and the HPV vaccine—correct answers to component questions.

Question	N	n (%)
How can you get infected with HPV		
By kissing	180	162 (90%)
By touch	180	24 (13.3%)
Sexual intercourse	180	138 (6.7%)
During natural childbirth	180	43 (23.9%)
By contact of infected blood with the blood of an uninfected person, e.g., using the same needle	180	142 (78.9%)
Who is at risk of HPV infection?		
Only women	180	146 (81.1%)
Only men	180	177 (98.3%)
Children	180	16 (8.9%)
Only homosexuals	180	180 (100%)
Both women and men, regardless of sexual orientation	180	142 (78.9%)
HPV infection predisposes to:		
Cancer of the genitourinary organs	180	71 (39.4%)
Cervical cancer	180	134 (74.4%)
Papillary lesions of the genital area	180	77 (42.8%)
Does HPV infection always lead to the manifestation of the disease?	180	134 (74.4%)
Do you know what the purpose of the Pap smear test is?	180	174 (96.7%)
What factors increase the risk of developing cervical cancer?		
Smoking cigarettes	180	54 (30%)
A family history of cervical cancer	180	120 (66.7%)
HPV infection	180	149 (82.8%)
A large number of sexual partners	180	107 (59.4%)
Lack of physical activity	180	173 (96.1%)
How can HPV infection be prevented, or the risk of HPV infection be reduced?		
By vaccination before sexual initiation	180	140 (77.8%)
By using condoms	180	114 (63.3%)
By limiting the number of sexual partners and by avoiding risky sexual behavior	180	127 (70.6%)
It is not possible to prevent HPV infection	180	178 (98.9%)
Mean percentage result (S.D.)	180	65.1 +/− 16.2
Is there a vaccine against HPV?	180	164 (91.1%)
Is the HPV vaccine available in Poland?	180	155 (86.1%)
For which sex are HPV vaccines registered in Poland?	180	124 (68.9%)
The target groups for the vaccine are:		
Girls around 12 years old	180	91 (50.6%)
Boys around 12 years old	180	165 (91.7%)
Young women before sexual initiation	180	98 (54.4%)
Young boys before sexual initiation	180	165 (91.7%)
Young women not infected with HPV	180	59 (32.8%)
Young men not infected with HPV	180	167 (92.8%)
The scientifically proven AEFI (Adverse events following immunization)	180	67 (37.2%)
Does HPV vaccination give 100 percent protection?	180	122 (67.8%)
Is the cost of the vaccine in Poland covered by the government?	180	81 (45%)
Mean percentage result (S.D.)	180	62.3 +/− 15.6

N = number of parents who answered the question.

3.3.1. Knowledge Regarding HPV

There were no significant statistical differences between the groups identified by the place of residence and the number of children. Considering the remaining characteristics (gender, age, education), parents with a higher education and women had more correct answers, which was statistically significant. Parents with a higher education had an overall higher test score and statistically more correct answers to questions about vaccine funding and vaccine availability in Poland and identified girls over the age of nine years as the target group for the vaccine. The number of correct answers decreased with the age of the parents.

3.3.2. Knowledge Regarding Vaccine

Women scored a statistically significant higher percentage of correct answers regarding the availability of the vaccine in Poland and a statistically significant higher percentage of correct answers regarding vaccine funding and identified young girls before sexual initiation as the target group for the vaccine.

There were more statistically significant differences for incorrect vaccine responses between the education groups. People with a higher education had overall higher test scores and statistically answered more questions correctly about preventing or reducing the possibility of an HPV infection and about identifying the routes of transmission of the virus (through sexual intercourse, during natural childbirth). Women correctly identified most of the cervical cancer risk factors. The number of correct answers decreased with the age of the parents.

3.3.3. Attitude towards Vaccination

The only factors differentiating the attitude towards vaccinations were knowledge and education. Parents with a test score in the third quartile indicated that the high effectiveness of the vaccine might influence their decision to vaccinate their children with the recommended vaccine. The remaining characteristics of the parents (sex, age, place of residence) did not significantly affect the attitude to vaccination. It was interesting that 55% of the parents would have vaccinated their children if the vaccination was covered by the government.

4. Discussion

This research is the first in Poland to assess the knowledge and attitudes of parents towards HPV vaccination. HPV vaccination may prevent diseases related to papillomaviruses, including cervical cancer. Research in this field has been conducted worldwide for many years [19–33], and an interesting analysis was conducted by Lopez et al. [18].

It should be emphasized, however, that the attitude of parents may be influenced by many factors, and one of the key influencing factors in Poland is the lack of recommendations and financing by the National Health Fund.

According to a study by Gerend et al., people recommended by the NHF to be vaccinated against HPV were forty times more likely to get vaccinated [34]. This is also confirmed by other studies [35–38].

The lack of recommendation and funding may have a negative impact on parents' attitudes, especially when the price of the vaccine is high. In these studies, over one-third of the respondents indicated the high price of the HPV vaccine as a possible reason for refusing to vaccinate their children.

However, it should be emphasized that in countries with recommendations and a reimbursement scheme, the problem of HPV vaccination is much more complex. As many as 28% of parents refuse to vaccinate in the USA, and 8% delay vaccination. The motivation of both groups for this type of behavior differs significantly. Parents who refused vaccinations gave reasons such as fear of promiscuity, lower vaccine efficacy expected, and higher expected side effects. Parents who delay vaccination do not rule out later vaccination after learning more about the vaccine [39]. In the study by Brabin et al., friends and school nurses (35% each) and teachers (20%) also influenced the views of girls about the HPV virus and HPV vaccination [40].

The state of parental knowledge has a crucial influence on the immunization of children. The study by Fishman et al. proved that mothers with more knowledge about HPV were not willing to vaccinate themselves or their daughters [41]. The present study found that the only factors that affect attitudes to vaccination are knowledge and education. The remaining characteristics of parents do not significantly affect the attitude to vaccination.

Lack of support from parents due to their fear of encouraging girls to engage in risky sexual behavior is also emphasized in the literature, reducing the motivation to vaccinate. Factors increasing parental acceptance of vaccination include HIV testing in the past, having an older daughter, having had more sexual partners, and having a family member with cancer [42]. The most common concerns indicated by parents in the available studies are related to vaccine safety, post-vaccination sexual promiscuity, moral problems related to sexuality, denial that the daughter is at risk, conservative and religious views, lack of knowledge, and unknown side effects [43].

An interesting aspect is a conversation with their children about HPV vaccinations as an introduction to sexuality. In the study by Marlow et al., mothers of the girls stated the age of their daughters at which they would like to start discussions with them about vaccinations, sex, cervical cancer, sexually transmitted diseases, HPV, and HPV vaccination (Table 7). The study shows that the age of the girls at which mothers would like to talk to them about HPV vaccines is statistically higher than the age of the girls at which mothers talk to them about general immunization, sex, and even higher for general discussions about HPV vaccines, the HPV virus, and sexually transmitted diseases [44].

Table 7. Average age of the discussion between parents and children on HPV-related topics (76).

Subject	Mean	S.D.	Statistical Difference between a Conversation about HPV Immunization and Other Topics of Conversation
Reason for vaccination	9.58	1.72	$t = -24.46, p < 0.0001$
Sex	10.61	1.73	$T = -8.07, p < 0.0001$
Cervical cancer	11.04	1.69	n.s. (not significant)
HPV vaccine	11.08	1.61	
HPV	11.18	1.60	$T = 4.00, p < 0.0001$
STDs	11.38	1.57	$T = 7.27, p < 0.0001$

The price of the vaccine is often discussed in the aspect of barriers that reduce vaccination. In the analysis, the low price of the vaccine was not a determinant for vaccinating children (0 answers). Most parents decided to vaccinate their child after a doctor recommended the vaccine or because the vaccine was very effective. However, in the case of HPV vaccination, more than one-third of the respondents indicated the high price of the HPV vaccine as a possible reason for not taking up vaccination (over two-thirds indicated possible side effects).

In the literature, concerns about the cost of the vaccine include costs to be borne by the parents and by healthcare professionals, and costs of the vaccine to be borne by the healthcare insurer [45]. Therefore, to increase vaccination availability in developing countries, vaccine companies have negotiated to lower the price of a single dose to 4.50–4.60 USD [46,47]. For comparison, in Poland, the price of a single dose of Cervarix and Silgard varies around 440 zloty for a single dose (around 110 USD). The price of the vaccine also affects the choice of the vaccine. Often, patients opt for a bivalent vaccine due to the lower cost.

This research is the first attempt in Poland to identify the most important barriers to the effective implementation of an HPV vaccination program, and thus to the prevention of diseases connected with this virus. The presented analysis may be of assistance in the implementation of HPV vaccination programs in Poland.

5. Conclusions

Parents' knowledge of the HPV virus is insufficient and depends on sex, age, and education and is independent of place of residence and the number of children. The parents' knowledge about the HPV vaccine is low and independent of the place of residence, the number of children, and depends on age, sex, and education. Further studies need to be carried out to provide information regarding pro-vaccine motivation tools.

Author Contributions: Conceptualization, K.S. and S.M.; methodology, S.M.; formal analysis, K.S.; investigation, K.S., A.D., S.D. and S.M.; resources, K.S. and S.M.; writing—original draft preparation, K.S., A.D., S.D. and S.M.; writing—review and editing, K.S. and A.D.; supervision, S.M.; project administration, K.S. and S.M. All authors have read and agreed to the published version of the manuscript.

Funding: This research received no external funding.

Institutional Review Board Statement: This study was conducted according to the guidelines of the Declaration of Helsinki and approved by the Ethics Committee of the Medical University of Warsaw (AKBE/123/16).

Informed Consent Statement: Informed consent was obtained from all subjects involved in the study.

Data Availability Statement: Not applicable.

Conflicts of Interest: The authors declare no conflict of interests.

Appendix A

Questionnaire

1. Have you ever heard of the human papillomavirus (HPV) before?
Select one answer

- Yes
- No
- I don't remember

2. How did you learn about HPV?
Select one answer

- From a social campaign
- From a doctor
- From a leaflet in a medical facility
- From the press or TV
- From friends
- From the Internet

3. How can you get infected with HPV?
You can tick several options

- By kissing
- By touch
- Through sexual intercourse
- During natural childbirth
- By contact of infected blood with the blood of an uninfected person, e.g., using the same needle
- I do not know

4. Who is at risk of HPV infection?
You can tick several options

- Only women

- Only men
- Children
- Only homosexuals
- Both women and men, regardless of sexual orientation
- I do not know

5. HPV infection predisposes to:
You can tick several options

- Cancer of the genitourinary organs (vagina, penis, anus, vulva)
- Cervical cancer
- Head and neck cancer
- Papillary lesions of the genital area
- Respiratory papillomatosis
- I do not know

6. Does HPV infection always lead to the manifestation of the disease?
Select one answer

- Yes
- No
- I do not know

7. Do you know what the purpose of the Pap smear test is?
Select one answer

- Yes
- No
- I do not know

8. What factors increase the risk of developing cervical cancer?

- You can tick several options
- Smoking cigarettes
- A family history of cervical cancer
- HPV infection
- A large number of sexual partners
- Lack of physical activity
- I do not know

9. How can HPV infection be prevented, or the risk of HPV infection be reduced?
You can tick several options

- By vaccination before sexual initiation
- By using condoms
- By limiting the number of sexual partners and by avoiding risky sexual behavior
- It is not possible to prevent HPV infection
- I do not know

10. Is there a vaccine against HPV?
Select one answer

- Yes
- No
- I do not know

11. Is the HPV vaccine available in Poland?
Select one answer

- Yes
- No
- I do not know

12. For which sex are HPV vaccines registered in Poland?
Select one answer

- For women
- For men
- For both women and men
- I do not know

13. The target groups for the vaccine in Poland are:
You can tick several options

- Young women/girls around 12 years old
- Young men/boys around 12 years old
- Young women before sexual initiation
- Young men before sexual initiation
- Young women not infected with HPV
- Young men not infected with HPV
- All women, regardless of age
- All men, regardless of age
- I do not know

14. The scientifically proven AEFI of HPV vaccination include:
Select one answer

- Pain at the site of vaccination and fainting after vaccination
- Autism, ADHD and other central nervous system disorders caused by thiomersal (ethyl mercury compound used as a preservative in the vaccine)
- An anaphylactic reaction in children allergic to proteins connected with the cultivation of vaccine viruses in chicken embryos
- All of the above
- None of the above

15. Does HPV vaccination give 100 percent protection against cervical cancer?
Select one answer

- Yes
- No
- I don't know

16. Is the cost of the vaccine in Poland covered by the government?
Select one answer

- Yes, 100%
- Yes, 50%
- Yes, but I do not know how much is covered by the government
- No
- I do not know

17. What do you think about childhood vaccinations:
Select only one answer

- I believe they are very much needed
- I believe they are unnecessary
- I consider them dangerous to health

18. Do you have a child/children?
Select only one answer

- Yes
- No

19. Please enter the age of the child/children:
If you have more than one child, please state the age of all your children

- Child 1:
- Child 2:
- Child 3:
- Child 4:
- Child 5:

20. Please select the gender of your child (ren)
Please select only one answer per line

- Male Female
- Child 1:
- Child 2:
- Child 3:
- Child 4:
- Child 5:

21. Have you vaccinated your child (ren) with obligatory vaccinations?
Select only one answer

- Yes, I have vaccinated them with all obligatory vaccinations
- Yes, but only with selected vaccinations
- No, neither
- I do not remember

22. Why did you not vaccinate your/their child/children?
Select only one answer

- Because vaccinations are dangerous to your health
- I did not know about such an obligation
- I forgot and the doctor didn't remind me
- Difficult access to medical services

23. Did you vaccinate your child (s) with the vaccines recommended but optional (additionally payable)?
Select only one answer

- Yes
- No
- I do not remember

24. What influenced your decision to vaccinate your child/you with the vaccine recommended but optional?
Select multiple answers

- Opinion about the vaccine on the Internet
- Vaccine safety
- Low price of the vaccine
- The vaccine is highly effective
- Positive doctor's statement about the vaccine
- Opinion of friends about the vaccine

25. Please select the opinion with which you agree.
Select multiple answers

- Vaccinating my child against HPV may contribute to unsafe sexual behavior
- Having my child vaccinated against HPV may contribute to prior sexual initiation
- It would be good to talk to your child about the HPV vaccine as an introduction to a conversation about human sexuality
- I do not agree with any of the above opinions

26. Have you vaccinated your children against HPV?
Select only one answer

- Yes
- No

27. What influenced your decision to vaccinate your child/you with the vaccine against HPV?

Select multiple answers

- Opinion about the vaccine on the Internet
- Vaccine safety
- Low price of the vaccine
- The vaccine is highly effective
- Positive doctor's statement about the vaccine
- Opinion of friends about the vaccine

28. Are you willing to vaccinate your children against HPV? Select only one answer

- Yes
- No
- I do not know yet

29. What factors may influence your decision not to vaccinate yours? Children against HPV?

Select multiple answers

- The high price of the vaccine
- Side effects of the vaccine
- Fear that the vaccine may cause children to engage in risky behavior sexual
- Reluctance to make children aware of human sexuality
- I believe this vaccine is unnecessary
- I believe this vaccine is ineffective
- I believe this vaccine is dangerous to health

30. Would you vaccinate your child against HPV if vaccination was covered by the government?

Select only one answer

- Yes
- No
- I do not know

31. Please enter your gender:

Select only one answer

- Woman
- Man

32. Please enter your age:

33. Please provide your education:

Select only one answer

- Primary
- Vocational
- Secondary
- Higher

34. Size of the place of residence

Select only one answer

- village
- city up to 20,000 inhabitants
- city from 20,000 up to 100,000 inhabitants
- city from 100,000 up to 500,000 inhabitants
- city above 500,000 inhabitants

35. How old are you?
36. Please select your gender:
- Female
- Male

References

1. Bernard, H.-U.; Burk, R.D.; Chen, Z.; van Doorslaer, K.; zur Hausen, H.; de Villiers, E.-M. Classification of papillomaviruses (PVs) based on 189 PV types and proposal of taxonomic amendments. *Virology* **2010**, *401*, 70–79. [CrossRef] [PubMed]
2. Graham, S.V. The human papillomavirus replication cycle, and its links to cancer progression: A comprehensive review. *Clin. Sci.* **2017**, *131*, 2201–2221. [CrossRef]
3. Van Doorslaer, K.; Chen, D.; Chapman, S.; Khan, J.; McBride, A.A. Persistence of an Oncogenic Papillomavirus Genome Requires cis Elements from the Viral Transcriptional Enhancer. *mBio* **2017**, *8*, e01758-17. [CrossRef] [PubMed]
4. Chan, C.K.; Aimagambetova, G.; Ukybassova, T.; Kongrtay, K.; Azizan, A. Human Papillomavirus Infection and Cervical Cancer: Epidemiology, Screening, and Vaccination—Review of Current Perspectives. *J. Oncol.* **2019**, *2019*, 3257939. [CrossRef] [PubMed]
5. Lei, J.; Ploner, A.; Elfström, K.M.; Wang, J.; Roth, A.; Fang, F.; Sundström, K.; Dillner, J.; Sparén, P. HPV Vaccination and the Risk of Invasive Cervical Cancer. *N. Engl. J. Med.* **2020**, *383*, 1340–1348. [CrossRef] [PubMed]
6. de Martel, C.; Plummer, M.; Vignat, J.; Franceschi, S. Worldwide burden of cancer attributable to HPV by site, country and HPV type. *Int. J. Cancer* **2017**, *141*, 664–670. [CrossRef]
7. Cohen, P.A.; Jhingran, A.; Oaknin, A.; Denny, L. Cervical cancer. *Lancet* **2019**, *393*, 169–182. [CrossRef]
8. Jary, A.; Teguete, I.; Sidibé, Y.; Kodio, A.; Dolo, O.; Burrel, S.; Boutolleau, D.; Beauvais-Remigereau, L.; Sayon, S.; Kampo, M.; et al. Prevalence of cervical HPV infection, sexually transmitted infections and associated antimicrobial resistance in women attending cervical cancer screening in Mali. *Int. J. Infect. Dis.* **2021**, *108*, 610–616. [CrossRef]
9. Bruni, L.; Albero, G.; Serrano, B.; Mena, M.; Gómez, D.; Muñoz, J.; Bosch, F.X.; de Sanjosé, S. *Human Papillomavirus and Related Diseases in the World. Summary Report*; ICO/IARC HPV Information Centre: Barcelona, Spain; Lyon, France, 2019.
10. World Health Organization. Human papillomavirus vaccines: WHO position paper, October 2014. *Wkly. Epidemiol. Rec.* **2014**, *39*, 465–491.
11. World Health Organization. Human papillomavirus vaccines: WHO position paper, May 2017. *Wkly. Epidemiol. Rec.* **2017**, *92*, 241–268.
12. Gargano, J.; Meites, E.; Watson, M.; Unger, E.; Markowitz, L. Chapter 5: Human Papillomavirus (HPV). In *Manual for the Surveillance of Vaccine-Preventable Diseases*; Centers for Disease Control and Prevention: Atlanta, GA, USA, 2017.
13. Bruni, L.; Saura-Lázaro, A.; Montoliu, A.; Brotons, M.; Alemany, L.; Diallo, M.S.; Afsar, O.Z.; LaMontagne, D.S.; Mosina, L.; Contreras, M.; et al. HPV vaccination introduction worldwide and WHO and UNICEF estimates of national HPV immunization coverage 2010–2019. *Prev. Med.* **2021**, *144*, 106399. [CrossRef] [PubMed]
14. Agencja Oceny Technologii Medycznych i Taryfikacji. *Profilaktyka Zakażeń Wirusem Brodawczaka Ludzkiego (HPV) w Ramach Programów Polityki Zdrowotnej*; AOTMiT: Warsaw, Poland, 2019.
15. Dubé, E.; Laberge, C.; Guay, M.; Bramadat, P.; Roy, R.; Bettinger, J. Vaccine hesitancy: An overview. *Hum. Vaccines Immunother.* **2013**, *9*, 1763–1773. [CrossRef] [PubMed]
16. Sekhon, M.; Cartwright, M.; Francis, J.J. Acceptability of healthcare interventions: An overview of reviews and development of a theoretical framework. *BMC Health Serv. Res.* **2017**, *17*, 88. [CrossRef] [PubMed]
17. Betsch, C.; Schmid, P.; Korn, L.; Steinmeyer, L.; Heinemeier, D.; Eitze, S.; Küpke, N.K.; Böhm, R. Impfverhalten psychologisch erklären, messen und verändern. *Bundesgesundheitsblatt Gesundh. Gesundh.* **2019**, *62*, 400–409. [CrossRef]
18. López, N.; Garcés-Sánchez, M.; Panizo, M.B.; de la Cueva, I.S.; Artés, M.T.; Ramos, B.; Cotarelo, M. HPV knowledge and vaccine acceptance among European adolescents and their parents: A systematic literature review. *Public Health Rev.* **2020**, *41*, 10. [CrossRef]
19. Alberts, C.J.; van der Loeff, M.F.; Hazeveld, Y.; de Melker, H.E.; van der Wal, M.F.; Nielen, A.; El Fakiri, F.; Prins, M.; Paulussen, T.G. A longitudinal study on determinants of HPV vaccination uptake in parents/guardians from different ethnic backgrounds in Amsterdam, the Netherlands. *BMC Public Health* **2017**, *17*, 220. [CrossRef]
20. Grandahl, M.; Tydén, T.; Westerling, R.; Nevéus, T.; Rosenblad, A.; Hedin, E.; Oscarsson, M. To Consent or Decline HPV Vaccination: A Pilot Study at the Start of the National School-Based Vaccination Program in Sweden. *J. Sch. Health* **2017**, *87*, 62–70. [CrossRef] [PubMed]
21. Borena, W.; Luckner-Hornischer, A.; Katzgraber, F.; Holm-von Laer, D. Factors affecting HPV vaccine acceptance in west Austria: Do we need to revise the current immunization scheme? *Papillomavirus Res.* **2016**, *2*, 173–177. [CrossRef]
22. Oddsson, K.; Gudmundsdottir, T.; Briem, H. Attitudes and knowledge among parents or guardians of 12-year-old girls about HPV vaccination—A population-based survey in Iceland. *Eur. J. Gynaecol. Oncol.* **2016**, *37*, 837–841.
23. Voidăzan, S.; Tarcea, M.; Morariu, S.H.; Grigore, A.; Dobreanu, M. Human Papillomavirus Vaccine—Knowledge and Attitudes among Parents of Children Aged 10–14 Years: A Cross-sectional Study, Tîrgu Mureş, Romania. *Cent. Eur. J. Public Health* **2016**, *24*, 29–38. [CrossRef]

24. Giambi, C.; D'Ancona, F.; Del Manso, M.; De Mei, B.; Giovannelli, I.; Cattaneo, C.; Possenti, V.; Declich, S.; Local Representatives for VALORE. Exploring reasons for non-vaccination against human papillomavirus in Italy. *BMC Infect. Dis.* **2014**, *14*, 545. [CrossRef] [PubMed]
25. Wegwarth, O.; Kurzenhäuser-Carstens, S.; Gigerenzer, G. Overcoming the knowledge-behavior gap: The effect of evidence-based HPV vaccination leaflets on understanding, intention, and actual vaccination decision. *Vaccine* **2014**, *32*, 1388–1393. [CrossRef] [PubMed]
26. Gefenaite, G.; Smit, M.; Nijman, H.W.; Tami, A.; Drijfhout, I.H.; Pascal, A.; Postma, M.J.; Wolters, B.A.; van Delden, J.J.M.; Wilschut, J.C.; et al. Comparatively low attendance during Human Papillomavirus catch-up vaccination among teenage girls in the Netherlands: Insights from a behavioral survey among parents. *BMC Public Health* **2012**, *12*, 498. [CrossRef]
27. Dahlström, L.A.; Tran, T.N.; Lundholm, C.; Young, C.; Sundström, K.; Sparén, P. Attitudes to HPV vaccination among parents of children aged 12–15 years—A population-based survey in Sweden. *Int. J. Cancer* **2010**, *126*, 500–507. [CrossRef] [PubMed]
28. Morison, L.A.; Cozzolino, P.J.; Orbell, S. Temporal perspective and parental intention to accept the human papillomavirus vaccination for their daughter. *Br. J. Health Psychol.* **2010**, *15*, 151–165. [CrossRef] [PubMed]
29. de Visser, R.; McDonnell, E. Correlates of parents' reports of acceptability of human papilloma virus vaccination for their school-aged children. *Sex. Health* **2008**, *5*, 331–338. [CrossRef] [PubMed]
30. Lenselink, C.H.; Gerrits, M.M.; Melchers, W.J.; Massuger, L.F.; van Hamont, D.; Bekkers, R.L. Parental acceptance of Human Papillomavirus vaccines. *Eur. J. Obstet. Gynecol. Reprod. Biol.* **2008**, *137*, 103–107. [CrossRef]
31. Stretch, R.; Roberts, S.A.; McCann, R.; Baxter, D.; Chambers, G.; Kitchener, H.; Brabin, L. Parental attitudes and information needs in an adolescent HPV vaccination programme. *Br. J. Cancer* **2008**, *99*, 1908–1911. [CrossRef]
32. Brabin, L.; Roberts, S.A.; Farzaneh, F.; Kitchener, H.C. Future acceptance of adolescent human papillomavirus vaccination: A survey of parental attitudes. *Vaccine* **2006**, *24*, 3087–3094. [CrossRef]
33. Brabin, L.; Roberts, S.A.; Kitchener, H.C. A semi-qualitative study of attitudes to vaccinating adolescents against human papillomavirus without parental consent. *BMC Public Health* **2007**, *7*, 20. [CrossRef]
34. Gerend, M.A.; Madkins, K.; Phillips, G., II; Mustanski, B. Predictors of Human Papillomavirus Vaccination Among Young Men Who Have Sex With Men. *Sex. Transm. Dis.* **2016**, *43*, 185–191. [CrossRef] [PubMed]
35. Zimet, G.D.; Rosberger, Z.; Fisher, W.A.; Perez, S.; Stupiansky, N.W. Beliefs, behaviors and HPV vaccine: Correcting the myths and the misinformation. *Prev. Med.* **2013**, *57*, 414–418. [CrossRef] [PubMed]
36. Rosenthal, S.L.; Weiss, T.W.; Zimet, G.D.; Ma, L.; Good, M.B.; Vichnin, M.D. Predictors of HPV vaccine uptake among women aged 19–26: Importance of a physician's recommendation. *Vaccine* **2011**, *29*, 890–895. [CrossRef] [PubMed]
37. Laz, T.H.; Rahman, M.; Berenson, A.B. An update on human papillomavirus vaccine uptake among 11–17 year old girls in the United States: National Health Interview Survey, 2010. *Vaccine* **2012**, *30*, 3534–3540. [CrossRef] [PubMed]
38. Ylitalo, K.R.; Lee, H.; Mehta, N.K. Health care provider recommendation, human papillomavirus vaccination, and race/ethnicity in the US National Immunization Survey. *Am. J. Public Health* **2013**, *103*, 164–169. [CrossRef]
39. Gilkey, M.B.; Calo, W.A.; Marciniak, M.W.; Brewer, N.T. Parents who refuse or delay HPV vaccine: Differences in vaccination behavior, beliefs, and clinical communication preferences. *Hum. Vaccines Immunother.* **2017**, *13*, 680–686. [CrossRef] [PubMed]
40. Brabin, L.; Roberts, S.A.; Stretch, R.; Baxter, D.; Elton, P.; Kitchener, H.; McCann, R. A survey of adolescent experiences of human papillomavirus vaccination in the Manchester study. *Br. J. Cancer* **2009**, *101*, 1502–1504. [CrossRef] [PubMed]
41. Fishman, J.; Taylor, L.; Kooker, P.; Frank, I. Parent and Adolescent Knowledge of HPV and Subsequent Vaccination. *Pediatrics* **2014**, *134*, e1049–e1056. [CrossRef]
42. Gerend, M.A.; Lee, S.C.; Shepherd, J.E. Predictors of human papillomavirus vaccination acceptability among underserved women. *Sex. Transm. Dis.* **2007**, *34*, 468–471. [CrossRef]
43. Gamble, H.L.; Klosky, J.L.; Parra, G.R.; Randolph, M.E. Factors Influencing Familial Decision-Making Regarding Human Papillomavirus Vaccination. *J. Pediatr. Psychol.* **2010**, *35*, 704–715. [CrossRef]
44. Marlow, L.A.V.; Waller, J.; Wardle, J. Parental attitudes to pre-pubertal HPV vaccination. *Vaccine* **2007**, *25*, 1945–1952. [CrossRef] [PubMed]
45. Holman, D.M.; Benard, V.; Roland, K.B.; Watson, M.; Liddon, N.; Stokley, S. Barriers to Human Papillomavirus Vaccination Among US Adolescents: A Systematic Review of the Literature. *JAMA Pediatr.* **2014**, *168*, 76–82. [CrossRef] [PubMed]
46. Gulland, A. Drug companies agree to cut price of HPV vaccine to developing countries to increase accessibility. *BMJ Br. Med. J.* **2013**, *346*, f3025. [CrossRef] [PubMed]
47. Anonymous. Price breaks for HPV vaccines may aid prevention. *Cancer Discov.* **2013**, *3*, Of9. [CrossRef]

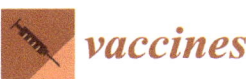

Review

The Efficacy of Therapeutic DNA Vaccines Expressing the Human Papillomavirus E6 and E7 Oncoproteins for Treatment of Cervical Cancer: Systematic Review

Ayazhan Akhatova [1], Chee Kai Chan [2,3], Azliyati Azizan [2,4] and Gulzhanat Aimagambetova [2,*]

[1] School of Medicine, Nazarbayev University, Kabanbay Batyr 53, Nur-Sultan 010000, Kazakhstan; ayazhan.akhatova@nu.edu.kz
[2] Department of Biomedical Sciences, School of Medicine, Nazarbayev University, Kabanbay Batyr 53, Nur-Sultan 010000, Kazakhstan; cchan@kean.edu (C.K.C.); aazizan@touro.edu (A.A.)
[3] Department of Biology, College of Science and Technology, Wenzhou-Kean University, Wenzhou 325000, China
[4] Department of Basic Sciences, College of Osteopathic Medicine, Touro University Nevada, Henderson, NV 89014, USA
* Correspondence: gulzhanat.aimagambetova@nu.edu.kz

Abstract: Cervical cancer is recognized as a serious public health problem since it remains one of the most common cancers with a high mortality rate among women despite existing preventative, screening, and treatment approaches. Since Human Papillomavirus (HPV) was recognized as the causative agent, the preventative HPV vaccines have made great progress over the last few years. However, people already infected with the virus require an effective treatment that would ensure long-term survival and a cure. Currently, clinical trials investigating HPV therapeutic vaccines show a promising vaccine-induced T-cell mediated immune response, resulting in cervical lesion regression and viral eradication. Among existing vaccine types (live vector, protein-based, nucleic acid-based, etc.), deoxyribonucleic acid (DNA) therapeutic vaccines are the focus of the study, since they are safe, cost-efficient, thermostable, easily produced in high purity and distributed. The aim of this study is to assess and compare existing DNA therapeutic vaccines in phase I and II trials, expressing HPV E6 and E7 oncoproteins for the prospective treatment of cervical cancer based on clinical efficacy, immunogenicity, viral clearance, and side effects. Five different DNA therapeutic vaccines (GX-188E, VGX-3100, pNGVL4a-CRT/E7(detox), pNGVL4a-Sig/E7(detox)/HSP70, MEDI0457) were well-tolerated and clinically effective. Clinical implementation of DNA therapeutic vaccines into treatment regimen as a sole approach or in combination with conservative treatment holds great potential for effective cancer treatment.

Keywords: cervical cancer; cervical intraepithelial neoplasia; HPV; E6 oncoprotein; E7 oncoprotein; therapeutic vaccine; DNA vaccine; DNA therapeutic vaccine

1. Introduction

Cervical cancer is a largely preventable cancer of the cervix, which is the narrow part of the lower uterus that connects to the vagina. According to the World Health Organization (WHO) statistics, cervical cancer became the fourth most frequent cancer in women in 2018, with 570,000 cases, which represent 6.6% of all female cancers worldwide [1]. Similarly, cervical cancer is the 2nd most common type of cancer among females, and the 4th most common cause of cancer-related deaths (8.5%) among women in Kazakhstan [1].

Previous studies have established the strong causative association between persistent infection with certain high-risk Human Papillomavirus (HPV) types and the development of cervical cancer [2]. HPV is a small, non-enveloped deoxyribonucleic acid (DNA) tumor virus, which primarily affects human vaginal and oral mucosa [2]. There are more than

100 HPV subtypes, which differ by less than 3% of their genome [3]. The most prevalent oncogenic subtypes in both symptomatic (50–70%) and asymptomatic (20–30%) women diagnosed with invasive cervical cancer are HPV-16 and HPV-18 [3].

About 90% of deaths from cervical cancer occurred in low- and middle-income countries largely due to the lack of proper prevention, early diagnosis, and effective screening [1]. In 2018, WHO started a new campaign to decrease the incidence rate, with the aim to eventually eradicate cervical cancer [4]. The campaign included three key steps, which are vaccination of 90% of girls by 15 years of age, screening provision of 70% of women by 35 years of age and again by 45, and treatment of 90% of women with diagnosed cervical neoplasia [5]. Ideally, if all countries accomplished the requirements of the campaign by 2030, it is expected to decrease the incidence of new cases by 40% and 5 million related deaths by 2050 [1]. However, it is now estimated that the annual number of new cases of cervical cancer would be increasing to 700,000, and the number of deaths would reach 400,000 by 2030 [4]. Such an increase is explained by the uneven provision of screening and vaccination among countries, since these actions have occurred mostly in high-income settings [4]. In high-income countries, screening programs cover 60% of the female population, while, in lower-middle-income countries, the figure is only 20% [4]. Although preventative measures are expected to be effective in the elimination of cervical cancer in the long term, the situation now requires a short-term solution for those already in need of better treatment and care.

Nowadays, early-stage cervical intraepithelial lesions (CIN) are treated by means of surgical resection of cancerous tissue, which include conization, loop electrical excision procedure (LEEP), and radical hysterectomy [6]. These already traumatizing procedures can be coupled with radiotherapy or chemotherapy for the purpose of treatment enhancement and prevention of relapse [6]. Since radiotherapy and cytotoxic chemotherapy target not only cancerous tissue but surrounding tissues as well, patients often suffer constitutional side effects such as fatigue, loss of appetite, nausea, hair loss, or adverse events (AEs) that negatively impact patient's quality of life like anemia, neutropenia, thrombocytopenia, neuropathy, nephro-/hepatotoxicity, premature menopause, and infertility [6]. Therefore, it is necessary to provide less toxic and traumatic treatment options, especially for patients with comorbidities. After surgical excision, quadrivalent HPV vaccination could be used for CIN2+ cervical lesions to reduce the risk of recurrent disease [7].

Therapeutic vaccines such as TheraCys, PROVENGE, and IMLYGIC used for the treatment of urothelial carcinoma in situ, prostate cancer, and advanced melanoma respectively with promising results [8]. These cancer vaccines showed greater median overall survival compared to the conservative chemotherapy approaches, resulting in the United States Food and Drug Administration (FDA) approval [8]. The development of effective therapeutic vaccines for precancerous cervical lesions and cervical cancer treatment and their implementation into clinical practice would be a huge improvement in gynecologic oncology.

Currently, HPV therapeutic vaccines under investigation include live vector vaccines (bacterial and viral vectors), subunit vaccines (peptides and protein-based vaccines), plant peptide/protein-based vaccines, nucleic acid vaccines (DNA and ribonucleic acid (RNA) replicon-based vaccines), and cell-based vaccines (dendritic cell-based vaccines and adoptive cell transfer) [2]. Among these subtypes, we are particularly interested in DNA therapeutic vaccines, since they are safe, cost-efficient, thermostable, easily produced in high purity, and distributed [2]. Unlike live vector vaccines, DNA therapeutic vaccines do not evoke neutralizing antibody production, thus allowing for repeated vaccination [9]. T cell-mediated immune response is achieved by targeting HPV E6 and E7 proteins, as they are solely responsible for the malignant transformation of cervical tissue [9]. Moreover, in a study by Daayana et al., strong adaptive immune responses to E6 and E7 were reported, and it was shown to be greater than previously reported immune responses to therapeutic HPV vaccines [2,10]. Thus, the immunogenicity of DNA vaccines expressing the HPV E6 and E7 oncoproteins needs to be further investigated. Currently, the majority of DNA therapeutic vaccines are undergoing clinical trials to evaluate their safety and stability.

Therefore, the aim of this article is to assess and compare existing DNA therapeutic vaccines, which are evaluated in phase I and II trials, expressing HPV E6 and E7 oncoproteins for the prospective treatment of cervical cancer based on clinical efficacy, immunogenicity, viral clearance, and side effects.

2. Materials and Methods

This systematic review was conducted according to the Preferred Reporting Items for Systematic Reviews (PRISMA) statement [11]. The study was registered in the PROSPERO database and confirmed with a registration code of CRD42021251476.

Systematic Literature Search and Eligibility Criteria

Articles were manually searched using databases as PubMed/MEDLINE, Google Scholar, and clinicaltrials.gov published in English from the year 2010.

The search was performed using the following keywords: "cervical cancer", "cervical intraepithelial neoplasia", "HPV", "HPV-positive", "E6 and E7 oncoproteins", "therapeutic vaccine", "DNA vaccine", and "DNA therapeutic vaccine". We used the medical subject heading (MeSH) term "Uterine Cervical Neoplasms" (MeSH Unique ID D002583) as major topic and "Vaccines" (MeSH Unique ID D014612), "E6 protein, HPV type 18" (MeSH Unique ID C052603) and "E7 protein, HPV type 16" (MeSH Unique ID C059731).

The search was narrowed by using "Cervical cancer OR Cervical Intraepithelial Lesion AND DNA therapeutic vaccines", "DNA therapeutic vaccines AND E6 OR/AND E7 oncoproteins". The selected studies were independently reviewed for inclusion eligibility by two reviewers (Akhatova and Aimagambetova) using standardized data collection forms. The following data were collected from the studies: the author, year of publication, number of study participants, vaccine administration strategies, and the main outcomes (clinical efficacy, viral clearance, immunogenicity, adverse events). Any discrepancy in the assessment of articles was resolved by discussion and consensus, as well as input from the third and fourth reviewers (Chan and Azizan).

The articles were selected to meet the following eligibility requirements to be included in the study: (1) research article, (2) human subject research, and (3) the study of DNA therapeutic vaccines targeting HPV E6 and E7 oncoproteins. The presence of the following did not allow for the study to be included: (1) reviews and case reports, (2) irrelevance to cervical cancer or CIN, (3) mouse model studies, (4) articles on preventative HPV vaccines, and (5) the use of the inappropriate methodology. Abstracts lacking full information about predefined criteria were excluded without further review.

The types of studies included were phase I and phase II clinical trials that were initiated and completed between 2003 and 2017, studying the clinical efficacy of DNA therapeutic vaccines expressing HPV E6 and E7 oncoproteins for the treatment of cervical intraepithelial lesions of grades 2 and 3 both newly diagnosed and recurrent malignancies. The treatment of the lesion may or may not be followed by conization or loop electrosurgical excision procedure. The study population was female patients aged 18 or older with histopathologically diagnosed CIN of grades 2 and 3, known to be caused by HPV 16 and/or HPV 18 based on polymerase chain reaction (PCR) amplification results. The main outcomes of the review were clinical efficacy based on the lesion regression, viral load reduction, immunogenicity, in particular, HPV E6 and E7 specific CD8+ T cell response, and AEs after vaccination.

3. Results

3.1. Study Identification and Selection

During this study, 120 articles were identified through PubMed/MEDLINE and Google Scholar searching platforms (Figure 1).

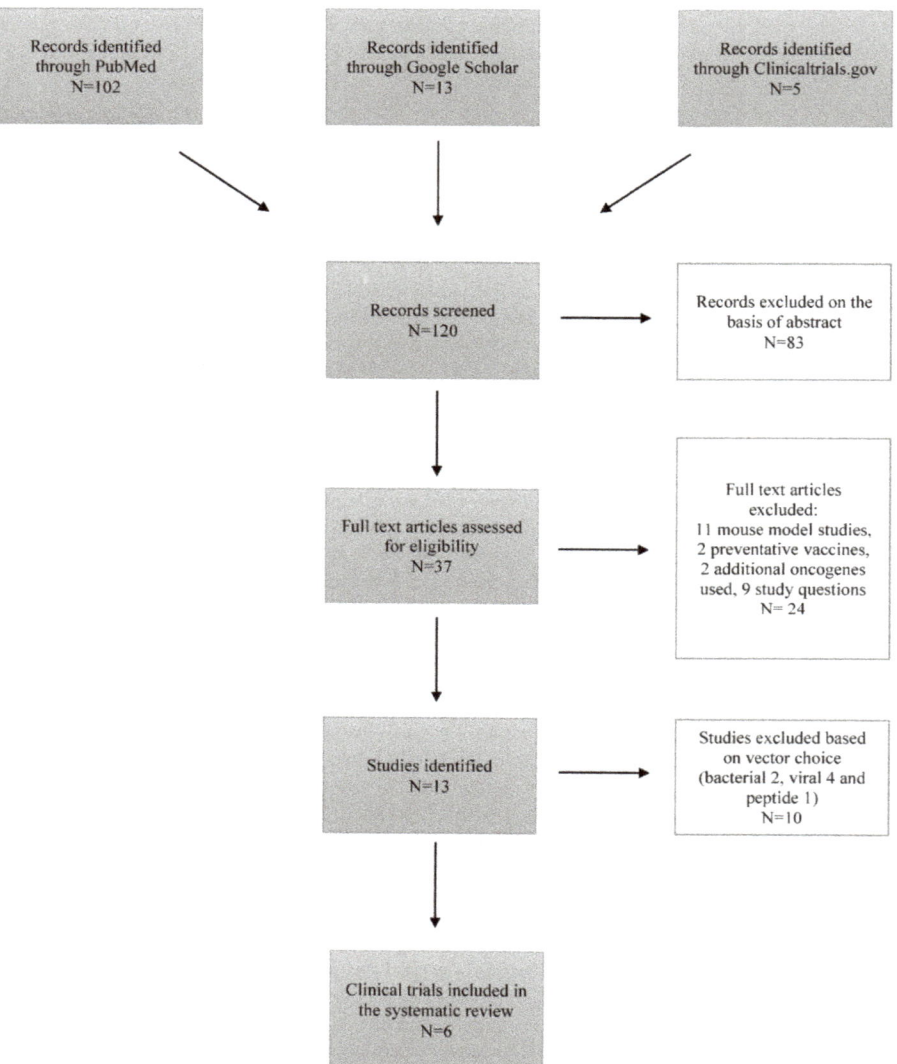

Figure 1. Flow-chart diagram of study selection.

Eighty-three articles were excluded based on the abstract, representing literature reviews. From the remaining 37 articles, 24 articles were excluded at this stage: 11 studies were mouse model-based, 9 studies were not addressing the study question, 2 studies were regarding the preventative vaccines, and 2 studies included additional oncogenes in the development of therapeutic vaccines. We included 6 studies performed between 2003 and 2017 in our systematic review after the exclusion of 7 articles studying the effects of therapeutic vaccines with either viral, bacterial, or peptide vectors [12–17]. These six studies represented the work completed in the United States of America, Korea, Estonia, South Africa, India, Canada, Australia, and Georgia [12–17] (Table 1).

Table 1. Clinical trials.

Vaccine	Trial Design	Pt.(N)	Site/Stage	Study Type	Vaccine Type	Additional Therapies	HPV Positivity Assessment	Study Duration/Location	Study Status	ClinicalTrials.Gov Identifier
GX-188E [12]	Subjects—19–50 years old women with HP diagnosed with CIN3 from an HPV type 16/18 (+), randomly assigned to treatment groups and received either 1 or 4 mg of GX-188E IM by EP in the deltoid muscle. Drug administration was performed 3 × in total during study period at visits 2, 3, and 5 (weeks 0, 4, and 12). At weeks 14 and 20 after the initial GX-188E administration, the efficacy of GX-188E was evaluated by CB and HPV DNA test. After 20 weeks of study, patients were provided with the option of entering the extension study for total of 36 weeks. Primary outcome: the rate of participants with HP regression to CIN ≤ 1 at V7 [13]. Secondary outcome: the rate of participants whose result inverted negative in HPV DNA test, the rate of HPV 16, E7-specific ELISPOT responder, cytological changes of the cervical lesions, the rate of AEs and solicited AEs, data in physical examination, vital signs, ECG, clinical lab test results related to investigational product, mean value of visual analogue scale on pain intensity, Plt-3L serum concentration.	72	CIN 3	Prospective, randomized, multicenter, open-label, phase II trial	HPV 16/E7 DNA therapeutic vaccine (Genexine, Inc.), consisting of a tissue plasminogen activator signal sequence, an FMS- like tyrosine kinase 3 ligand, and shuffled E6 and E7 genes of HPV type 16/18, as described previously	None.	PCR identification	Trial conducted at 4 Korean sites: the Catholic University of Seoul St. Mary's Hospital (Seoul, South Korea), the Cheil Hospital (Seoul, South Korea), the Korea University Guro Hospital (Seoul, South Korea), and the Keimyung University and Dongsan Hospital (Daegu, South Korea) for 36 weeks. Study Start date: July 2014. Study Completion date: March 2016.	Completed.	NCT02139267
GX-188E [13]	Subjects—20–50 year old women with HP diagnosed with HPV16/18-associated CIN3 were vaccinated in a series of three injections IM using EP device in deltoid muscle at weeks 0, 4 and 12. A standard 3+3 dose escalation scheme was followed and dose levels of 1, 2 and 4 mg (2 + 2 mg) were tested within 36 weeks of follow up. Primary outcome: determination ofMTD, clinical lab test results, vital signs. Secondary outcome: the expression levels of GX-188E in blood, immunologic reactogenicity by measuring HPV 16 and E7-specific T cell response by ELISPOT, and changes of the involved lesions and HPV infection status.	11	CIN 3	Open label, single center, dose-escalation, phase I study	A plasmid DNA encoding E6 and E7 proteins of HPV 16 or E7 genes fragmented into two parts (C-terminal and N-terminal regions) with a small overlapping sequence (encoding 16 amino acids). The fused DNA sequences including tpa, Flt3L and shuffled E6/E7 genes were inserted in high expression vector, pGX27 produced in E. coli DH5alpha under cGMP condition.	None.	PCR identification.	Cheil General Hospital & Women's Healthcare Center, Seoul, Korea for total of 36 weeks. Study start date: November 2012. Study Completion Date: February 2014.	Completed.	NCT01634503
VGX-3100 [14]	Subjects—18–55 years old women with HP confirmed HPV 16/18-positive CIN 2/3 randomized to receive 6 mg VGX-3100 (3 mg plasmid targeting HPV 16 E6 and E7, and 3 mg plasmid targeting HPV 18 E6 and E7) or placebo (1 mL), given IM at weeks 0, 4, and 12 weeks, followed by EP with CELLECTRA-5P. Randomization was stratified by age (<25 and >25 years) and CIN2 vs. CIN3. Primary outcome: number of participants with HP regression to CIN1 or normal pathology 36 weeks after first dose. Secondary outcome: number of participants with virologically proven clearance of HPV 16 or 18 in combination with HP regression of cervical lesions to ≤CIN1.	167	CIN 2/3	Multicentre, randomized, double-blind, placebo-controlled phase 2b trial with masked endpoint acquisition and adjudication.	Two DNA plasmids encoding optimised synthetic consensus E6 and E7 genes of HPV-16 and HPV-18, using a proprietary design strategy, SynCon (Inovio Pharmaceuticals, Plymouth Meeting, PA, USA).	At the week 36 primary endpoint visit, patients with colposcopic evidence of residual disease underwent standard therapeutic resection.	Linear Array HPV assay (Roche, Basel, Switzerland).	Trial conducted at 36 academic centres and private gynaecology practices in the USA, Estonia, South Africa, India, Canada, Australia, and Georgia. Study Start date: April 2011. Study Completion date: April 2015.	Completed.	NCT01304524
pNGVL4a-CRTE7(detox) [15]	Subjects ≥ 19 years old women with HP confirmed HPV16 associated CIN 2/3 were enrolled and administered pNGVL4a-CRT-E7(detox) by either PMED/IM, or IL injection at study weeks 0, 4 and 8. LEEP or cold knife conization was performed at week 15. Patients were assessed for the safety and feasibility of vaccine administration, the clinical response, and the induction of an immune response to the vaccine antigen. Primary outcome: the feasibility and toxicity of vaccination in women with CIN2/3 caused by HPV16, evaluate the effect of vaccination on histology, comparison of immunogenicity of three different routes of administration: PMED, IM, and IL. Secondary outcome: changes in HPV VL, cellular immune response, humoral immune response, local tissue immune response, and correlated measures of immune response.	132	CIN2/3	Interventional, non-randomized, open label, phase I study	pNGVL4a expression vector containing coding sequences for HPV16 E7 linked to CRT. The E7 sequence in this construct has been modified at aa24 and 27, which abrogates its transforming potential. CRTis a 46 kDa calcium-binding chaperonin related to the family of HSПs.	A standard therapeutic resection of the cervical squamocolumnar junction (either a cold knife conization or a LEEP) was performed at study week 15, seven weeks after the third vaccination.	HPV16-specific TaqMan kinetic PCR amplification.	University of Alabama at Birmingham, Johns Hopkins Outpatient Center, Johns Hopkins Bayview Medical Center (US). Study start date: September 2009. Study Completion date: July 2016.	Completed.	NCT00988559

Table 1. Cont.

Vaccine	Pt.(N)	Site/Stage	Study Type	Trial Design	Vaccine Type	Additional Therapies	HPV Positivity Assessment	Study Duration/Location	Study Status	Clinicaltrials.Gov Identifier
pNGVL4a-Sig/E7(detox)/HSP70 [16]	16	CIN2/3	Intervent, single-site, open label, phase I dose escalation study	Subjects–18–50 years old women with HP confirmed HPV16 + CIN2/3 received 3 vaccinations with 1 of 3 doses of study vaccine, 0.5, 1.0, or 3.0 mg IM at weeks 0, 4, and 8, and standard therapeutic resection of the cervical SCJ at week 15. *Primary outcome:* the feasibility and toxicity of pNGVL4a-Sig/E7(detox)/HSP70 DNA vaccine in preventing the cervical cancer in HPV16+ CIN2/3; the effect of the vaccine on the histology of cervical tissue specimens from these patients. *Secondary outcome:* the changes in lesion size and HPV VL, cellular, humoral, and local tissue immune responses, correlated measures of immune response with clinical response, correlated response with those observed in the preclinical model.	A closed circular DNA plasmid expressing HPV16 E7 mutated at aa 24 and 26, linked to coding for Sig and HSP70.	Patients underwent standard cone or LEEP resection of the SCJ at week 15, and had a postoperative exam at week 19.	HPV16-specific TaqMan real-time PCR method.	Sidney Kimmel Comprehensive Cancer Center at Johns Hopkins. *Study Start date:* November 2003. *Study Completion date:* January 2010.	Completed.	NCT00121173
MEDI0457 (INO-3112) [7]	10	SCC, AC, or ASCC of the cervix, stage IB-IVB	Intervent, non-randomized, open label, phase 1/2a study	Subjects–18–70 years old women with inoperable cervical cancer, stage IB-IVB, HPV16/18+. Patients were stratified into 2 cohorts: (1) newly diagnosed cancers; (2) persistent or recurrent cervical cancer. After chemoradiation, patients received MEDI0457 immediately followed by EP with the CELLECTRA 5P device given every 4 weeks for a total of 4 doses. *Primary outcome:* safety and tolerability of immunotherapy with MEDI0457 when delivered IM followed by EP in study patients. *Secondary outcome:* cellular and humoral immune responses to HPV 16/18 E6/E7 and treatment response as measured by clinical examination and PET/CT imaging after CRT and DNA vaccination.	Combined plasmids encoding modified, nonconcogenic E6 and E7 viral oncoproteins of HPV16 and HPV18 (VGX-3100) with a plasmid encoding IL-12 (INO-9012).	CRT must have been completed within 10 weeks of initiation. Intracavitary or interstitial brachytherapy was delivered weekly. Weekly cisplatin chemotherapy (40 mg/m²) was administered on day 1 of EBRT and given during weeks 1 to 5 of standard EBRT and during the parametrial boost.	ThinPrep testing for HPV PCR amplification.	University of Chicago Medical Center, University of Michigan, Columbia University Medical Center. *Study Start date:* June 2014. *Study Completion date:* September 2017.	Completed.	NCT02172911

Abbreviations: histopathological—HP; intramuscularly—IM; electroporation—EP; cervical biopsy—CB; adverse events—AEs; maximum tolerated dose—MTD; particle-mediated epidermal delivery—PMED; cervical intralesional—IL; positron emission tomography—PET; computer tomography—CT; calreticulin—CRT; heat shock proteins—HSPs; squamocolumnar junction—SCJ; viral load—VL; chemoradiotherapy—CRT; squamous cell carcinoma—SCC; adenocarcinoma—AC; adenosquamous cell carcinoma—ASCC; loop electrosurgical excision procedure—LEEP; external beam radiation therapy—EBRT.

Therapeutic vaccines were evaluated based on clinical efficacy (histopathological regression of the lesion to CIN < 1), viral clearance, immunogenicity, and adverse events after the vaccination. Subjects, female patients aged 18 or older with histopathologically diagnosed cervical intraepithelial neoplasia of grades 2 and 3, known to be caused by HPV 16 and/or HPV 18, received DNA therapeutic vaccines in different dose formulations and were evaluated generally within 20 weeks (36 weeks in extended trial groups) for the effects of vaccines mentioned above. Study populations ranged from 10 patients to 167, median age mostly being 21–30, except for Hasan et al. (2020) study, where the median age of participants was 51.50 years old due to more advanced stages of cancer [17].

3.2. Outcomes

3.2.1. Clinical Efficacy

Clinical efficacy was evaluated according to the histopathological regression to CIN $\leq$1, which is less than one-third of the thickness of the cervical epithelium, on a colposcopy-guided biopsy 15, 20, or 36 weeks after the first injection. All six studies [12–17] report tumor size decrease to some extent (Table 2).

GX-188 E in phase I trial by Kim et al. [13] showed a 78% success rate of complete response both histologically and virologically. The same vaccine in the phase II trial by Choi et al. (2019) resulted in histopathological regression to CIN < 1 in 52% of patients 20 weeks and 67% of patients 36 weeks after the first dose [12]. MEDI0457 by Hasan et al. showed 87.5% of complete response to the vaccine and 1 patient had a partial response to the treatment [17]. pNGVL4a-CRT/E7(detox) [15] and pNGVL4a-Sig/E7(detox)/HSP70 [16] vaccines both showed a similar response rate of around 30%.

3.2.2. Viral Load Clearance

Viral load was measured by means of PCR amplification to assess the clearance of HPV DNA from the cervical biopsy after vaccination. Choi et al. established that HPV clearance was associated with the histopathologic regression as 77% of regressors had no trace of HPV DNA, while only 12% of non-regressors had no viral load in the tissue biopsy [12]. Kim et al. results show that GX-188E takes time to clear off the virus [13]. MEDI0457 [17] and VGX-3100 [14] report the association between viral clearance and tumor size reduction, whilst pNGVL4a-CRT/E7(detox) [15] did not result in any difference between pre- and post-treatment viral load.

3.2.3. Immunogenicity

Immunogenicity is one of the key features of the therapeutic vaccines as it represents the potential of the vaccine to induce virus-specific T cell response, in particular HPV E6 and E7 specific CD8+ T cell immune response. IFN-γ response was measured by means of *ex vivo* ELISpot assay with cryopreserved and thawed peripheral blood mononuclear cells (PBMCs) at pre- and post-treatment stages. The vaccine response is considered positive when the increase in T-cell frequency was at least three times greater compared to the study entry measurement. GX-188E both in phase I [13] and phase II [12] studies showed a significant increase in IFN-γ response, which was correlated with the histopathologic regression and viral clearance. Moreover, an E6 specific response was more pronounced than E7 specific [12,13]. VGX-3100 induced 9.5 times greater IFN-γ response in the treatment group compared to the placebo, which lasted as long as 24 weeks post-vaccination [14]. On the contrary, MEDI0457 induced a greater response to E7, particularly in newly diagnosed cohort 1 that persisted up to 48 weeks [17]. In cohort 1, 4 of 7 patients exhibited IFNγ-producing spots exceeding 100 SFU/10^6 PBMC, whereas no patients produced similar responses in cohort 2 [17]. pNGVL4a-CRT/E7(detox) and pNGVL4a Sig/E7(detox)/HSP70 showed minimal dose-dependent immune response, which was remarkable from the unvaccinated group [15,16].

Table 2. Comparison of the trials' results.

Vaccine	Clinical Efficacy (Histopathology, Colposcopy, Tumor Size)	Viral Clearance	Immunogenicity (E6 and E7 Specific CTL Activity)	Adverse Events/Toxicity	Additional Findings	Limitations
GX-188E, [12]	HP regression to CIN < 1 in 33/64 patients (52%) at V7, and 35/52 (67%) at V8 (Visit 8, week 36). Lesions that cover <50% showed better efficacy than the ones >50% after GX-188E injection, 63% vs. 41% (V7; χ2 test; P 14 0.133.	Of the patients with HP regression, 73%, (24/33) exhibited HPV clearance at V7 and 77% (27/35) exhibited clearance at V8. Of the nonresponders, 16% (5/31) exhibited HPV clearance at V7 (Visit 7, week 20) and 12% (2/17) exhibited clearance at V8. HPV clearance and HP regression were significantly associated at the V7 (OR 14 13.867; 95% confidence interval (CI), 4.070—47.249; $p < 0.001$] and V8 visits (OR 14 25.313; 95% CI, 4.750–14.883; $p < 0.001$).	A higher percentage of patients (16/25) with HP regression exhibited >3-fold increase in IFN-γ ELISpot responses compared with the group without HP regression (χ^2 test (P 14 0.028), but 7 of 22 nonresponders developed more than 3-fold increase in these responses. Patients with HPV clearance (n 14 26) presented significant increases in IFN-γ ELISpot responses compared with those without clearance (n 14 21; fold changes were 28 and 10, respectively; t test; P 14 0.002).	GX-188E: well- tolerated. The AEs relating to the injection site-pain, erythema, induration, and swelling/edema in both groups; pain was the most common AE (occurring in 94.4% and 100.0% in the 1 and 4 mg GX-188E groups, respectively). One patient was lost to follow up due to pregnancy (1 mg GX-188E group).	HPV sequence variants: HP regression in 42% (11/26) of the CIN3 patients with HPV variants, whereas 75% (12/16) occurred in those without any of the three variants. 1 vs. 4 mg: 1 mg was found to have better efficacy at V7 and V8, (χ2 test; P 14 0.006 and P 14 0.027, respectively) HLA types: HLA- A02 was associated with HP regression at V7 (20 weeks after the first injection; P 14 0.032; OR 14 2.381; 95% CI, 1.064–5.327), but not at V8 (36 weeks after the first injection, P 14 0.404; OR 14 1.490; 95% CI, 0.582–3.811.	Lack of control / placebo group. The selection bias-patients recruited into the study were diagnosed with CIN 3 only. The attrition bias-20/72 participants withdrew from the study due to various reasons. The confirmation bias—in the discussion part, authors concluded that immunologic response and HP regression had weak association. However, earlier in the results they mentioned an association between HP regression and systemic immune response.
GX-188E [13]	At 8 weeks post last vaccination (VFI). 6/9 patients were free of lesions—2 patients from each cohort (A01 and A03 from 1 mg cohort, A05 and A06 from 2 mg cohort, A07 and A08 from 4mg cohort). GX-188E vaccination led to the clinically and virologically meaningful complete response rate of 78% (7/9).	At week 12, 5/9 patients showed viral clearance. At week 20, 6/9 patients showed viral clearance. At week 36, 7/9 patients showed viral clearance.	All subjects exhibited a marked increase in the vaccine- induced E6- and E7-specific IFN-g ELISPOT response compared with the background level before vaccination. Vaccine-induced cellular immune responses became progressively stronger in all patients during GX-188E vaccination. The response against the E6 antigen was more vigorous than against E7 as determined by the magnitude of response (69–89% against E6 versus 11–31% against E7 at VFI). GX-188E: vaccination-induced E6/E7-specific memory T-cell response can be maintained for at least 24 weeks post vaccination. Apart from patient A04, GX-188E vaccine elicited activation of both HPV16-specific CD4 and CD8 T cells. The amount of Th1 effector cytokines, such as IFN-γ, IL-2 and tumour necrosis factor α (TNF-α) increased after vaccination in most of the patients (median 49.9·, 13·- and 22.9·-fold increases for IFN-γ, IL-2, and TNF-α, respectively).	AEs associated with GX-188E: vaccination–chills, injection site pain, swelling and hypoaesthesia in 19/49 patients. AEs–headache, rhinitis and fatigue in 7/49 of the cases could be potentially associated with the vaccine.	6/7 responders carrying HLA-A*02 exhibited high polyfunctional CD8+ T-cell responses as well as complete regression of CIN3. Among the two non-responders, patient A04 with HLA-A*26 and -A*30 did not induce HPV-specific CD8+ T-cell responses at all.	Too small study population, which does not allow for generalization of the results and drawing conclusions. No stratification by age, ethnicity, monoinfection/mixed infection. Randomization or masking of the population was not introduced as well. No control group. All patients had CIN 3 – both severe dysplasia and carcinoma in situ The confirmation bias)-no consideration of spontaneous regression.
VGX-3100 [14]	HP regression in 53/107 patients (49.5%) in treatment group, 11/36 (30.6%) in placebo group; (PPD) 19.0, 95% CI 1.4-36.6; $p = 0.034$). Modified intention-to-treat analyses: HP regression in 55/114 patients (48.2%) in treatment group, 12/40 (30%) in placebo group, (percentage point difference 18.2, 1·3–34·4; $p = 0.034$) Post-hoc efficacy analyses: HP regression to normal in 43/107 patients (40.2%) in treatment group, 6/36 (16.7%) of placebo recipients (PPD 23.5, 95% CI 4.4–37.0; $p = 0.012$).	Viral clearance occurred in 56/107 patients (52.3%) in treatment group, 9/35 (25.7%) in placebo group (percentage point difference 26·6, 95% CI 6·8–42·2; $p = 0.006$). Among those with HP regression, viral clearance was more likely among VGX-3100 recipients (about 80%) than among placebo recipients (about 50%).	In post-hoc immunological analyses, T-cell responses to HPV-16 and HPV-18 E6 and E7 peaked at week 14 for VGX-3100 recipients, with 9.5 times greater median response than in placebo ($p < 0.001$). VGX-3100 elicited significantly increased frequencies of antigen-specific, activated CD8+ T cells, identified by cell surface expression of CD137, that also expressed perforin compared with placebo ($p = 0.001$). VGX-3100 recipients with HP regression and viral clearance developed antibody responses to both HPV-16 and HPV-18 E7 that were significantly higher than for non-responders, at the time of peak response (post-dose 3) but also as early as post-dose 2 and as late as weeks 24.	Injection site erythema—88/125, 78.4% in treatment group, 57.1% in placebo group. 4 patients discontinued due to AEs— 2 injection site pain, 1 muscoluapapular reaction, 1 allergic reaction. No serious AEs reported.	None	Skewing of the population towards more severe disease and older age. 92.8% of the participants had genotypes of HPV 16+ at the entry. The attrition bias-18 patients in treatment group and 6 patients in control group were excluded from the study due to different reasons. HPV genotyping, which was based on the cervical swabs, included the possibility of only HPV16 or/and HPV18. Therefore, mixed infection study group could be underestimated. The confirmation bias-Vaccination induced HP regression and viral clearance in about 40% of women with CIN2/3 positive for HPV-16 or HPV-18, whereas surgical excision would have eliminated the dysplastic tissue in 85–90% of women.

Table 2. *Cont.*

Vaccine	Clinical Efficacy (Histopathology, Colposcopy, Tumor Size)	Viral Clearance	Immunogenicity (E6 and E7 Specific CTL Activity)	Adverse Events/Toxicity	Additional Findings	Limitations
pNGVL4a-CRT/E7(detox) [13]	HP regression in 8/32 patients (30%). Remaining 70% of patients had persistent CIN 2/3. • 1 patient had regression to CIN1. • 7 patients had no residual CIN.	No differences between pre- and post-vaccination viral loads in any of the treatment cohorts.	Immune response to E7 was minimal and was not significantly different than response to E6. Intraepithelial CD8+ T cell infiltrates increased after vaccination in intralesional administration cohort ($p = 0.013$).	Total vaccine specific AEs in 22/32 patients (69%). 50% of IM vaccination patients, 80% of PMED patients, and 75% of intralesional vaccination patients experienced AEs. Most common—constitutional and injection site grade 1 or less AEs. No grade 3 or 4 AEs. No vaccine-related serious AEs. 1 bleeding after LEEP, 3 pregnancies unrelated to vaccine.	None	This was a small phase 1 trial designed to primarily evaluate the feasibility and safety of pNGVL4a-CRT/E7(detox). Only HPV 16 positive CIN patients were included in the study. The majority of these patients were Caucasians. Patients were required to have a hemoglobin of 9 g/dL or greater. The selection bias-anemia is considered strong prognostic factor. The ND10 PMED has a reduced number of components to ease large-scale manufacturability, compared to previously used ND5.5. This could potentially lead to discrepancies in results due to device error.
pNGVL4a-Sig/E7(detox)/HSP70 [4]	No HP progression was observed. 3/9 patients (33%) had complete histologic regression of disease at week 15 in the highest dose cohort.	NA	E7 specific T cell response was identified in 3/15 patients: • 1 patient-response increased subsequent to vaccination at week 15 • 1 patient-stable response • 1 patient-declined response. E6 specific T cell response: 5/15 patients. Overall, responses to E6 were not of greater absolute magnitude in regressors compared with non-regressors at either of the two time points. ($p = 0.4228$ and $p = 0.4994$, respectively). At 6 months response to E7 was detected in 5/9 patients (55.6%) in highest dose cohort.	Transient local reactogenicity was reported in 5/15 (33%). Systemic symptoms (malaise, myalgia, headaches) after vaccination were also reported by 5/15 subjects. No dose-limiting toxicities were observed.	None	This was a small phase 1 study—15 patients only. No masking. Follow up period was 19 weeks, whereas the average follow-up period in selected studies was 36 weeks. Vaccine targets specifically HPV16 E7 oncoprotein, without HPV 18, or E6 oncoprotein. Local and systemic AEs were assessed by patients, which may result in self-reporting bias such as social desirability or recall bias.
MEDI0457 [17]	All cohort 1 patients remain alive with no evidence of disease clinically or by PET/CT. Of the cohort 2 patients: • 1 died • 1 had persistent disease • 1 remains free of disease. The estimated PFS at 12 months was 88.9% overall, 100% in cohort 1, and 50% in cohort 2. 7/8 patients achieved a complete response (6/7 in cohort 1 and 1/3 in cohort 2), and 1 (cohort 1) achieved partial response (decreased or stable hypermetabolic activity after CRT+MEDI0457) after completion of the immunization series.	All patients cleared detectable HPV DNA at week 16 after immunizations. 5/6 patients cleared HPV RNA by in situ hybridization at the completion of immunization.	8 patients had detectable cellular or humoral immune responses after chemoradiation and MEDI0457. 6 patients showed increased IFN-γ responses over baseline against HPV16 E6 and E7. 5 patients showed increased IFN-γ responses against HPV16 E6 and E7. Anti-HPV responses were numerically greater in cohort 1 (23.3 SFU/10^6 PBMC to 369 SFU/10^6 PBMC) compared to cohort 2 (6.7 SFU/10^6 PBMC to 63.3 SFU/10^6 PBMC). 6/10 patients exhibited de novo sero-responses to HPV16 antigens, and 6/10 patients exhibited de novo sero-responses to HPV18 antigens.	Vaccine related AEs in 8 patients-grade 1 injection site bruising (n = 2), injection site pain (n = 2). Treatment related AEs occurred in 8 patients, mainly grades 1 or 2. Grade >3 AEs in 4 patients–abdominal pain and pneumonia in cohort 1; pathologic fracture, anemia, intestinal perforation (grade 5). AEs were followed after chemoradiation and 3 doses of INO3112.	Expression of PD-L1 on panCK+ tumor cells, CD68+ macrophages, and CD8+ T cells in serial biopsy specimens: • post-CRT and post-CRT+MEDI0457 showed decreased epithelial cells, consistent with tumor regression. • PD-L1 was detectable on panCK+ tumor cells and CD68+ cells at pre-CRT and post-CRT biopsies. • PD-L1 was detectable on CD8+ T cells. Compared with pre-CRT and post-CRT time points, post-CRT β MEDI0457 biopsies were associated with decreased PD-L1+CD8+, PD-L1+CD8+, and PD-L1+CD68+ subpopulations.	Too small study (n = 10) population, which does not allow for generalization of the results and drawing conclusions. Study included several histologic diagnoses–squamous cell carcinoma, adenocarcinoma, adenosquamous cell carcinoma of the cervix with various prognosis. The confirmation bias-patients received a vaccine 2 to 4 weeks after chemoradiation, which could impact the vaccine effect on organism. It is unclear whether longer period of recovery would result in better outcome. Dosing and timing regimen of MEDI0457 was based on studies of preinvasive cancer, thus the applicability of the regimen for invasive cancer types is questionable [1]. There was no control group of "chemoradiation only" in order to assess the sole effect of vaccination.

Abbreviations: —histopathological-HP; percentage point difference—PPD; progression—free survival—PFS; positron emission tomography—PET; computer tomography—CT; adverse events—AEs; particle-mediated epidermal delivery—PMED; human leukocyte antigens-HLA; chemoradiotherapy—CRT; —intramuscularly—IM; electroporation—EP; cervical biopsy—CB; maximum tolerated dose—MTD; cervical intralesional—C-RT; calreticulin—IL; heat shock proteins—HSPs; squamocolumnar junction—SCJ; viral load—VL.

3.2.4. Toxicity/Adverse Events

Overall, all vaccines were well-tolerated without vaccine-related serious adverse events. The most common adverse events were injection site pain and erythema, as well as constitutional symptoms (malaise, myalgia, and headache) [12–17]. No serious adverse events (Grade 3/4) related to the vaccination were reported. No dose-limiting toxicities were observed.

4. Discussion

This systematic review summarizes the findings of phase I and phase II clinical trials investigating the treatment of patients with histopathologically diagnosed CIN associated with HPV 16 or/and HPV 18 with DNA therapeutic vaccines. Six studies have demonstrated immunologic response in the form of lesion size regression, viral clearance, and increased T cell response of five different DNA vaccines–GX-188E (phase I and phase II), VGX-3100, pNGVL4a-CRT/E7 (detox), pNGVL4a-Sig/E7 (detox)/HSP70, MEDI0457. Vaccines were plasmid DNA encoding for either non-oncogenic E6/E7 or both, and chaperonin proteins such as HSP 70 and Calreticulin for the enhancement of the uptake by antigen-presenting cells, and MHC class I processing and presentation. MEDI0457 [17] had the same plasmid formulation as VGX-3100 [14] combined with plasmid encoding IL-12. All vaccines were well tolerated by patients, leading to only grade 1 or less systemic and local side effects.

Previous reviews have studied various existing therapeutic vaccines including live vectors, plant-based, protein, whole cell, and combinatorial vaccines [18]. This is the first systematic review of DNA therapeutic vaccines against cervical cancer expressing HPV16 and HPV18 E6 and E7 oncogenes. The feasibility of production, storage, and transportation, cost-effectiveness, the capability of multiple immunizations, and targeting different co-stimulatory genes provided the rationale for the study of DNA therapeutic vaccines [18]. However, comparatively weak immunogenicity and the risk of integration into the host genome are the main concerns, which could be addressed by modification of E6 and E7 to abolish its transformative capacity [18]. There are approaches of boosting the potency of DNA vaccines, such as increasing the number of antigen-expressing dendritic cells (DCs) by using a gene gun delivery method, enhancing antigen processing and presentation in dendritic cells via codon optimization, and improving the DCs and T-cell interaction [18]. These strategies were used in our selected studies, which led to increased antigen-specific, activated CD8+ T cell response in all of them. Patients with CIN2/3 were more likely to induce E6 and E7 specific CD8+ immune response, according to the IFNgamma ELISPOT results, compared to the invasive cervical cancer [17]. According to Hasan et al., diminished immune response in more advanced disease stages is associated with immune exhaustion, the effect of chemoradiation and selection of patients with diminished immunity against HPV [17]. The strongest evidence of the immunogenicity of DNA therapeutic vaccine VGX-3100 was observed by the increased intensity of CD8+ infiltrates in histopathologically regressed patients compared to the placebo group with regressed lesions [14].

DNA therapeutic vaccines were also assessed based on their clinical efficacy, i.e., the ability to induce cervical lesion regression. The regression to $\leq$CIN1 among study participants was observed in all studies with significantly varying degrees. The study of VGX-3100 vaccine with both treatment and placebo groups showed a response rate of 49.5% vs. 30.6%, respectively [14]. Meanwhile, GX-188E vaccine has resulted in histopathological regression in 67% of patients in both phase I study and phase II studies [12,13]. Choi et al. [12] have observed an enhanced response to GX-188E over time up to 83% among those with cervical lesions <50%, probably due to the enhanced memory T cell-driven therapeutic effect. The difference in clinical benefit between VGX-3100 and GX-188E could be explained with the recruitment of CIN3 HPV-positive patients only, the lack of placebo group, and the small number of participants in the latter. pNGVL4a-CRT/E7 (detox) and pNGVL4a-Sig/E7 (detox)/HSP70 had the lowest clinical efficacy of approximately 30% response rate among all [15,16]. However, the effect of these two vaccines on the lesion regression is questionable, as this rate is similar to spontaneous remission rate over a 15-week period [15].

It was established that women, after excision of the cervical lesion, are more likely to have a relapse; therefore, viral clearance is a key factor of vaccine efficacy [18]. VGX-3100, GX-188E, and MEDI0457 effectively cleared detectable HPV DNA, which was significantly associated with histopathological regression [12–14,17]. In contrast, pNGVL4a-CRT/E7 (detox) has not resulted in viral load reduction [15].

Nevertheless, there are several limitations to this study. Firstly, limited data exist on the topic of DNA therapeutic vaccines, as not a single therapeutic vaccine against cervical cancer was approved. All these clinical trials were in either the phase I or phase II stage of assessing the efficacy and safety in humans. Secondly, the majority of studies enrolled a small number of participants without masking, stratification, or the control group, which poses a potential risk for bias. As vaccines investigated in this study had different structural designs, it was not feasible to make a statistical analysis of vaccine outcomes; therefore, qualitative analysis was performed overall.

5. Conclusions

As it was stated by WHO, a global strategy to accelerate the elimination of cervical cancer, 90–70–90 targets for prevention, screening, and treatment are the key to success. Preventative bivalent and quadrivalent HPV vaccines have undergone significant advancement in development and implementation. However, these preventative vaccines do not elicit a therapeutic effect but could be used as an adjuvant to surgical treatment. DNA therapeutic vaccines represent a potentially safe and novel approach to cervical cancer treatment. The main goal of this review was to discuss the effectiveness of existing DNA therapeutic vaccines against cervical cancer expressing HPV 16/18 oncoproteins E6 and E7. The idea of DNA therapeutic vaccines is inducing an adaptive immune response and immunologic memory via the expression of tumor antigens and activation of antigen-presenting cells.

DNA therapeutic vaccines are currently undergoing clinical trials to improve the potency of therapeutic vaccines and clinical efficacy using strategies as a modifying route of administration, adjuvant therapy, prime-boost regimen, and co-administering with other drugs for a synergistic effect. Nowadays, despite the treatment of locally advanced disease with chemoradiation, patients have a high recurrence rate and a poor 5-year survival rate, estimated at 50% and 70%, respectively. In contrast, the MEDI0457 vaccine, which contained VGX-3100 plasmid coupled with an IL-12 expression plasmid to promote T-cell function, evaluated the disease progression-free survival (PFS) at 12 months, which was estimated as 88.9% overall. These findings strengthen the hypothesis that DNA therapeutic vaccines could effectively induce *de novo* or boost existing immune responses. Moreover, studies have shown that using femtosecond laser treatment could also improve transfection efficiency administered intradermally and into the lesion *in vivo*. Thus, continuous efforts to improve the efficacy of DNA therapeutic vaccines and implementation of therapeutic vaccines into a treatment regimen as a sole approach or in combination with conservative treatment may greatly improve the current situation.

Author Contributions: A.A. (Ayazhan Akhatova)—data collection; A.A. (Ayazhan Akhatova) and G.A.—compiled, analyzed, and reviewed the data. A.A. (Ayazhan Akhatova) and G.A. prepared the manuscript draft. C.K.C. and A.A. (Azliyati Azizan) reviewed the final manuscript. All authors reviewed and approved the final article. All authors have read and agreed to the published version of the manuscript.

Funding: There is no funding source to declare.

Institutional Review Board Statement: Due to the nature of the study (systematic review), ethical approval is not required.

Informed Consent Statement: Not applicable.

Data Availability Statement: The datasets used and/or analyzed during the current study available from the corresponding author on reasonable request.

Acknowledgments: The authors would like to acknowledge the Nazarbayev University School of Medicine for the support that enabled the completion of this review.

Conflicts of Interest: The authors have no conflict of interest to declare.

References

1. World Health Organization. Cervical Cancer. Available online: https://www.who.int/health-topics/cervical-cancer#tab=tab_1 (accessed on 21 September 2021).
2. Chabeda, A.; Yanez, R.J.R.; Lamprecht, R.; Meyers, A.E.; Rybicki, E.P.; Hitzeroth, I.I. Therapeutic vaccines for high-risk HPV-associated diseases. *Papillomavirus Res.* **2018**, *5*, 46–58. [CrossRef] [PubMed]
3. Ibeanu, O.A. Molecular pathogenesis of cervical cancer. *Cancer Biol. Ther.* **2011**, *11*, 295–306. [CrossRef] [PubMed]
4. Canfell, K. Towards the global elimination of cervical cancer. *Papillomavirus Res.* **2019**, *8*, 100170. [CrossRef] [PubMed]
5. Canfell, K.; Kim, J.J.; Brisson, M.; Keane, A.; Simms, K.T.; Caruana, M.; Burger, E.A.; Martin, D.; Nguyen, D.; Bénard, É.; et al. Mortality impact of achieving WHO cervical cancer elimination targets: A comparative modelling analysis in 78 low-income and lower-middle-income countries. *Lancet* **2020**, *395*, 591–603. [CrossRef]
6. Johnson, C.A.; James, D.; Marzan, A.; Armaos, M. Cervical cancer: An overview of pathophysiology and management. *Semin. Oncol. Nurs.* **2019**, *35*, 166–174. [CrossRef] [PubMed]
7. Ghelardi, A.; Parazzini, F.; Martella, F.; Pieralli, A.; Bay, P.; Tonetti, A.; Svelato, A.; Bertacca, G.; Lombardi, S.; Joura, E.A. SPERANZA project: HPV vaccination after treatment for CIN2+. *Gynecol. Oncol.* **2018**, *151*, 229–234. [CrossRef] [PubMed]
8. DeMaria, P.J.; Bilusic, M. Cancer Vaccines. *Hematol. Oncol. Clin. N. Am.* **2019**, *33*, 199–214. [CrossRef] [PubMed]
9. Cheng, M.A.; Farmer, E.; Huang, C.; Lin, J.; Hung, C.F.; Wu, T.C. Therapeutic DNA Vaccines for Human Papillomavirus and Associated Diseases. *Hum. Gene Ther.* **2018**, *29*, 971–996. [CrossRef] [PubMed]
10. Daayana, S.; Elkord, E.; Winters, U.; Pawlita, M.; Roden, R.; Stern, P.L.; Kitchener, H.C. Phase II trial of imiquimod and HPV therapeutic vaccination in patients with vulvar intraepithelial neoplasia. *Br. J. Cancer* **2010**, *102*, 1129–1136. [CrossRef] [PubMed]
11. Page, M.J.; McKenzie, J.E.; Bossuyt, P.M. The PRISMA 2020 statement: An updated guideline for reporting systematic reviews. *Br. Med. J.* **2021**, *372*, n71. [CrossRef] [PubMed]
12. Choi, Y.J.; Hur, S.Y.; Kim, T.J.; Hong, S.R.; Lee, J.K.; Cho, C.H.; Park, K.S.; Woo, J.W.; Sung, Y.C.; Suh, Y.S.; et al. A phase II, Prospective, Randomized, Multicenter, open-label study of GX-188E, an HPV DNA vaccine, in patients with Cervical Intraepithelial Neoplasia 3. *Clin. Cancer Res.* **2019**, *26*, 1616–1623. [CrossRef] [PubMed]
13. Kim, T.J.; Jin, H.T.; Hur, S.Y.; Yang, H.G.; Seo, Y.B.; Hong, S.R.; Lee, C.W. Clearance of persistent HPV infection and cervical lesion by therapeutic DNA vaccine in CIN3 patients. *Nat. Commun.* **2014**, *5*, 5317. [CrossRef] [PubMed]
14. Trimble, C.L.; Morrow, M.P.; Kraynyak, K.A.; Shen, X.; Dallas, M.; Yan, J.; Edwards, L.; Parker, R.L.; Denny, L.; Giffear, M.; et al. Safety, efficacy, and immunogenicity of VGX-3100, a therapeutic synthetic DNA vaccine targeting human papillomavirus 16 and 18 E6 and E7 proteins for cervical intraepithelial neoplasia 2/3: A randomised, double-blind, placebo-controlled phase 2b trial. *Lancet* **2015**, *386*, 2078–2088. [CrossRef]
15. Alvarez, R.D.; Huh, W.K.; Bae, S.; Lamb, L.S., Jr.; Conner, M.G.; Boyer, J.; Wang, C.; Hung, C.F.; Sauter, E.; Paradis, M.; et al. A pilot study of pNGVL4a-CRT/E7(detox) for the treatment of patients with HPV16+ cervical intraepithelial neoplasia 2/3 (CIN2/3). *Gynecol. Oncol.* **2016**, *140*, 245–252. [CrossRef] [PubMed]
16. Trimble, C.L.; Peng, S.; Kos, F.; Gravitt, P.; Viscidi, R.; Sugar, E.; Pardoll, D.; Wu, T.C. A phase I trial of a human papillomavirus DNA vaccine for HPV16+ cervical intraepithelial neoplasia 2/3. *Clin. Cancer Res.* **2009**, *15*, 361–367. [CrossRef] [PubMed]
17. Hasan, Y.; Furtado, L.; Tergas, A.; Lee, N.; Brooks, R.; McCall, A.; Golden, D.; Jolly, S.; Fleming, G.; Morrow, M.; et al. A Phase 1 Trial Assessing the Safety and Tolerability of a Therapeutic DNA Vaccination Against HPV16 and HPV18 E6/E7 Oncogenes After Chemoradiation for Cervical Cancer. *Int. J. Radiat Oncol. Biol. Phys.* **2020**, *107*, 487–498. [CrossRef] [PubMed]
18. Hung, C.-F.; Ma, B.; Monie, A.; Tsen, S.-W.; Wu, T.-C. Therapeutic human papillomavirus vaccines: Current clinical trials and future directions. *Expert Opin. Biol. Ther.* **2008**, *8*, 421–439. [CrossRef] [PubMed]

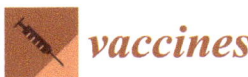

Systematic Review

Pharmacists' Perceived Barriers to Human Papillomavirus (HPV) Vaccination: A Systematic Literature Review

Oluwafemifola Oyedeji [1], Jill M. Maples [2,*], Samantha Gregory [2], Shauntá M. Chamberlin [3], Justin D. Gatwood [4], Alexandria Q. Wilson [5], Nikki B. Zite [2] and Larry C. Kilgore [2]

1. Department of Public Health, The University of Tennessee, Knoxville, TN 37996, USA; oonaade@vols.utk.edu
2. Department of Obstetrics and Gynecology, Graduate School of Medicine, The University of Tennessee, Knoxville, TN 37920, USA; SGregory1@utmck.edu (S.G.); NZite@utmck.edu (N.B.Z.); LKilgore@utmck.edu (L.C.K.)
3. Department of Family Medicine, Graduate School of Medicine, The University of Tennessee, Knoxville, TN 37920, USA; SChamberlin@utmck.edu
4. Department of Clinical Pharmacy and Translational Science, College of Pharmacy, University of Tennessee Health Science Center, Nashville, TN 37211, USA; jgatwood@uthsc.edu
5. Preston Medical Library, Graduate School of Medicine, The University of Tennessee, Knoxville, TN 37920, USA; AQWilson@utmck.edu
* Correspondence: jmaple13@uthsc.edu or JMaples1@utmck.edu

Abstract: About 45:000 cancers are linked to HPV each year in the United States alone. The HPV vaccine prevents cancer and is highly effective, yet vaccination coverage remains low. Pharmacies can play a meaningful role in increasing HPV vaccination access due to their availability and convenience. However, little is known about pharmacists' perceived barriers to HPV vaccination. The objective of this systematic review was to summarize existing literature on perceived barriers to administering HPV vaccination reported by pharmacists. Barriers identified from selected studies were synthesized and further grouped into patient, parental, (pharmacist's) personal, and system/organization barrier groups. Six studies were included in this review. The cost of the HPV vaccine, insurance coverage and reimbursement were commonly reported perceived barriers. Adolescent HPV vaccination barriers related to parental concerns, beliefs, and inadequate knowledge about the HPV vaccine. Perceived (pharmacist's) personal barriers were related to lack of information and knowledge about HPV vaccine and recommendations. At the system/organization level, barriers reported included lack of time/staff/space; difficulty in series completion; tracking and recall of patient; perceived competition with providers; and other responsibilities/vaccines taking precedence. Future strategies involving pharmacy settings in HPV-related cancer prevention efforts should consider research on multilevel pharmacy-driven interventions addressing barriers.

Keywords: Human Papillomavirus; barriers; pharmacists; vaccination

Citation: Oyedeji, O.; Maples, J.M.; Gregory, S.; Chamberlin, S.M.; Gatwood, J.D.; Wilson, A.Q.; Zite, N.B.; Kilgore, L.C. Pharmacists' Perceived Barriers to Human Papillomavirus (HPV) Vaccination: A Systematic Literature Review. *Vaccines* 2021, *9*, 1360. https://doi.org/10.3390/vaccines9111360

Academic Editor: Gloria Calagna

Received: 1 November 2021
Accepted: 16 November 2021
Published: 19 November 2021

Publisher's Note: MDPI stays neutral with regard to jurisdictional claims in published maps and institutional affiliations.

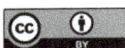

Copyright: © 2021 by the authors. Licensee MDPI, Basel, Switzerland. This article is an open access article distributed under the terms and conditions of the Creative Commons Attribution (CC BY) license (https://creativecommons.org/licenses/by/4.0/).

1. Introduction

Human Papillomavirus (HPV) is estimated to be the cause of 70% oropharynx, vaginal, and vulvar cancers, 60% of penile cancers, and 90% of anal and cervical cancers [1]. HPV-associated cancers are the only known cancers that can be prevented by receiving a vaccine. Yet, there are over 45,000 newly diagnosed HPV-related cancers in the United States each year [1]. The HPV vaccine has been shown to be safe and highly effective [2]. The Centers for Disease Control and Prevention (CDC) established HPV vaccination as a public health priority, yet vaccination coverage rates are less than the Healthy People 2020 goal that 80% of adolescents complete the vaccine series [3,4]. Nationally in 2017, less than 66% of adolescents received the first dose of the HPV vaccine, and only about 49% completed the series [5]. The HPV vaccine dosing schedule consists of a series of two or three doses, depending on the age of the patient at the start of the schedule [6]. For example, a patient that is under the age of 15 is recommended to receive two doses of the HPV vaccine administered 6–12 months apart. A patient starting the vaccine series on or after the 15th birthday is recommended to receive three doses of the HPV vaccine [6]. In this dosing schedule, the second vaccine should be administered 1–2 months after the first dose, and the third dose should be administered 6 months after the first dose [6].

Community pharmacies have the potential to play a meaningful role in increasing HPV vaccination rates. The President's Cancer Panel [7] and National Vaccine Advisory Committee [8] released statements urging the increase in uptake of HPV vaccination rates by using pharmacies as a strategic site. Pharmacies are conveniently located for most families, including those in rural communities. In fact, most residents in the United States (91%) live within five miles of a pharmacy [9]. Additionally, pharmacies are typically open for extended hours and on weekends. Given the expanding scope of practice and evolving role of the pharmacist and pharmacy as playing a vital role in public health, due to their accessibility, cost-efficacy, and ability to provide education and shared responsibility, along with patient acceptance, they have been identified as crucial partners in vaccination administration [10].

During the ongoing COVID-19 pandemic, the U.S. Department of Health and Human Services (HHS) declared that pharmacists are allowed to administer childhood vaccines for children that are three years and above [11]. Most state laws also allow pharmacists to administer HPV vaccine to patients, with some states having varying age restrictions and/or prescription requirements (only two states do not allow pharmacists to administer the HPV vaccine at all) [12]. Pharmacists provide a convenient option for patients to receive the HPV vaccine. However, little is known about the current perceptions and barriers to administrating HPV vaccination among pharmacists. Therefore, this review aims to systematically examine the literature on pharmacists' perceived barriers to administering the HPV vaccine as a mechanism for improving HPV vaccination uptake.

2. Methodology

This systematic review was conducted following the Preferred Reporting Items for Systematic Reviews and Meta-Analyses statement (PRISMA) [13].

2.1. Search Strategy

Electronic searches were created and completed by a research team member and health sciences librarian (A.W.) experienced with systematic searches in the following databases: PubMed [NLM], Web of Science [Thomson Reuters], Cochrane Central Register of Controlled Trials [Wiley], and Scopus [Elsevier]. The search strategy was created first in PubMed (Appendix A), and then translated for each database platform as applicable. MeSH terms and keywords were used to search concepts related to Human Papillomavirus, vaccines, barriers, and pharmacists. The searches were performed on 18 September 2020. Results were restricted to English language. There were no restrictions set on the year of publication for inclusion. Duplicate references were removed using Rayyan software [14]. The references cited in the included articles were reviewed for additional relevant articles.

2.2. Study Selection & Data Extraction

The titles and abstracts were first screened independently for eligibility by two researchers (S.G., O.O.). Then, the same researchers reviewed the full text of selected abstracts for further eligibility. Conflicts were resolved by a third researcher (J.M.M.). Study inclusion criteria include: (1) primary research article including qualitative, quantitative, and mixed-method studies, (2) reported outcome included perceived barrier to administering HPV vaccine (3) study population included pharmacists, pharmacy students, pharmacy technicians, and pharmacist representatives. Studies were excluded if the study objectives were unrelated to HPV vaccination. Two co-authors (O.O., J.M.M.) abstracted and synthesized all findings. Barrier type categorization was adapted from the findings reported in the included studies [15–17]. Some barriers extended, at least partially, across other barrier types. All barrier type classifications were discussed among co-authors, and a

3. Results

3.1. Literature Search and Study Characteristics

The electronic database searches yielded 444 articles; 292 titles and abstracts were selected, and 13 full-text studies were reviewed for inclusion. In the end, 6 out of 13 studies were selected for this review using the exclusion and inclusion criteria [15–20]. Figure 1 illustrates the PRISMA diagram detailing the search and selection process. Four of the studies [15,16,18,20] examined barriers related to HPV vaccine alone, while the remaining two studies [17,19] included other vaccines in addition to HPV. All included studies were carried out in the United States; however, geographical location and pharmacy setting differ across studies (Table 1). Table 2 presents an overview of the study designs, methodologies, and data reporting. While all the studies utilized a cross-sectional study design, the methodologies and results reporting varied widely across studies (Table 2). Table 3 presents a summary of the key findings for the included studies. These findings were further grouped by level of barrier into patient, parental, (pharmacist's) personal, and system/organization barrier groups, which were adapted from the findings reported in the included studies (Table 4) [15–17]. Some barriers extended, at least partially, across other barrier types. For example, "financially-related" (or cost) barriers were reported across multiple barrier types [15,17–20]. To the patient a "financially-related" (or cost) barrier may be the out-of-pocket cost of the vaccine, which is distinct from the "financially-related" (or cost) barrier at the systems/organizational level, which may be more related to the financial burden of stocking the vaccine.

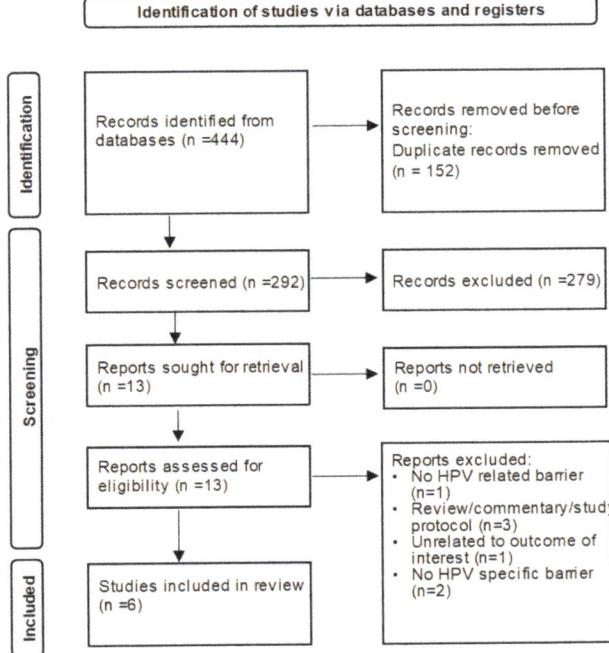

Figure 1. PRISMA diagram showing search and selection.

Table 1. Characteristics of included studies.

Author, Publication Year	Sample Size	Study Population Characteristics	Pharmacy Setting	Vaccines Examined
Berce et al., 2020 [17]	236	Pharmacists located in Wisconsin (USA). 79% worked in pharmacies that were primarily located in urban counties (79%), 7% were in rural counties and 14% were located in multiple counties and/or in both rural and urban areas	Health system community (29%), chain community (27%), independent (26%), ambulatory care clinic (11%), inpatient (7%)	HPV, Influenza, Zoster, Pneumococcal, Tdap/Td, DTap, Hepatitis A and B, Hepatitis A, Meningococcal, MMR, Varicella, Polio and others
Hastings et al., 2017 [15]	154	One participant represented each pharmacy which included pharmacy owners, managers, or staff pharmacists located in Alabama (USA)	Chain pharmacy (53%), and independently owned (47%)	HPV
Islam et al., 2019 [18]	40	Pharmacists from 8 states (Alabama, Indiana, California, Maine, Kentucky, Tennessee, Texas, and Washington) in the USA that previously or currently were administering HPV, Meningococcal, Tdap or TD vaccines to adolescents	Chain (78%), independent (13%), grocery (5%), big box retailer (5%)	HPV
Ryan et al., 2020 [16]	11	Pharmacists in 7 rural counties in Iowa (USA)	Independently owned (100%)	HPV
Skiles et al., 2011 [19]	24	Pharmacy association directors or designees from all 50 states in the USA were targeted (92% were pharmacists)	Information not reported	HPV, Tdap, Influenza
Tolentino et al., 2018 [20]	240	Community pharmacists in Utah (USA)	Community/outpatient (80%), ambulatory care clinic (10%), community outpatient and inpatient (8%), other (3%)	HPV

Td-Tetanus/Diphtheria, Tdap-Tetanus/Diphtheria/Pertussis, MMR- Measles/Mumps/Rubella, Other- Typhoid, Yellow fever, Japanese Encephalitis and not otherwise stated.

Table 2. Overview of included study methodologies and data reporting.

Author, Publication Year	Study Design	Data Collection Tool	Data Reporting
Berce et al., 2020 [17]	Cross-sectional survey design using an anonymous electronic survey	Modified version of a previous national physician survey [21] on barriers to adult vaccination which asks respondents to classify multiple potential barriers to immunization on a 4-point response scale.	Barriers were grouped by pharmacies that provide and do not provide immunization.
Hastings et al., 2017 [15]	Cross-sectional survey design using a modified version of Dillman's Tailored Design Method of survey administration [22]	A 65-item survey that took approximately 15 min to complete. Measures were categorized into 5 sections: 1. key informant and pharmacy site demographic characteristics; 2. general vaccination services and strategies used to increase HPV vaccine uptake; 3. pharmacists' perceptions of HPV and the vaccine; 4. perceived system barriers to the provision of HPV vaccinations; and 5. perceived parental reasons for HPV vaccine hesitancy. Most of the questions were 5-point Likert-type rating scales. Questions measuring HPV and the vaccine perceptions were adapted from an existing instrument. Questions assessing system barriers were informed by previous research.	Descriptive statistics were used to describe participants characteristics, vaccine practices, barriers and attitudes.
Islam et al., 2019 [18]	Cross-sectional study design using semi-structed interview to complete a survey	Survey items included 52 close-ended questions and 24 open-ended questions to examine pharmacists insights into administering vaccines. Interviews lasted 30–60 min.	Semi-qualitative responses were analyzed using thematic analysis, to create response categories and then coded using descriptive frequency statistics.

Table 2. Cont.

Author, Publication Year	Study Design	Data Collection Tool	Data Reporting
Ryan et al., 2020 [16]	Cross-sectional study design using interview.	Interview guide using questions and concepts adapted from a previous project that included the following topics: the role of rural, independent pharmacists in HPV vaccine promotion and uptake; willingness to educate parents, refer patient, and administer the HPV vaccine; priority of HPV vaccine promotion, and vaccination barriers and facilitators in the pharmacy and the community	Interview responses were analyzed using thematic analysis.
Skiles et al., 2011 [19]	Cross-sectional study design using telephone interviews to complete a survey	Survey questions asked about immunization practices, vaccine beliefs, minor consent issues, and minor consent laws. Responses to the attitude and/or belief questions were measured on a 5-point Likert scale.	Attitude and belief responses were collapsed to a dichotomous response for analysis. Differences in attitudes across vaccines were tested using score test on the basis of the generalized estimating equation for the generalized linear model.
Tolentino et al., 2018 [20]	Cross-sectional study design using an anonymous electronic survey	A 73-item survey adapted from an HPV vaccination survey previously conducted with Utah primary care providers that asked about HPV vaccination knowledge, attitudes about the HPV vaccine, behavior for recommending the vaccines (HPV, influenza, meningococcal disease, Tdap), and barriers for adolescents' vaccination. Survey questions were multiple choice, true/false, and Likert scale.	Descriptive statistics were used to analyze the demographics of pharmacists, as well as their knowledge and attitudes regarding the HPV vaccine, vaccine recommendation levels and strategies, and self-identified barriers to vaccine recommendations. Content analyses were used to identify the themes.

Table 3. Key findings of included studies.

Author	Summary of Findings
Skiles et al. [19]	96% reported that financial challenge is a barrier to HPV vaccination access for adolescents ($p < 0.001$); 75% of participants reported that access to HPV vaccine is moderately to extremely difficult ($p = 0.030$); 67% reported that ACIP recommendations are moderately to extremely controversial in the community ($p < 0.001$)
Hastings et al. [15]	Participants reported the following as very/extremely likely to be a system-related barrier to HPV vaccination: lack of demand (56.5%), failure of cost coverage by insurance (54.8%), vaccine expiration before use (54.1%), difficulty ensuring patients are completing the necessary 3 doses (39.9%), and lack of adequate reimbursement (38.4%). Participants reported that they somewhat agree/strongly agree that the following are parent-related barriers to HPV vaccination: lack of education (86.6%) safety concerns (78.7%), reluctancy to talk about sexuality/sexually transmitted infections (76%), concerns that agreeing to vaccination means they support premarital sex (67.3%), concerns about efficacy of vaccine (64.6%), cost (53.3%), believe that their children are not at risk (67.3%), believe that their children are too young (65.3%), concern that children will practice riskier sexual behaviors (58.7%).
Berce et al. [17]	Insurance and time/priority were reported as largest barrier. Compared with those that do not immunize, financial barrier was larger among those that do immunize ($p = 0.022$). Barriers reported among those that do immunize included patients having insurance coverage for vaccines (90%), patients refusal due to financial reasons (89%), patients refusing vaccine (89%), determining insurance reimbursement (87%), other responsibilities taking precedence (84%), patient refusal due to perceived safety issues (79%), lack of staff (78%), remembering to screen patients (76%), having enough demand to justify the cost of stocking vaccines (71%), upfront cost of buying vaccines and supplies (55%), adequate compensation for administration (72%), and adequate compensation for product (68%) and supplies (58%) purchase. Barriers reported among those that do not immunize included other responsibilities taking precedence over vaccinating (94%), patient refusal (72%), patient refusal due to perceived safety issues (67%), determining insurance reimbursement (66%), lack of staff (61%), remembering to screen patients (60%), patient having insurance coverage (57%) and adequate compensation for administration (53%).

Table 3. Cont.

Author	Summary of Findings
Ryan et al. [16]	Barriers were grouped into personal and organizational barrier. Personal barriers included sensitivity on the subject of HPV infection, lack of information, safety concerns, misinformation about HPV vaccination coverage and access. Organization barriers include lack of time and staff, liability issues relating to adverse effect after vaccination, low number of adolescents coming to the pharmacy, and competition with local health care providers.
Tolentino et al. [20]	Barriers reported included lack of parental knowledge, parental concerns/opposition, lack of educational materials for parents, high copay, lack of demand from parents, lack of time and space, high priority for other vaccines compared with HPV, and lack of incentive for series completion.
Islam et al. [18]	Major barriers to providing HPV vaccines to adolescents included the following: parental consent (28%), tracking and recall of patients (17%), stigma about vaccination among parents (17%), education/vaccination promotion (17%), cost of vaccination (11%), potential adverse reactions (11%).

Table 4. Summary of key barriers grouped by level of barrier.

Author, Year	Barrier Levels			
	Patient	Parental	Personal	System/Organization
Skiles et al., 2011 [19]	• Financial barriers • Access to HPV vaccination is difficult		• Belief that ACIP recommendations are controversial	
Hastings et al., 2017 [15]	• Too few patients who want the HPV vaccine	• Safety concerns about HPV vaccine • Concerns that agreeing to vaccination means they are condoning premarital sex • Efficacy concerns about HPV vaccine • Lack of education/understanding about HPV infection • Parental belief that their children are not at risk for HPV infection • Reluctancy to discuss sexuality/sexually transmitted infections • Parental belief that their children are too young for the vaccine • Concern that their children will practice riskier sexual behaviors if they receive the vaccine • Parental belief that the cost of vaccine is high		• Lack of coverage of vaccination cost by some insurance companies • Vaccine expiration before use • Difficulty ensuring series completion • Lack of adequate reimbursement
Tolentino et al., 2018 [20]		• Lack of parental knowledge • Parental concerns/opposition • Lack of demand from parents		• Lack of time and space • High priority for other vaccines compared with HPV • Lack of incentive for series completion • High copay • Lack of educational materials for parents

Table 4. *Cont.*

Author, Year	Barrier Levels			
	Patient	Parental	Personal	System/Organization
Islam et al., 2019 [18]		• Parental consent • Perceived stigma about vaccination among parents of adolescents	• Potential adverse reaction	• Tracking and recall of patients • Cost of vaccination • Education/promotion of vaccination
Berce et al., 2020 [17]	• Patient refusing vaccine • Patient refusal due to perceived safety issues • Patients having insurance coverage for vaccine • Patient refusing vaccines for financial reasons			• Other responsibilities taking precedence over vaccinating • Determining if patient's insurance with reimburse • Having enough staff to provide vaccine • Remembering to screen patients for needed vaccine • Adequate compensation for vaccine administration • Adequate compensation for vaccine product purchase • Adequate compensation for supplies purchase. • Upfront cost of buying vaccines and supplies • Having enough demand to justify the cost of stocking some or all recommended vaccines
Ryan et al., 2020 [16]	• Low number of adolescents coming to the pharmacy		• Sensitivity of subject • Lack of information • Safety concerns • Misinformation	• Lack of time, staff and space • Liability issues • Competition with local health care providers

3.2. Barrier Levels

Patient: Four out of the six included studies reported patient-related barriers [15–17,19]. The most commonly reported barriers at the patient level were inadequate demand [15,16] and patient refusal [17]. Reasons for patient refusal reported in one of the studies included perceived safety concerns and financial reasons [17]. Other barriers included patients lacking insurance coverage [17] and difficulty overcoming financial barriers for an adolescent [19].

Parental: Three studies included parent-related barriers [15,18,20]. Across these studies, certain parental concerns and perceptions were reported as pharmacists perceived barriers to HPV vaccination. This included safety and efficacy concerns about the HPV vaccine [15], concerns that agreeing to vaccination means they are condoning premarital sex [15], and concerns that their children will engage in riskier sexual behaviors if they receive the vaccine [15]. Parental beliefs that their children are not at risk for HPV infection and that children are not old enough for the HPV vaccine were also reported as barriers [15]. Other key parent-related barriers reported include inadequate demand from parents [20], parental believe the cost is too high [15], perceived stigma about vaccination among parents of adolescents [18], parental consent [18], lack of knowledge [20], and inadequate education/understanding about HPV infection [15].

(Pharmacist's) Personal: Three studies reported pharmacist's personal barriers to HPV vaccination. [16,18,19]. In one of the studies, lack of information was reported as a barrier [16]. This included inadequate knowledge to educate and recommend the HPV vaccine and also a lack of information on subjects such as cost and storage of the vaccine [16]. Misinformation among pharmacists regarding HPV vaccination and administration was also reported as a barrier [16]. For instance, one pharmacist believed (incorrectly) that the HPV vaccination coverage in their (rural) area was good [16]. Another example of misinformation was evidenced by a pharmacist stating that Medicaid does not allow pharmacists to provide the HPV vaccine to those under 18, even with a prescription [16]. A third example of misinformation was evidenced by a pharmacist stating that adolescents are supposed to receive the HPV vaccine only at their doctor's office [16]. The perception that HPV infection/mode of transmission is a sensitive subject was also cited as a barrier [16]. Other personal barriers include safety concerns about the potential adverse reaction after receiving the HPV vaccine [16,18], and the belief that the Advisory Committee on Immunization Practices (ACIP) recommendations are controversial [19].

System/Organization: Five out of the six studies reviewed reported system/organization level barriers [15–18,20]. Three of these studies reported lack of time and staffing as barriers to HPV vaccine administration [16,17,20]. For example, often times only one pharmacist may be present, which could result in major interruptions in work flow to stop and administer an HPV vaccine [16]. Two studies reported that a lack of physical space was also a barrier [16,20]. For example, a lack of consulting space to accommodate both parent and adolescent for HPV vaccine counseling and/or administration is a barrier [16]. Financial barriers related to vaccination cost, insurance reimbursement, and compensation were also frequently cited [15,17,18,20]; this included lack of insurance coverage of vaccine costs [15], difficulty in knowing whether insurance will reimburse for vaccine [17], and adequate compensation for vaccine purchase/supplies purchase/vaccine administration [17]. Other cost-related barriers included upfront cost of buying vaccine/supplies and lack of demand to justify cost of stocking vaccines [17].

At the organization level, other responsibilities/vaccines taking precedence over HPV vaccination was also reported as a barrier [17,20]. Other reported barriers were related to series completion which included lack of incentives for series completion [15,17], tracking and recall of patients [18], and remembering to screen patients for vaccine [17].

In one study, concerns that it may appear that pharmacists are in competition with health care providers to administer the vaccine was seen as a barrier [16]. Liability issues relating to adverse effects after vaccination [16], lack of educational materials to provide to parents [20]; and inadequate vaccine promotion/education were also reported as barriers [18].

4. Discussion

Community pharmacies could potentially play an important role in improving HPV vaccination rates due to their availability and accessibility. This review presents a summary of the literature on pharmacists' perceived barriers to providing the HPV vaccine in a pharmacy setting. Based on the findings from the six included studies, pharmacists' perceived barriers to HPV vaccination uptake exist at the patient, parental, pharmacist's (personal), and system/organization levels. The existence of reported barriers at different levels suggests that efforts at improving HPV vaccination rates among pharmacies should be targeted at these levels.

Barriers related to the cost of the HPV vaccine and insurance coverage were frequently cited in the articles reviewed for this paper [15,17–20]. This is in concert with previous studies where vaccine cost and lack of insurance coverage have also been reported as specific barriers to HPV vaccination among health care providers [23,24]. Other studies have also reported that financial reasons may be a parental barrier for HPV vaccination for their children [25]. In fact, one study found that a lower proportion of parents were willing to vaccinate their children if the vaccine was not covered by insurance [25]. A number of options are available to cover the cost of HPV vaccine. Under the Affordable Care Act (ACA), most private insurance plans in the United States are required to cover immunizations recommended by ACIP without consumer cost-sharing [7]. Additionally, the Vaccine for Children (VFC) program is a federally funded program in the United States that covers vaccine costs for eligible children below 19 years of age (eligibility criteria include Medicaid-eligible, uninsured, underinsured, and American Indian or Alaska Native) [26]. A study among physicians reported that those participating in VFC program were less likely to indicate cost as a barrier to HPV vaccination [24,27]. Previous research showed that the VFC program led to increased vaccination for certain vaccines [28]. However, barriers such as state laws (only 34 states allow pharmacies to participate in VFC), inadequate reimbursement to cover actual costs, administrative burden and low demand from eligible persons may affect pharmacies' participation in VFC or willingness to carry all vaccines [7,29]. Other sources that cover HPV vaccine cost in the United

States include Merck assistance programs [30], Medicaid and Children's Health Insurance Program (CHIP) [31]. Promotion and public education on these little or no-cost options for HPV vaccination could improve access.

Parents play an important role in HPV vaccination for their adolescent children. Results from this review showed that pharmacists perceived parental concerns, beliefs, and lack of knowledge as barriers to HPV vaccination [15,18,20]. Similar findings were reported from a study that examined perceived barriers to HPV vaccination among health care providers; the authors reported parental beliefs and misconceptions as a major barrier to HPV vaccination [32]. About one-third of parents in previous research reported that they were willing to allow their children to get the HPV vaccine in a pharmacy setting [33]. Likewise, another study showed that 44% of parents are willing to get an HPV vaccine from pharmacies for their children [34]. Improving parental awareness and clarity that pharmacists offer HPV vaccines for children may facilitate series completion [33]. Also, strategies to educate parents on the importance of the HPV vaccine and demystify misconceptions may positively influence parental decision to vaccinate their children. This may include additional training for pharmacists on ways to educate and provide effective HPV vaccine recommendations to parents [15].

Partnerships and collaboration agreements between health care providers and pharmacists, including strong provider recommendation and referral to pharmacies for subsequent HPV vaccine doses may increase parental awareness and vaccine uptake [33]. Physicians could help improve parental awareness as parents may prefer to learn about the availability of pharmacists to provide the HPV vaccination from their children's physicians [33]. However, there is a lack of uniformity across states in the US and diverging opinions regarding authority to administer vaccines to children and adolescents that complicates the theoretical partnerships and collaboration agreements between health care providers and pharmacists. For instance, laws and regulations granting pharmacists the authority to administer HPV vaccine to all or certain adolescent age groups vary across states [12]. Also, there is a lack of consensus among professional organizations, like the American Academy of Pediatrics (AAP), and the US Department of Health and Human Services regarding whether pharmacists should be authorized to administer vaccines to children and adolescents [11,35]. In 2020, AAP released a statement that their organization believes that children should receive vaccines from a pediatrician, which opposes HHS authorization that allows pharmacists to administer childhood vaccines [36].

Three studies included in this review reported personal barriers among pharmacists to HPV vaccine administration [16,18,19]. The personal barriers were not religious or moral, but related primarily to inadequate knowledge to provide recommendations for HPV vaccination, or educate patients about the HPV vaccine (considering the sensitivity of HPV-related subject) [16,19]. This is promising as additional training on HPV vaccine recommendation strategies, coverage, and administration for practicing pharmacists, as well as student pharmacists, could help improve the pharmacists' knowledge and comfort level in educating and administering the HPV vaccine [37].

At the organization level, remembering to screen [17] as well as tracking and recall of patients were identified as barriers to HPV vaccination [18]. In one of the studies reviewed, only 33 percent of participants reported that they utilized their state's Immunization Information Systems (IIS) [18]. IIS can ensure timely immunization, clinical decision support, records consolidation, and data exchange among health care providers [38]. However, the operating and reporting for IIS requirements vary by state [39]. Another key organization level barrier reported was other responsibilities/vaccines taking precedence [17,20] over HPV vaccination and lack of time/staff/space [16,17,20]. The decision to prioritize and offer HPV vaccines by pharmacies may depend on the goals of the organization/management and may differ between independent versus chain pharmacies.

While the purpose of this review was to summarize existing literature related to the perceived barriers to administering HPV vaccination reported by pharmacists, some of the studies reported facilitators of HPV vaccination suggested by study participants [16,18,20].

Most frequently suggested facilitator was education about HPV vaccine [16,18,20]. As reported in one of the studies, education may involve providing education to patient/parent, pharmacists, and health care providers [20]. Another suggested way to improve HPV vaccination is advertising specifically through mass/social media [16,20]. Pharmacist providing stronger recommendation to patients about getting HPV vaccination was also reported as potential facilitator of HPV vaccination [20]. Partnership involving health care providers, schools [16,20] and public health organization [16] was reported as a facilitator. For instance, doctors may recommend that their patient get the HPV vaccine in a pharmacy or schools holding vaccine clinics [20]. Other facilitators reported by pharmacists include ease of accessibility of community pharmacies [16], clear guidelines from pharmacy/corporate management [18], vaccine promotion within and outside the pharmacy [18], adequate insurance coverage for vaccination [20], and state legislative authority to provide vaccination [18].

Evidence-based strategies to improve HPV vaccination rates that have previously been implemented in other settings, such as in primary care, may help to improve HPV vaccination in pharmacies. For instance, previous studies suggest that reminder and recall systems [40] and decision support systems [41] may be effective in improving HPV vaccination, which potentially could facilitate series completion. Alternatively, successful evidence-based strategies implemented in pharmacy settings to improve other vaccines could also be adapted to improving HPV vaccination rates. In one study, pharmacy-based interventions, including newspaper press releases, use of flyer advertisement, and personalized letters about herpes zoster infection and vaccination were shown to improve herpes zoster vaccination rates [42]. In another study, individuals who received a phone call intervention from pharmacists were more likely to receive their second dose of the recombinant zoster vaccine, thereby facilitating series completion [43]. Further research is needed to explore interventions unique and specific to improving HPV vaccination and series completion in pharmacies.

To our knowledge, this is the first study to review previously reported perceptions of barriers to HPV vaccine administration among pharmacists. Numerous commentaries and professional organizations suggest that pharmacies could play an important role in improving HPV vaccine uptake. The studies included in this review varied greatly in terms of study design, which made the synthesis of findings challenging. The search strategy employed to identify eligible studies for this review, encompassed publications on studies conducted worldwide. However, all the eligible studies included in this review were conducted in the United States. The perceived barriers that pharmacists experience may vary geographically within and outside of the United States. Therefore, generalizability of results may be limited. Nevertheless, many of these barriers are, to some extent, universal and therefore may provide direction for those investigating HPV vaccination barriers in different health care delivery systems. This literature search yielded only a few studies, which indicates that additional research is needed to explore pharmacist's perceived barriers, especially at the system/organization levels. Because most of the studies included in this review relied primarily on quantitative survey-based data collection methods, it limits the ability to thoroughly understand pharmacists' perceived barriers to HPV vaccine administration. A more comprehensive understanding of barriers to HPV vaccine administration is needed, especially to better understand how these barriers may impact various pharmacies in utilizing differing immunization delivery practices. Future work should include in-depth qualitative analyses of barriers among pharmacists practicing in a wide variety of settings.

In conclusion, pharmacies present an opportunity to increase HPV vaccination rates. Targeted public health efforts to increase HPV vaccination among pharmacies should consider a multilevel approach. Future strategies involving pharmacy settings in HPV-related cancer prevention efforts should consider research on pharmacy-driven interventions that addresses the barriers to administering the HPV vaccine at various levels.

Author Contributions: Conceptualization, J.M.M. and O.O.; methodology, A.Q.W., O.O. and J.M.M.; formal analysis, O.O., S.G. and J.M.M.; writing—original draft preparation, O.O., S.G. and A.Q.W.; writing—review and editing, J.M.M., S.M.C., J.D.G., N.B.Z. and L.C.K.; visualization, O.O.; supervision, J.M.M., L.C.K. and N.B.Z.; project administration, J.M.M.; funding acquisition, L.C.K., N.B.Z. and J.M.M. All authors have read and agreed to the published version of the manuscript.

Funding: This research was funded by the University of Tennessee Medical Center Cancer Institute Research Grant Awarded to L.C.K., N.B.Z., J.M.M.

Institutional Review Board Statement: Not applicable.

Informed Consent Statement: Not applicable.

Data Availability Statement: Not applicable.

Conflicts of Interest: Justin Gatwood reports vaccine-related research funding provided by Merck & Co. and GlaxoSmithKline.

Appendix A. PubMed Search Strategy

(Papillomavirus Infections[Mesh]) OR (HPV[tw] OR "human papilloma virus"[tw] or "human papillomavirus"[tw])

AND

(Immunization[Mesh] OR "Vaccination"[Mesh] OR "Immunization Programs"[Mesh] OR "Mass Vaccination"[Mesh] OR "Papillomavirus Vaccines"[Mesh]) OR (vaccin*[tw] OR immunization[tw])

AND

(Pharmacies[Mesh] OR "Pharmacy Technicians"[Mesh] OR "Pharmacy Residencies"[Mesh] OR "Students, Pharmacy"[Mesh] OR "Pharmacists"[Mesh] OR "Community Pharmacy Services"[Mesh]) OR (pharmac*[tw])

AND

barrier*[tw] OR challenge*[tw] OR constrain*[tw] OR difficult*[tw] OR interfer*[tw] OR obstruct*[tw] OR problem*[tw] OR restrain*[tw] OR restrict*[tw]

References

1. Centers for Disease Control and Prevention. *Cancers Associated with Human Papillomavirus, United States—2013–2017*; USCS Data Brief; Centers for Disease Control and Prevention: Atlanta, GA, USA, 2020. Available online: https://www.cdc.gov/cancer/uscs/about/data-briefs/no18-hpv-assoc-cancers-UnitedStates-2013-2017.htm (accessed on 9 April 2021).
2. Centers for Disease Control and Prevention. *Human Papillomavirus (HPV): HPV Vaccination is Safe and Effective*; Centers for Disease Control and Prevention: Atlanta, GA, USA, 2021. Available online: https://www.cdc.gov/hpv/parents/vaccinesafety.html (accessed on 18 August 2021).
3. Office of Disease Prevention and Health Promotion. *Immunization and Infectious Diseases: IID-11.4 Increase the Percentage of Female Adolescents Aged 13 through 15 Years Who Receive 2 or 3 Doses of Human Papillomavirus (HPV) Vaccine as Recommended*; Office of Disease Prevention and Health Promotion: Washington, DC, USA, 2020. Available online: https://www.healthypeople.gov/2020/data-search/Search-the-Data#objid=4657 (accessed on 25 April 2021).
4. Office of Disease Prevention and Health Promotion. *Immunization and Infectious Diseases: IID-11.5 Increase the Percentage of Male Adolescents Aged 13 through 15 Years Who Receive 2 or 3 Doses of Human Papillomavirus (HPV) Vaccine as Recommended*; Office of Disease Prevention and Health Promotion: Washington, DC, USA, 2020. Available online: https://www.healthypeople.gov/2020/data-search/Search-the-Data#objid=10676 (accessed on 25 April 2021).
5. Walker, T.Y.; Elam-Evans, L.D.; Yankey, D.; Markowitz, L.E.; Williams, C.L.; Mbaeyi, S.A.; Fredua, B.; Stokley, S. National, Regional, State, and Selected Local Area Vaccination Coverage Among Adolescents Aged 13-17 Years-United States, 2017. *Morb. Mortal. Wkly. Rep.* **2018**, *67*, 909–917. [CrossRef] [PubMed]
6. Centers for Disease Control and Prevention. *Human Papillomavirus (HPV): HPV Vaccine Schedule and Dosing*; Centers for Disease Control and Prevention: Atlanta, GA, USA, 2019. Available online: https://www.cdc.gov/hpv/hcp/schedules-recommendations.html (accessed on 18 August 2021).
7. President's Cancer Panel. *HPV Vaccination for Cancer Prevention: Progress, Opportunities, and a Renewed Call to Action. A Report to the President of the United States from the Chair of the President's Cancer Panel*; President's Cancer Panel: Bethesda, MD, USA, 2018. Available online: https://prescancerpanel.cancer.gov/report/hpvupdate/pdf/PresCancerPanel_HPVUpdate_Nov2018.pdf (accessed on 9 April 2021).

8. National Vaccine Advisory Committee. Overcoming Barriers to Low HPV Vaccine Uptake in the United States: Recommendations from the National Vaccine Advisory Committee: Approved by the National Vaccine Advisory Committee on 9 June 2015. *Public Health Rep.* **2016**, *131*, 17–25. [CrossRef]
9. National Association of Chain Drug Stores (NACDS). Face-to-Face with Community Pharmacies. Available online: https://www.nacds.org/pdfs/about/rximpact-leavebehind.pdf (accessed on 26 July 2021).
10. Shen, A.K.; Peterson, A. The pharmacist and pharmacy have evolved to become more than the corner drugstore: A win for vaccinations and public health. *Hum. Vaccines Immunother.* **2020**, *16*, 1178–1180. [CrossRef] [PubMed]
11. U.S. Department of Health and Human Services. HHS Expands Access to Childhood Vaccines during COVID-19 Pandemic. 2020. Available online: https://www.hhs.gov/about/news/2020/08/19/hhs-expands-access-childhood-vaccines-during-covid-19-pandemic.html (accessed on 19 April 2021).
12. National Alliance of State Pharmacy Associations. Pharmacist Immunization Authority. 2020. Available online: https://naspa.us/resource/pharmacist-authority-to-immunize/ (accessed on 19 April 2021).
13. Page, M.J.; McKenzie, J.E.; Bossuyt, P.M.; Boutron, I.; Hoffmann, T.C.; Mulrow, C.D.; Shamseer, L.; Tetzlaff, J.M.; Akl, E.A.; Brennan, S.E.; et al. The PRISMA 2020 statement: An updated guideline for reporting systematic reviews. *BMJ* **2021**, *372*. [CrossRef]
14. Ouzzani, M.; Hammady, H.; Fedorowicz, Z.; Elmagarmid, A. Rayyan—A web and mobile app for systematic reviews. *Syst. Rev.* **2016**, *5*, 210. [CrossRef] [PubMed]
15. Hastings, T.J.; Hohmann, L.A.; McFarland, S.J.; Teeter, B.S.; Westrick, S.C. Pharmacists' attitudes and perceived barriers to Human Papillomavirus (HPV) vaccination services. *Pharmacy* **2017**, *5*, 45. [CrossRef] [PubMed]
16. Ryan, G. Exploring opportunities to leverage pharmacists in rural areas to promote administration of Human Papillomavirus vaccine. *Prev. Chronic Dis.* **2020**, *17*. [CrossRef] [PubMed]
17. Berce, P.C.; Bernstein, R.S.; MacKinnon, G.E.; Sorum, S.; Martin, E.; MacKinnon, K.J.; Rein, L.E.; Schellhase, K.G. Immunizations at Wisconsin Pharmacies: Results of a statewide vaccine registry analysis and pharmacist survey. *Vaccine* **2020**, *38*, 4448–4456. [CrossRef]
18. Islam, J.Y.; Gruber, J.F.; Kepka, D.; Kunwar, M.; Smith, S.B.; Rothholz, M.C.; Brewer, N.T.; Smith, J.S. Pharmacist insights into adolescent Human Papillomavirus vaccination provision in the United States. *Hum. Vaccines Immunother.* **2019**, *15*, 1839–1850. [CrossRef] [PubMed]
19. Skiles, M.P.; Cai, J.; English, A.; Ford, C.A. Retail pharmacies and adolescent vaccination—An exploration of current issues. *J. Adolesc. Health* **2011**, *48*, 630–632. [CrossRef]
20. Tolentino, V.; Unni, E.; Montuoro, J.; Bezzant-Ogborn, D.; Kepka, D. Utah pharmacists' knowledge, attitudes, and barriers regarding Human Papillomavirus vaccine recommendation. *J. Am. Pharm. Assoc.* **2018**, *58*, S16–S23. [CrossRef]
21. Hurley, L.P.; Bridges, C.B.; Harpaz, R.; Allison, M.A.; O'Leary, S.T.; Crane, L.A.; Brtnikova, M.; Stokley, S.; Beaty, B.L.; Jimenez-Zambrano, A.; et al. US physicians' perspective of adult vaccine delivery. *Ann. Intern. Med.* **2014**, *160*, 161–170. [CrossRef] [PubMed]
22. Dillman, D.A. *Mail and Internet Surveys: The Tailored Design Method*; Wiley & Sons: New York, NY, USA, 1999.
23. Holman, D.M.; Benard, V.; Roland, K.B.; Watson, M.; Liddon, N.; Stokley, S. Barriers to Human Papillomavirus vaccination among US adolescents: A systematic review of the literature. *JAMA Pediatrics* **2014**, *168*, 76–82. [CrossRef] [PubMed]
24. McCave, E.L. Influential factors in HPV vaccination uptake among providers in four states. *J. Community Health* **2010**, *35*, 645–652. [CrossRef]
25. Barnack, J.L.; Reddy, D.M.; Swain, C. Predictors of Parents' Willingness to Vaccinate for Human Papillomavirus and Physicians' Intentions to Recommend the Vaccine. *Women's Health Issues* **2010**, *20*, 28–34. [CrossRef]
26. Centers for Disease Control and Prevention. Vaccine For Children (VFC) Program. 2016. Available online: https://www.cdc.gov/vaccines/programs/vfc/about/index.html (accessed on 18 August 2021).
27. Malo, T.L.; Hassani, D.; Staras, S.A.; Shenkman, E.A.; Giuliano, A.R.; Vadaparampil, S.T. Do Florida Medicaid providers' barriers to HPV vaccination vary based on VFC program participation? *Matern. Child Health J.* **2013**, *17*, 609–615. [CrossRef]
28. Walsh, B.; Doherty, E.; O'Neill, C. Since the start of the vaccines for children program, uptake has increased, and most disparities have decreased. *Health Aff.* **2016**, *35*, 356–364. [CrossRef]
29. Dullea, E.; Knock, K. Successes and Barriers to Pharmacists' Participation in the Vaccines for Children (VFC) Program in the US. Immunize Colorado. 2020. Available online: https://teamvaccine.com/2020/08/04/successes-and-barriers-to-pharmacists-participation-in-the-vaccines-for-children-vfc-program-in-the-u-s/ (accessed on 20 April 2021).
30. Merck Helps. Gardasil 9. Available online: https://www.merckhelps.com/GARDASIL%209 (accessed on 18 August 2021).
31. The Henry J. Kaiser Family Foundation. The HPV Vaccine: Access and Use in the U.S. 2018. Available online: https://files.kff.org/attachment/fact-sheet-the-hpv-vaccine-access-and-use-in-the-u-s (accessed on 18 August 2021).
32. Javanbakht, M.; Stahlman, S.; Walker, S.; Gottlieb, S.; Markowitz, L.; Liddon, N.; Plant, A.; Guerry, S. Provider perceptions of barriers and facilitators of HPV vaccination in a high-risk community. *Vaccine* **2012**, *30*, 4511–4516. [CrossRef]
33. Calo, W.A.; Gilkey, M.B.; Shah, P.; Marciniak, M.W.; Brewer, N.T. Parents' willingness to get Human Papillomavirus vaccination for their adolescent children at a pharmacy. *Prev. Med.* **2017**, *99*, 251–256. [CrossRef] [PubMed]
34. Shah, P.D.; Calo, W.A.; Marciniak, M.W.; Golin, C.E.; Sleath, B.L.; Brewer, N.T. Service quality and parents' willingness to get adolescents HPV vaccine from pharmacists. *Prev. Med.* **2018**, *109*, 106–112. [CrossRef]

35. American Academy of Paediatrics. AAP: HHS Action on Pharmacy Vaccination 'Misguided'. 2020. Available online: https://www.aappublications.org/news/2020/08/19/immunization081920 (accessed on 26 April 2021).
36. American Academy of Paediatrics. American Academy of Pediatrics Opposes HHS Action on Childhood Vaccines; Calls It 'Incredibly Misguided'. 2020. Available online: https://services.aap.org/en/news-room/news-releases/aap/2020/american-academy-of-pediatrics-opposes-hhs-action-on-childhood-vaccines-calls-it-incredibly-misguided/ (accessed on 26 April 2021).
37. Omecene, N.E.; Patterson, J.A.; Bucheit, J.D.; Andersot, A.N.; Rogers, D.; Goode, J.V.; Caldas, L.M. Implementation of pharmacist-administered pediatric vaccines in the United States: Major barriers and potential solutions for the outpatient setting. *Pharm. Pract.* **2019**, *17*. [CrossRef]
38. Centers for Disease Control and Prevention. Immunization Information Systems. 2019. Available online: https://www.cdc.gov/vaccines/programs/iis/about.html (accessed on 18 August 2021).
39. Martin, D.W.; Lowery, N.E.; Brand, B.; Gold, R.; Horlick, G. Immunization information systems: A decade of progress in law and policy. *J. Public Health Manag. Pract.* **2015**, *21*, 296. [CrossRef] [PubMed]
40. Rand, C.M.; Brill, H.; Albertin, C.; Humiston, S.G.; Schaffer, S.; Shone, L.P.; Blumkin, A.K.; Szilagyi, P.G. Effectiveness of centralized text message reminders on Human Papillomavirus immunization coverage for publicly insured adolescents. *J. Adolesc. Health* **2015**, *56*, S17–S20. [CrossRef] [PubMed]
41. Fiks, A.G.; Grundmeier, R.W.; Mayne, S.; Song, L.; Feemster, K.; Karavite, D.; Hughes, C.C.; Massey, J.; Keren, R.; Bell, L.M.; et al. Effectiveness of decision support for families, clinicians, or both on HPV vaccine receipt. *Pediatrics* **2013**, *131*, 1114–1124. [CrossRef] [PubMed]
42. Wang, J.; Ford, L.J.; Uroza, S.F.; Jaber, N.; Smith, C.T.; Randolph, R.; Lane, S.; Foster, S.L. Effect of pharmacist intervention on herpes zoster vaccination in community pharmacies. *J. Am. Pharm. Assoc.* **2013**, *53*, 46–53. [CrossRef]
43. Tyler, R.; Kile, S.; Strain, O.; Kennedy, C.A.; Foster, K.T. Impact of pharmacist intervention on completion of recombinant zoster vaccine series in a community pharmacy. *J. Am. Pharm. Assoc.* **2021**, *61*, S12–S16. [CrossRef]

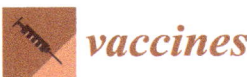

Article

Effectiveness of a Community-Based Organization—Private Clinic Service Model in Promoting Human Papillomavirus Vaccination among Chinese Men Who Have Sex with Men

Zixin Wang [1,*], Yuan Fang [2], Paul Shing-fong Chan [1], Andrew Chidgey [3], Francois Fong [4], Mary Ip [1] and Joseph T. F. Lau [1,*]

1. JC School of Public Health and Primary Care, Faculty of Medicine, The Chinese University of Hong Kong, Hong Kong, China; pchan@link.cuhk.edu.hk (P.S.-f.C.); mitk@cuhk.edu.hk (M.I.)
2. Department of Early Childhood Education, The Education University of Hong Kong, Hong Kong, China; lunajoef@gmail.com
3. AIDS Concern, Hong Kong, China; andrew.childgey@aidsconcern.org.hk
4. Neohealth, Hong Kong, China; drfong@neohealth.com.hk
* Correspondence: wangzx@cuhk.edu.hk (Z.W.); jlau@cuhk.edu.hk (J.T.F.L.)

Abstract: This study evaluated the effectiveness of the community-based organization (CBO)-private clinic service model in increasing human papillomavirus (HPV) vaccination uptake among unvaccinated men who have sex with men (MSM) in Hong Kong during a 12-month follow-up period. A CBO-private clinic model was implemented to promote HPV vaccination among Chinese MSM. A CBO with good access to MSM approached MSM aged 18–45 years who had never received an HPV vaccination, invited them to receive an online health promotion, and referred them to receive HPV vaccination at gay-friendly private clinics. A baseline survey and a follow-up evaluation at Month 12 were conducted. A total of 350 participants completed the baseline survey. Among 274 participants who were followed up at Month 12, 46 (16.8%) had taken up at least one dose of HPV vaccination. After adjusting for significant baseline characteristics, the perceived susceptibility (AOR:1.25, $p = 0.002$) and perceived severity (AOR:1.21, $p = 0.003$) of HPV and HPV-related diseases, perceived benefits (AOR:1.16, $p = 0.03$), self-efficacy to receive HPV vaccination (AOR:1.37, $p = 0.001$), and behavioral intention to take up HPV vaccination at baseline (AOR:6.99, $p < 0.001$) significantly predicted HPV vaccination uptake. The process evaluation of the program was positive. The CBO-private clinic service model was helpful in increasing HPV vaccination uptake among MSM.

Keywords: HPV vaccination; men who have sex with men; online health promotion; outcome and process evaluation

1. Introduction

Across countries, men who have sex with men (MSM) have a much higher risk of contracting human papillomavirus (HPV) and its related diseases (e.g., genital warts and penile cancers) than the general male population [1–4]. As reported by a meta-analysis, the overall prevalence of genital HPV infection was very high among both human immunodeficiency virus (HIV)-negative (63.9%) and HIV-infected MSM (92.6%) [5]. Moreover, MSM's risk of genital warts and anal cancers were much higher than the general population [6,7]. The prevalence of genital warts was 13.2–58.6% among MSM [6,7]. The overall prevalence of high-grade anal histological lesions was 23.9% among HIV-infected MSM and 15.2% among HIV-negative MSM [5]. The HPV-related cancer risk was the highest among HIV-infected MSM, which accounted for 9.9% of the MSM population in China in 2016 [8]. Slow clearance and increased persistence of high-risk HPV might explain why HIV-infected MSM are more susceptible to HPV and its related diseases compared with HIV-negative MSM [9–13]. A previous study showed that men with HIV infection had lower high-risk HPV clearance [9]. In-vitro studies showed increased expression of HPV E1

Citation: Wang, Z.; Fang, Y.; Chan, P.S.-f.; Chidgey, A.; Fong, F.; Ip, M.; Lau, J.T.F. Effectiveness of a Community-Based Organization—Private Clinic Service Model in Promoting Human Papillomavirus Vaccination among Chinese Men Who Have Sex with Men. *Vaccines* **2021**, *9*, 1218. https://doi.org/10.3390/vaccines9111218

Academic Editor: Gloria Calagna

Received: 27 September 2021
Accepted: 15 October 2021
Published: 20 October 2021

Publisher's Note: MDPI stays neutral with regard to jurisdictional claims in published maps and institutional affiliations.

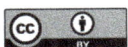

Copyright: © 2021 by the authors. Licensee MDPI, Basel, Switzerland. This article is an open access article distributed under the terms and conditions of the Creative Commons Attribution (CC BY) license (https://creativecommons.org/licenses/by/4.0/).

and L1 viral gene in the presence in HIV trans-activator of transcription (tat) protein [10]. HIV-tat protein was shown to enhance HPV transcription during HPV replication [11]. Moreover, uncontrolled HIV infection might increase the persistence of high-risk HPV through altered cell-mediated immunity, local molecular interactions, and reduced tight junction function [12,13]. In Hong Kong, among MSM with an experience of HPV screening, 25% were diagnosed with HPV infection [14].

HPV vaccination is highly effective in preventing vaccine-type genital warts and cancers among MSM [15,16] and other HPV-related diseases [17]. HPV vaccination provides maximum benefit if a person receives it before he/she is sexually active, and its efficacy is lower for MSM aged up to 45 years who have an HPV infection [18,19]. However, the Advisory Committee on Immunization Practices of the United States Centers for Disease Control and Prevention (CDC) recommends that people having an HPV infection should still receive HPV vaccination if they are in the appropriate age group because vaccination may protect them against high-risk HPV types that they have not yet acquired [20].

The CDC recommends MSM aged ≤45 years to receive the HPV vaccination [21,22]. In the United Kingdom, national programs provide free HPV vaccination for MSM aged up to 45 years attending sexual health and HIV clinics [23,24]. In 2017, the Victorian Government of Australia rolled out a free time-limited HPV vaccination catch-up program for MSM aged up to 26 years [25]. Relatively high HPV vaccination uptake was observed among MSM in national programs in developed countries, ranging from 37.6% in the United States [26], 42.6% in Australia [25], 49.1% in England [27], to 63.7% in Scotland [24]. However, in Hong Kong, there is no free or subsidized HPV vaccination program for MSM or other male populations. HPV vaccination uptake among the male population is very low in Hong Kong [28–30].

A randomized controlled trial (RCT) was conducted between 2017 and 2019 among MSM in Hong Kong to evaluate online intervention promoting HPV vaccination [31]. The results showed that watching a 5-min online video based on the Health Belief Model [32] and receiving brief motivational interviewing (MI) through telephone was effective in improving HPV vaccination uptake over a 24-month study period [31].

Community-based organization (CBO) in Hong Kong has a good position of promoting HPV vaccination among local MSM. First, half of MSM usually received HIV prevention services provided by local CBO (e.g., 45.5–51.5% of the HIV testing and counseling services) [29,33]. Second, it is easier to promote HPV vaccination by CBO staff, as it is naturally for MSM to receive HIV/sexually transmitted infections (STI)-related information from them. Participants may feel less stigmatized and embarrassed. Third, we found that a cue to action, a construct of the HBM [32], was strongly associated with the acceptability of HPV vaccination among local MSM.

Suggestion from peer CBO workers can serve as a strong cue to action [29]. Moreover, these CBOs have been working closely with gay-friendly private clinics providing STI screening and treatment for MSM. A CBO having good access to local MSM adapted the online intervention developed by the aforementioned RCT and initiated a CBO-private clinic service model promoting HPV vaccination for MSM in August 2019. The CBO approached MSM using its network, provided online intervention promoting HPV vaccination, and referred interested participants to gay-friendly private clinics in its service network for vaccination uptake. This study evaluated the effectiveness of the CBO-private clinics service model in increasing HPV vaccination uptake among unvaccinated MSM in Hong Kong during a 12-month follow-up period. Baseline factors predicting HPV vaccination uptake were investigated and process evaluation was performed.

2. Materials and Methods

2.1. Study Design

This longitudinal study was conducted from August 2019 to April 2021. All participants completed a telephone survey before they received online interventions promoting HPV vaccination, and completed another telephone survey 12 months after the baseline survey. There was no control or comparison group. The flowchart diagram was shown in Figure 1. The study was registered at ClinicalTrial.gov (NCT04815837).

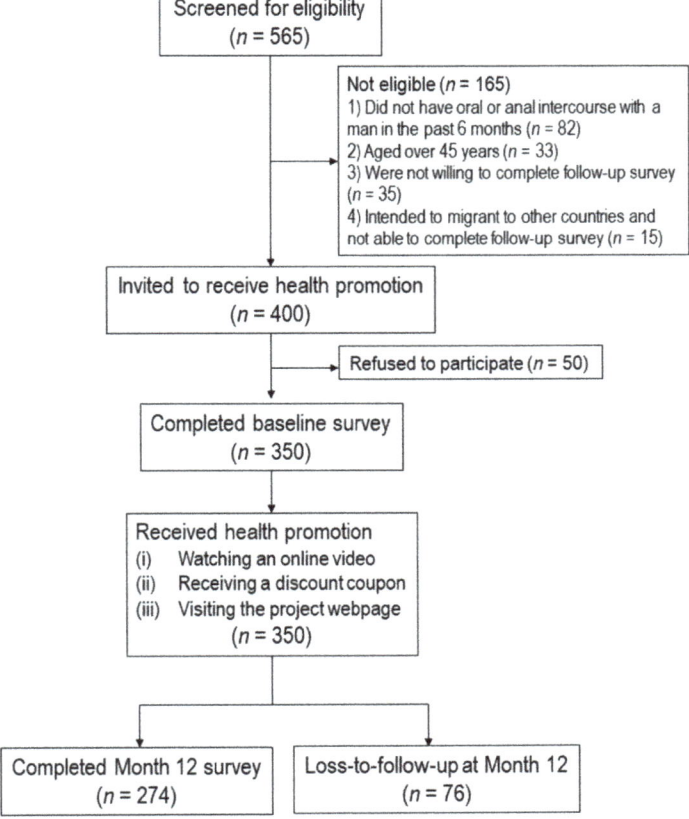

Figure 1. Flowchart diagram.

2.2. Participants

Inclusion criteria were: (1) Hong Kong Chinese speaking males aged 18–45 years old, (2) self-reported having had oral or anal intercourse with at least one man in the last six months, (3) never received HPV vaccination, and (4) willing to complete a follow-up telephone survey 12 months after the baseline survey.

2.3. Sampling and Data Collection

Trained staff of a CBO providing HIV-related services recruited participants through multiple sources, including outreaching in gay bars or saunas in Hong Kong, online recruitment, and referrals made by peers and other CBOs. Detailed recruitment procedures were reported in a published paper [14]. Interested participants contacted fieldworkers through WhatsApp, telephone, email, or other means. Participants were guaranteed anonymity during the study, and had the right to end participation in the study at any time. Their refusal or withdrawal from the study would not affect their access to any future services. Verbal instead of written informed consent was obtained due to maintaining anonymity, and the fieldworkers signed a form pledging that the participants had been fully informed about the study. Multiple forms of contact information were obtained to make appointments for conducting the baseline and Month 12 telephone interview. A HK$25 (approximately US$3.2) supermarket or café coupon was mailed to participants as compensation of their time after they completed each survey. Ethics approval was obtained from the Survey and Behavioral Research Ethics Committee of the Chinese University of Hong Kong (reference number: KPF18HLF22).

2.4. Baseline Telephone Survey and Health Promotion

By appointment, the CBO staff conducted the 15-min baseline survey by telephone. All participants received the following health promotion components:

(1) Watching an online video promoting HPV vaccination for MSM: The online video developed by our team in a previous RCT was modified for this study [31]. The modifications included: (i) cost of HPV vaccination was updated based on the recent market rate, and (ii) information of collaborative clinics (e.g., location and contacts) were added. The video was guided by the HBM [32].

In the video, a peer MSM talked about the risk of having penile or anal cancers among MSM, the severe consequences of HPV-related diseases, high efficacy, and long protection duration of HPV vaccination. The video also contained flashes of scary images of genital warts and penile and anal cancers to increase the perceived severity. The peer MSM also emphasized that HPV vaccination was a worthy long-term investment for their health. He demonstrated the procedures for receiving HPV vaccination in one of the collaborative private clinics, which was convenient, caring, privacy guaranteed, and non-judgmental. Participants could not fast-forward or skip any part of the video.

(2) Each participant was sent a discount coupon through SMS/WhatsApp and could enjoy a 10% discount for taking up three doses of HPV vaccines at a collaborative private clinic.

(3) Participants could access the project webpage by scanning the Quick Response (QR) code on the discount coupon. Through the webpage, participants could: (i) watch the aforementioned online video; (ii) read the description of the project, knowledge, and benefits of HPV vaccination, information about HPV/HPV-related diseases that increased the perceived susceptibility and perceived severity; (iii) access a discussion forum containing positive feedbacks of peers who have taken up HPV vaccination. These testimonials provided cue to action supporting HPV vaccination; and (iv) obtain the contact information of the project staff and information about the collaborative private clinics.

(4) Five reminders were sent to participants by SMS/WhatsApp at Month 1, 2, 4, 6, and 8.

2.5. Facilitating HPV Vaccination Uptake in Collaborative Private Clinics

During the project period, two types of HPV vaccines were available for males (Gardasil 4-valent and 9-valent vaccines). For participants who decided to take the vaccine in the collaborative private clinics, they could sign up on the project webpage by filling up their contacts and preferable timeslots. The CBO staff would contact them by telephone or WhatsApp to facilitate appointment making to take up HPV vaccination at collaborative private clinics at a 10% discount from the market rate (about HK$4200 or US$542 for three doses). Participants could also directly contact the collaborative clinics to make an appointment. The project did not limit participants' choice for taking up HPV vaccination in other places.

2.6. Month 12 Follow-up Telephone Survey

Participants were invited to complete a follow-up telephone survey 12 months after the baseline survey. Up to five calls were made at different timeslots during weekdays and/or weekends before considering a participant as a dropout.

2.7. Measurements

2.7.1. Primary Outcome

The primary outcome of the study was the validated uptake of any doses of HPV vaccination within a 12-month follow-up period. To validate HPV vaccination uptake, the participants were requested to send the project staff an image of their receipt without personal identification after they received each dose of HPV vaccines. The same approach to validate HPV vaccination uptake was used in a previous study [31]. Vaccinated participants were asked about the location and cost of HPV vaccination uptake, whether they experienced side-effects after vaccination, and the severity of those side-effects.

2.7.2. Baseline Characteristics

Various baseline information was collected, such as socio-demographics, sexual orientation, HIV or STI prevention service utilization, history of HIV and other STIs, and queried sexual behaviors, which included anal intercourse with male regular and non-regular sex partners and male sex workers, condomless anal intercourse (CAI) with men, multiple male sex partnerships, sexualized drug use (SDU), and so on. Regular male sex partners (RP) were defined as lovers and/or stable boyfriends, while non-regular male sex partners (NRP) were defined as casual sex partners. In this study, SDU was defined as the use of any psychoactive substance before or during sexual intercourse [34,35].

Six items measured knowledge related to HPV and HPV vaccination. A composite variable was constructed by counting the number of correct responses (ranged from 0 to 6). Five scales assessed perceptions based on the HBM, including a three-item Perceived Susceptibility Scale, four-item Perceived Severity Scale, four-item Perceived Benefit Scale, five-item Perceived Barrier Scale, two-item Cue to Action Scale, and two-item Perceived Self-Efficacy Scale. These scales were modified from those used in a previous study among MSM in Hong Kong [31].

2.7.3. Process Evaluation

At Month 12, participants were asked to evaluate the health promotion (e.g., whether the contents were clear and attractive). Participants who have taken up HPV vaccination were asked additional questions rating their satisfaction of the services provided by the collaborating clinics.

2.8. Statistical Analysis

The difference in baseline characteristics between participants who completed Month 12 follow-up and dropouts were compared by using chi-square tests (for categorical variables) or Mann–Whitney U tests (for continuous variables). The subsequent analysis was performed with data from those who had completed both surveys. We used the validated uptake of any doses of HPV vaccination during the follow-up period as the dependent variable and baseline background characteristics (e.g., socio-demographics, sexual orientation, and history of HIV and other STIs) as independent variables.

Crude odds ratios (OR) predicting that the dependent variable were obtained using logistic regression models. After adjustment for those variables with $p < 0.05$ in the univariate analysis, the association between knowledge and perceptions related to HPV and HPV vaccination and the dependent variable were then assessed by adjusted odds ratios (AOR). Each AOR was obtained by fitting a single logistic regression model, which involved one of the perceptions and the significant background variables. SPSS version 21.0 (Chicago, IL, USA) was used for data analysis, and $p < 0.05$ (two-sided) is considered as statistically significant.

3. Results

3.1. Baseline Characteristics

Four hundred of the 565 prospective participants were screened to be eligible, 50 of whom refused to participate in the study for time or other logistic reasons, and 350 (87.5%) completed the baseline survey and received health promotion. At Month 12, 274 (78.3%) completed the follow-up survey.

At baseline, about half of the participants were 18–30 years old (50.3%), and with a monthly personal income at least HK$20,000 (US$2565) (57.4%). The majority of the participants were currently single (75.7%), had attained tertiary education or above (86.6%), were employed full-time (82.9%), and identified themselves as homosexuals (91.1%). Among the participants, 1.7%, 8.9%, and 16.9% reported a history of HIV, HPV infection/genital warts, and other STI infection, respectively. In the past six months, 50.3% and 54.6% reported CAI with men and multiple male sex partnerships.

Regarding knowledge related to HPV or HPV vaccination, 48.9–95.7% gave correct responses to different items. The Cronbach alpha for the five scales based on the HBM were acceptable (0.61–0.85). Single factors for these scales by exploratory factor analysis, which explained 56.2–82.5% of the total variance. Apart from self-reported HIV sero-status ($p = 0.02$), anal intercourse with NRP ($p = 0.02$), and male sex workers ($p = 0.01$), no significant difference was found between participants who completed the Month 12 follow-up and dropouts (Table 1).

Table 1. Baseline characteristics of the participants.

	All Participants ($n = 350$)	Being Followed Up at Month 12 ($n = 274$)	Dropouts ($n = 76$)	p Values
	n (%)	n (%)	n (%)	
Socio-demographics				
Age group (years)				
18–24	48 (13.7)	34 (12.4)	14 (18.4)	0.34
25–30	128 (36.6)	106 (38.7)	22 (28.9)	
31–40	133 (38.0)	103 (37.6)	30 (39.5)	
>40	41 (11.7)	31 (11.3)	10 (13.2)	
Relationship status				
Currently single	265 (75.7)	210 (76.6)	55 (72.4)	0.44
Married or cohabited with a man	85 (24.3)	64 (23.4)	21 (27.6)	
Highest education level attained				
Secondary or below	47 (13.4)	37 (13.5)	10 (13.2)	0.94
Tertiary of above	303 (86.6)	237 (86.5)	66 (86.8)	
Employment status				
Full-time	290 (82.9)	229 (83.6)	61 (80.3)	0.50
Part-time/unemployed/retired/students	60 (17.1)	45 (16.4)	15 (19.7)	
Monthly personal income, HK$ (US$)				
<10,000 (1282)	37 (10.6)	27 (9.9)	10 (13.2)	0.28
10,000–19,999 (1282–2564)	106 (30.3)	87 (31.8)	19 (25.0)	
20,000–39,999 (2565–5128)	134 (38.3)	107 (39.1)	27 (35.5)	
40,000 (5129)	67 (19.1)	50 (18.2)	17 (22.4)	
Refuse to disclose	6 (1.7)	3 (1.1)	3 (3.9)	
Sexual orientation				
Homosexual	319 (91.1)	252 (92.0)	67 (88.2)	0.30
Bisexual	31 (8.9)	22 (8.0)	9 (11.8)	

Table 1. Cont.

	All Participants (n = 350)	Being Followed Up at Month 12 (n = 274)	Dropouts (n = 76)	p Values
	n (%)	n (%)	n (%)	
Lifestyles				
Smoking in lifetime				
No	257 (73.4)	203 (74.1)	54 (71.1)	0.60
Yes	93 (26.6)	71 (25.9)	22 (28.9)	
Drinking in the past year				
No	86 (24.6)	64 (23.4)	22 (28.9)	0.32
Yes	264 (75.4)	210 (76.6)	54 (71.1)	
History of HIV and other STIs and service utilization				
Self-reported HIV sero-status				
Negative	311 (88.9)	251 (91.6)	60 (78.9)	0.02
Positive	6 (1.7)	4 (1.5)	2 (2.6)	
Refuse to disclose	11 (3.1)	7 (2.6)	4 (5.3)	
Had never tested for HIV antibody	22 (6.3)	12 (4.4)	10 (13.2)	
History of HPV infection and/or genital warts (Yes)	31 (8.9)	27 (9.9)	4 (5.3)	0.21
History of other STIs (Yes)	59 (16.9)	47 (17.2)	12 (15.8)	0.78
Utilization of other HIV/STI prevention services (e.g., receiving free condoms, peer education and pamphlets, and attending seminars) (Yes)	81 (23.1)	69 (25.2)	12 (15.8)	0.09
Sexual behaviors in the past six months				
Anal intercourse with regular male sex partners (Yes)	293 (83.7)	230 (83.9)	63 (82.9)	0.83
Anal intercourse with non-regular male sex partners (Yes)	170 (48.6)	124 (45.3)	46 (60.5)	0.02
Anal intercourse with male sex workers (Yes)	9 (2.6)	4 (1.5)	5 (6.6)	0.01
Condomless anal intercourse with men (Yes)	176 (50.3)	142 (51.8)	34 (44.7)	0.27
Multiple male sex partnerships (Yes)	191 (54.6)	143 (52.2)	48 (63.2)	0.09
Sexual intercourse with female sex partners (Yes)	6 (1.7)	3 (1.1)	3 (3.9)	0.09
Condomless sex with female sex partners (Yes)	3 (0.9)	2 (0.7)	1 (1.3)	0.62
Sexualized drug use (use of psychoactive substances before or during sexual intercourse) (Yes)	20 (5.7)	17 (6.2)	3 (3.9)	0.45
Knowledge related to HPV or HPV vaccination				
Both males and females could be affected by HPV				
Yes [a]	335 (95.7)	264 (96.4)	71 (93.4)	0.11
No	5 (1.4)	2 (0.7)	3 (3.9)	
Do not know	10 (2.9)	8 (2.9)	2 (2.6)	
HPV infection could cause STI				
Yes [a]	317 (90.6)	248 (90.5)	69 (90.8)	0.79
No	8 (2.3)	7 (2.6)	1 (1.3)	
Do not know	25 (7.1)	19 (6.9)	6 (7.9)	
HPV infection could cause cancers among males				
Yes [a]	258 (73.7)	200 (73.0)	58 (76.3)	0.54
No	27 (7.7)	20 (7.3)	7 (9.2)	
Do not know	65 (18.6)	54 (19.7)	11 (14.5)	
HPV could be totally cured by available treatment				
Yes	62 (17.7)	48 (17.5)	14 (18.4)	0.93
No [a]	171 (48.9)	133 (48.5)	38 (50.0)	
Do not know	117 (33.4)	93 (33.9)	24 (31.6)	
Availability of effective HPV vaccination for males in Hong Kong				
Yes [a]	288 (82.3)	229 (83.6)	59 (77.6)	0.12
No	8 (2.3)	4 (1.5)	4 (5.3)	
Do not know	54 (15.4)	41 (15.0)	13 (17.1)	
Number of shots required to prevent HPV infection in males				
3 [a]	176 (50.3)	135 (49.3)	41 (53.9)	
Other answers/Do not know	174 (49.7)	139 (50.7)	35 (46.1)	
Number of correct responses, mean (SD)	4.4 (1.3)	4.4 (1.3)	4.4 (1.2)	0.91

Table 1. Cont.

	All Participants (n = 350)	Being Followed Up at Month 12 (n = 274)	Dropouts (n = 76)	p Values
	n (%)	n (%)	n (%)	
Perceptions related to HPV or HPV vaccination based on the HBM				
Perceived susceptibility to HPV (high/very high)				
Perceived risk of contracting HPV in lifetime	89 (25.4)	65 (23.7)	24 (31.6)	0.16
Perceived risk of contracting genital warts in lifetime	72 (20.6)	50 (18.2)	22 (28.9)	0.04
Perceived risk of having penile/anal cancers in lifetime	42 (12.0)	32 (11.7)	10 (13.2)	0.73
Perceived Susceptibility Scale [b], mean (SD)	8.2 (2.6)	8.1 (2.6)	8.8 (2.7)	0.35
Perceived severity of HPV-related diseases (agree/strongly agree)				
HPV infection would increase risk of HIV acquisition	106 (30.3)	81 (29.6)	25 (32.9)	0.58
HPV infection would cause penile or anal cancers	127 (36.3)	98 (35.8)	29 (38.2)	0.70
Genital warts would have severe harms on your health	182 (52.0)	140 (51.1)	42 (55.3)	0.52
Penile or anal cancers would have severe harms on your health	263 (75.1)	207 (75.5)	56 (73.7)	0.74
Perceived Severity Scale [c], mean (SD)	13.4 (3.1)	13.3 (3.2)	13.8 (2.7)	0.43
Perceived benefits of HPV vaccination (agree/strongly agree)				
HPV vaccination is highly effective in preventing HPV infection	273 (78.0)	210 (76.6)	63 (82.9)	0.24
HPV vaccination is highly effective in preventing genital warts	240 (68.6)	181 (66.1)	59 (77.6)	0.054
HPV vaccination is highly effective in preventing penile/anal cancers	214 (61.1)	166 (60.6)	48 (63.2)	0.68
HPV vaccination can protect you for a long time	193 (55.1)	149 (54.4)	44 (57.9)	0.59
Perceived Benefit Scale [d], mean (SD)	15.3 (2.5)	15.2 (2.6)	15.6 (2.1)	0.20
Perceived barriers of receiving HPV vaccination (agree/strongly agree)				
It is not worthy speeding HK$6000–7000 (US$774–903) to receive HPV vaccination	107 (30.6)	88 (32.1)	19 (25.0)	0.23
You would have severe side-effects after receiving HPV vaccination	37 (10.6)	30 (10.9)	7 (9.2)	0.66
Others would think you are having high-risk behaviors if you receive HPV vaccination	45 (12.9)	37 (13.5)	8 (10.5)	0.49
You would be stigmatized when you receive HPV vaccination	34 (9.7)	26 (9.5)	8 (10.5)	0.79
If you already infected with HPV, HPV vaccination could not protect you	111 (31.7)	88 (32.1)	23 (30.3)	0.76
Perceived Barrier Scale [e], mean (SD)	12.4 (3.1)	12.4 (3.1)	12.2 (3.5)	0.76
Perceived cue to action related to HPV vaccination (agree/strongly agree)				
Mass media suggest males to receive HPV vaccination	62 (17.7)	46 (16.8)	16 (21.1)	0.39
People who are important to you would suggest you to receive HPV vaccination	83 (23.7)	66 (24.1)	17 (22.4)	0.76
Cue to Action Scale [f], mean (SD)	4.9 (2.0)	4.8 (2.0)	5.2 (2.0)	0.14
Perceived self-efficacy related to HPV vaccination (agree/strongly agree)				
You are confident to receive HPV vaccination in the next year if you want	160 (45.7)	129 (47.1)	31 (40.8)	0.33
Receiving HPV vaccination in the next year is easy for you if you want	182 (52.0)	148 (54.0)	34 (44.7)	0.15
Perceived Self-efficacy Scale [g], mean (SD)	6.8 (2.0)	6.9 (2.0)	6.7 (2.0)	0.37

Table 1. Cont.

	All Participants (n = 350)	Being Followed Up at Month 12 (n = 274)	Dropouts (n = 76)	p Values
	n (%)	n (%)	n (%)	
Behavioral intention to take up HPV vaccination (likely/very likely)				
Likelihood of taking up three required doses of HPV vaccines in the next year	64 (18.3)	52 (19.0)	12 (15.8)	0.53

[a] Correct response. [b] Perceived Susceptibility Scale: three items, Cronbach's alpha: 0.85, one factor was identified by exploratory factor analysis, explaining for 77.2% of total variances. [c] Perceived Severity Scale: four items, Cronbach's alpha: 0.72, one factor was identified by exploratory factor analysis, explaining for 54.9% of total variances. [d] Perceived Benefit Scale: four items, Cronbach's alpha: 0.79, one factor was identified by exploratory factor analysis, explaining for 62.4% of total variances. [e] Perceived Barrier Scale: five items, Cronbach's alpha: 0.62, one factor was identified by exploratory factor analysis, explaining for 57.9% of total variances. [f] Cue to Action Scale: two items, Cronbach's alpha: 0.61, one factor was identified by exploratory factor analysis, explaining for 56.2% of total variances. [g] Perceived Benefit Scale: two items, Cronbach's alpha: 0.79, one factor was identified by exploratory factor analysis, explaining for 82.5% of total variances. HK: Hong Kong; HIV: human immunodeficiency virus; STI: sexually transmitted infection; and HPV: human papillomavirus.

3.2. HPV Vaccination Uptake

At Month 12, 46 participants self-reported having had taken up at least one dose of HPV vaccination (three doses: n = 13; two doses: n = 24; and one dose: n = 9). All of them were able to provide receipts for verification. The location for receiving HPV vaccination included the collaborative private clinics (28/46, 60.9%) and other private hospitals/clinics (18/46, 39.1%). The participants self-paid HK$2000–6800 (US$ 258–877; median: HK$4200 or US$542) to receive the vaccination. Most vaccinated participants reported no side effects (37/46, 80.4%). The reported side effects included pain at the injection site (5/46, 10.9%), fatigue (4/46, 8.7%), and dizziness (1/46, 2.2%). Most of these side effects were very mild or mild (8/9, 88.9%).

3.3. Factors Predicting HPV Vaccination Uptake

Among 274 participants who had completed both baseline and Month 12 surveys, a history of HPV infection and/or genital warts (OR: 6.02, 95%CI: 2.60, 13.94, p < 0.001) and utilization of HIV/STI prevention services other than HIV testing at baseline (OR: 1.98, 95%CI: 1.01, 3.89, p = 0.046) were associated with higher HPV vaccination uptake during the follow-up period (Table 2).

After adjusting for these significant baseline characteristics, four constructs of the HBM were associated with the dependent variable in expected directions. They were: (1) perceived higher risk of contracting HPV and HPV-related diseases (perceived susceptibility) (AOR: 1.25, 95% CI: 1.09, 1.43, p = 0.002), (2) perceived consequences of HPV-related diseases to be severer (AOR: 1.21, 95%CI: 1.07, 1.37, p = 0.003), (3) perceived benefits of HPV vaccination (AOR: 1.16, 95% CI: 1.01, 1.33, p = 0.03), and (4) perceived self-efficacy of taking up HPV vaccination (AOR: 1.37, 95%CI: 1.14, 1.65, p = 0.001). In addition, behavioral intention to take up HPV vaccination at baseline was also associated with higher uptake during the follow-up period (AOR: 6.99, 95% CI: 3.34, 14.60, p < 0.001) (Table 3).

Table 2. Baseline background characteristics predicting human papillomavirus vaccination uptake (among participants who completed Month 12 follow-up, $n = 274$).

	OR (95%CI)	p Values
Socio-demographics		
Age group (years)		
18–24	1.0	
25–30	0.80 (0.32, 2.03)	0.64
31–40	0.43 (0.16, 1.16)	0.10
>40	0.63 (0.18, 2.17)	0.46
Relationship status		
Currently single	1.0	
Married or cohabited with a man	0.77 (0.35, 1.68)	0.51
Highest education level attained		
Secondary or below	1.0	
Tertiary of above	1.78 (0.60, 5.29)	0.30
Employment status		
Full-time	1.0	
Part-time/unemployed/retired/students	0.57 (0.21, 1.54)	0.27
Monthly personal income, HK$ (US$)		
<10,000 (1282)	1.0	
10,000–19,999 (1282–2564)	1.53 (0.41, 5.80)	0.53
20,000–39,999 (2565–5128)	1.73 (0.47, 6.33)	0.41
40,000 (5129)	2.00 (0.50, 8.00)	0.33
Refuse to disclose	N.A.	N.A.
Sexual orientation		
Homosexual	1.0	
Bisexual	1.11 (0.36, 3.45)	0.86
Lifestyles		
Smoking in lifetime		
No	1.0	
Yes	0.88 (0.42, 1.84)	0.74
Drinking in the past year		
No	1.0	
Yes	0.96 (0.46, 2.03)	0.92
History of HIV and other STIs and service utilization		
Self-reported HIV sero-status		
Negative	1.0	
Positive	5.28 (0.72, 38.55)	0.10
Refuse to disclose	3.96 (0.85, 18.36)	0.08
Had never tested for HIV antibody	0.49 (0.06, 3.82)	0.49
History of HPV infection and/or genital warts		
No	1.0	
Yes	6.02 (2.60, 13.94)	<0.001
History of other STIs (Yes)		
No	1.0	
Yes	1.02 (0.44, 2.36)	0.96
Utilization of other HIV/STI prevention services (e.g., receiving free condoms, peer education and pamphlets, and attending seminars)		
No	1.0	
Yes	1.98 (1.01, 3.89)	0.046
Sexual behaviors in the past six months		
Anal intercourse with regular male sex partners		
No	1.0	
Yes	1.08 (0.45, 2.60)	0.87
Anal intercourse with non-regular male sex partners		
No	1.0	
Yes	1.55 (0.82, 2.93)	0.18
Anal intercourse with male sex workers		
No	1.0	
Yes	1.67 (0.17, 16.39)	0.66
Condomless anal intercourse with men		
No	1.0	
Yes	1.26 (0.66, 2.38)	0.49
Multiple male sex partnerships		
No	1.0	
Yes	1.91 (0.99, 3.69)	0.06
Sexual intercourse with female sex partners		
No	1.0	
Yes	N.A.	N.A.
Condomless sex with female sex partners		
No	1.0	
Yes	N.A.	N.A.
Sexualized drug use (use of psychoactive substances before or during sexual intercourse)		
No	1.0	
Yes	1.58 (0.49, 5.07)	0.45

OR: crude odds ratios; CI: confidence interval; HK: Hong Kong; HIV: human immunodeficiency virus; STI: sexually transmitted infection; HPV: human papillomavirus; and N.A.: not applicable.

Table 3. Factors predicting human papillomavirus vaccination uptake (among participants who completed Month 12 follow-up, $n = 274$).

	OR (95%CI)	p Values	AOR (95%CI)	p Values
Knowledge related to HPV or HPV vaccination				
Number of correct responses	1.29 (0.97, 1.70)	0.08	1.15 (0.86, 1.54)	0.35
Perceptions related to HPV or HPV vaccination based on the HBM				
Perceived Susceptibility Scale	1.31 (1.15, 1.49)	<0.001	1.25 (1.09, 1.43)	0.002
Perceived Severity Scale	1.19 (1.06, 1.33)	0.003	1.21 (1.07, 1.37)	0.003
Perceived Benefit Scale	1.19 (1.05, 1.36)	0.009	1.16 (1.01, 1.33)	0.03
Perceived Barrier Scale	0.88 (0.79, 0.98)	0.02	0.90 (0.80, 1.01)	0.07
Cue to Action Scale	1.16 (0.99, 1.36)	0.08	1.10 (0.93, 1.30)	0.26
Perceived Self-efficacy Scale	1.42 (1.19, 1.71)	<0.001	1.37 (1.14, 1.65)	0.001
Behavioral intention to take up HPV vaccination				
Likelihood of taking up three required doses of HPV vaccines in the next year				
Very unlikely/unlikely/neutral	1.0		1.0	
Likely/very likely	8.86 (4.38, 17.95)	<0.001	6.99 (3.34, 14.60)	<0.001

HPV: human papillomavirus; HBM: health belief model; OR: crude odds ratios; CI: confidence interval; and AOR: adjusted odds ratios, odds ratios adjusted for significant baseline background characteristics (i.e., history of HPV infection and/or genital warts, and utilization of other HIV/STI prevention services).

3.4. Reasons for Not Taking up HPV Vaccination

At Month 12, 228 unvaccinated participants were asked about their reasons for not taking up HPV vaccination. The most commonly mentioned reason was the high cost of HPV vaccination (128/228, 56.1%), followed by feeling unnecessary to receive such vaccination (79/228, 34.6%), concerns about COVID-19 transmission (73/228, 32.0%), and no time to do so (60/228, 26.3%).

3.5. Process Evaluation

Among 274 participants who completed the Month 12 survey, 72.3% and 38.7% believed the health promotion video was clear and attractive respectively. The participants thought the video was helpful in the following aspects, such as increasing awareness of benefits of HPV vaccination (73.4%), reducing barriers to receive HPV vaccination (46.0%), and increasing self-efficacy (56.2%) and intention (40.5%) to receive HPV vaccination.

Among 46 vaccinated participants, 50–95.7% rated "satisfactory" to the following services/features of the collaborating clinics: (1) convenience of the location of clinic (89.1%), (2) convenience of the arranged time slot for vaccination (95.7%), (3) waiting time between making appointment and receiving the first dose (84.8%), (4) level of privacy (69.6%), (5) staff's acceptance of MSM's subculture (50.0%), (6) explanation made by the staff of private clinics (73.9%), and (7) professionalism of the staff of private clinics (76.1%) (Table 4).

Table 4. Process evaluation of the health promotion and the procedures to receive human papillomavirus vaccination at private clinics.

	n	%
Process evaluation of the health promotion (among participants who completed the Month 12 follow-up evaluation, n = 274) (agree/strongly agree)		
The content of the health promotion is clear	198	72.3
The content of the health promotion is attractive	106	38.7
The health promotion has increased their understanding on benefit of HPV vaccination	201	73.4
The health promotion has reduced their barriers to take up HPV vaccination	126	46.0
The health promotion has increased their confidence to take up HPV vaccination	154	56.2
The health promotion has increased their willingness to take up HPV vaccination	111	40.5
Satisfaction with the following procedures to receive HPV vaccination at private clinics (among participants who had completed HPV vaccination during the follow-up period, n = 46) (satisfied/very satisfied)		
Convenience of the location of clinic	41	89.1
Convenience of the arranged time slot for vaccination	44	95.7
Waiting time between making appointment and receiving the first dose of HPV vaccination	39	84.8
Level of privacy	32	69.6
Private clinic staff's acceptance of MSM's subculture	23	50.0
Explanation made by the staff of the private clinic	34	73.9
Level of professionalism of the staff of the private clinic	35	76.1

HPV: human papillomavirus; and MSM: gay, bisexual, other men who have sex with men.

4. Discussion

It is important to transform research findings into regular services. We involved CBO and private clinics as key stakeholders at the planning stage. The implementation was smooth and concurred with routine services of CBO and private clinics. The evaluation results showed that the CBO-private clinic service model was helpful in increasing HPV vaccination uptake among MSM in Hong Kong, as 16.8% of participants being followed up at Month 12 had taken up at least one dose of HPV vaccination. We expected most of these participants would complete all three required doses in near future, as all of them settled the payment for the entire package when receiving the first dose and made appointments for receiving the remaining doses.

Although there was an increase in the cost of HPV vaccines (from HK$3800 or US$490 to HK$4200 or US$542) and there was no MI, the uptake rate was comparable to the intervention group (17.3%) in previous RCT [31]. However, the HPV vaccination uptake in this study was lower than those in the United States (19.4–45%) [36–39]. The difference could be partially explained by the cost of HPV vaccination, as it was free in the United States while it was charged at market price with a slight discount in this study. It was likely that COVID-19 had a negative impact on HPV vaccination uptake in this study, as one third of unvaccinated participants mentioned concerns about COVID-19 transmission as a reason of not taking up HPV vaccination at Month 12.

The findings also had some implications to health service and health care policy. Our results supported that HPV vaccination was accepted by local MSM at the market rate. Providing subsidized or free HPV vaccination would further increase the uptake rate. MSM in Australia and the United Kingdom responded well to pilot programs providing free HPV vaccination [23–25]. Hong Kong should consider a similar pilot program for MSM, which would largely increase HPV vaccination coverage in this group and reduce HPV-related disease burdens.

The planning of future programs can be facilitated by the experiences of the present study. We found that those with history of HPV infection and/or genital warts were more responsive to the health promotion as compared to MSM without such history. It is possible that MSM with such history would perceive a stronger need to protect themselves by taking up HPV vaccination. Future studies are needed to explore whether different strategies should be applied for MSM with and without prior experience of HPV infection/genital warts. We also found that the baseline measurement of perceived susceptibility, perceived severity, perceived benefit, perceived self-efficacy, and behavioral intention related to HPV vaccination significantly predicted HPV vaccination uptake during the project period.

Since our health promotion was standard and one-off, such findings suggested that some follow-ups should be implemented to modify these perceptions. Meta-analysis suggested that interventions tailored to one's stage of change (SOC) were more effective than non-stage-tailored, especially among less motivated individuals [40]. Studies also showed that people might move forward to a higher SOC, go back to a lower SOC, or stay in the same SOC after exposing to the health promotion [41]. Therefore, future programs should consider stage-tailored health promotion with multiple sessions, which might be helpful to strengthen the perceived threat of HPV and perceived benefit of HPV vaccination.

Moreover, asking people to provide where, when, and how they want to perform a behavior could increase the perceived self-efficacy [42]. The results of the process evaluation also provide insights for improving health promotion and procedures to receive HPV vaccination in future program. Future programs should consider crowdsourcing, which allows experts and target audience to share solutions together to increase the attractiveness of the contents [43]. Half of the MSM were not satisfied about HPV vaccination service providers' acceptance of their subculture. Interventions targeting service providers to enhance their knowledge about MSM's subculture is needed, and there were effective interventions in the literature [44]. Since the amount of HPV vaccination service providers would be relatively small, training to improve the situation should be feasible.

This study had the strengths of a relatively low dropout rate, validated primary outcome, and good process evaluation. However, it had several limitations. First, there was no control or comparison group. The aim of this study was to evaluate the effectiveness of the service model in real-world setting. Second, a selection bias existed, as we were not able to collect information from MSM who refused to join the project. They might have different characteristics comparing to participants. Third, attrition bias existed. The dropouts were more likely to be HIV positive or with unknown sero-status and had anal intercourse with NRP and male sex workers at the baseline. However, the bias should be limited as these baseline characteristics did not significantly predict HPV vaccination uptake during the project period.

Fourth, we did not ask for details about how COVID-19 influenced the participants' HPV vaccination. However, a previous study exploring the difficulties to access HIV-related services among MSM in Hong Kong during the same period provided some insights. Worrying about being exposed to a potentially COVID-19 infectious environment, experiencing disruptions in work due to COVID-19 and its control measures, and reduced connection to the MSM community during the pandemic were associated with increased difficulties in accessing HIV-related services in general [45]. Some of these factors might have negatively affected HPV vaccination among our participants. Finally, the study was based on a convenient sample of MSM, cautions should be taken when generalizing the results to MSM in Hong Kong.

5. Conclusions

The CBO-private clinic service model was helpful in increasing HPV vaccination uptake among MSM in Hong Kong. A larger-scale pilot program should be considered based on the experience of this project.

Author Contributions: Conceptualization: Z.W., A.C., F.F., J.T.F.L.; Methodology: Z.W., J.T.F.L., Data curation: Z.W., M.I., A.C. and F.F.; Formal analysis: Z.W. and Y.F.; Project administration: Z.W., M.I. Resources: Z.W., M.I., A.C., and F.F.; Supervision: Z.W. and M.I.; Writing—original draft preparation: Z.W., Y.F. and P.S.-f.C.; Writing—review and editing: Z.W., Y.F., P.S.-f.C. and J.T.F.L.; Funding acquisition: Z.W., and J.T.F.L. All authors have read and agreed to the published version of the manuscript.

Funding: This research was funded by the Knowledge Transfer Project Fund, the Chinese University of Hong Kong (grant number: KPF18HLF22).

Institutional Review Board Statement: The study was conducted according to the guidelines of the Declaration of Helsinki, and approved by the Survey and Behavioral Research Ethics Committee of the Chinese University of Hong Kong (reference number: KPF18HLF22 and date of approval: 18 March 2019).

Informed Consent Statement: Informed consent was obtained from all subjects involved in the study.

Data Availability Statement: The data presented in this study are available from the corresponding authors upon request. The data are not publicly available as they contain sensitive personal behaviors.

Acknowledgments: The authors would like to express their gratitude to all the participants for their engagement in this study.

Conflicts of Interest: The authors declare no conflict of interest.

References

1. World Health Organization. Human Papillomavirus Vaccines: WHO Position Paper, May 2017. Available online: http://apps.who.int/iris/bitstream/handle/10665/255353/WER9219.pdf;jsessionid=0F6E736DC1E29E420436DE39CD4551DD?sequence=1 (accessed on 13 May 2021).
2. Liu, F.F.; Hang, D.; Deng, Q.J.; Liu, M.F.; Xi, L.F.; He, Z.H.; Zhang, C.T.; Sun, M.; Liu, Y.; Li, J.J.; et al. Concurrence of oral and genital human papillomavirus infection in healthy men: A population-based cross-sectional study in rural China. *Sci. Rep.* **2015**, *5*, 15637. [CrossRef]
3. Hebnes, J.B.; Olesen, T.B.; Duun-Henriksen, A.K.; Munk, C.; Norrild, B.; Kjaer, S.K. Prevalence of Genital Human Papillomavirus among Men in Europe: Systematic Review and Meta-Analysis. *J. Sex. Med.* **2014**, *11*, 2630–2644. [CrossRef] [PubMed]
4. Zhang, X.J.; Yu, J.P.; Li, M.; Sun, X.Y.; Han, Q.; Li, M.; Zhou, F.; Li, Z.W.; Yang, Y.; Xiao, D.; et al. Prevalence and Related Risk Behaviors of HIV, Syphilis, and Anal HPV Infection Among Men who have Sex with Men from Beijing, China. *Aids Behav.* **2013**, *17*, 1129–1136. [CrossRef] [PubMed]
5. Machalek, D.A.; Poynten, M.; Jin, F.Y.; Fairley, C.K.; Farnsworth, A.; Garland, S.M.; Hillman, R.J.; Petoumenos, K.; Roberts, J.; Tabrizi, S.N.; et al. Anal human papillomavirus infection and associated neoplastic lesions in men who have sex with men: A systematic review and meta-analysis. *Lancet Oncol.* **2012**, *13*, 487–500. [CrossRef]
6. Jiang, J.; Cao, N.X.; Zhang, J.P.; Xia, Q.; Gong, X.D.; Xue, H.Z.; Yang, H.T.; Zhang, G.C.; Shao, C.G. High prevalence of sexually transmitted diseases among men who have sex with men in Jiangsu Province, China. *Sex. Transm. Dis.* **2006**, *33*, 118–123. [CrossRef] [PubMed]
7. D'Souza, G.; Wentz, A.; Wiley, D.; Shah, N.; Barrington, F.; Darragh, T.M.; Joste, N.; Plankey, M.; Reddy, S.; Breen, E.C.; et al. Anal Cancer Screening in Men Who Have Sex with Men in the Multicenter AIDS Cohort Study. *J. Acquir. Immune Defic. Syndr.* **2016**, *71*, 570–576. [CrossRef]
8. Qin, Q.Q.; Tang, W.M.; Ge, L.; Li, D.M.; Mahapatra, T.; Wang, L.Y.; Guo, W.; Cui, Y.; Sun, J.P. Changing trend of HIV, Syphilis and Hepatitis C among Men Who Have Sex with Men in China. *Sci. Rep.* **2016**, *6*, 31081. [CrossRef]
9. Geskus, R.B.; Gonzalez, C.; Torres, M.; Romero, J.D.; Viciana, P.; Masia, M.; Blanco, J.R.; Iribarren, M.; De Sanjose, B.; Hernandex-Novoa, B.; et al. Incidence and clearance of anal high-risk human papillomavirus in HIV-positive men who have sex with men: Estimates and risk factors. *AIDS* **2016**, *30*, 37–44. [CrossRef]
10. Kang, M.; Cu-Uvin, S. Association of HIV viral load and CD4 cell count with human papillomavirus detection and clearance in HIV-infected women initiating highly active antiretroviral therapy. *HIV Med.* **2012**, *13*, 372–378. [CrossRef]
11. Vernon, S.D.; Hart, C.E.; Reeves, W.C.; Icenogle, J.P. The HIV-1 tat protein enhances E2-dependent human papillomavirus 16 transcription. *Virus Res.* **1993**, *27*, 133–145. [CrossRef]
12. Scott, M.; Nakagawa, M.; Moscicki, A.B. Cell-mediated immune response to human papillomavirus infection. *Clin. Diagn. Lab. Immunol.* **2001**, *8*, 209–220. [CrossRef]
13. Tugizov, S.M.; Herrera, R.; Chin-Hong, P.; Veluppillai, P.; Greenspan, D.; Berry, J.M.; Pilcher, C.D.; Shiboski, C.H.; Jay, N.; Rubin, M.; et al. HIV-associated disruption of mucosal epithelium facilitates paracellular penetration by human papillomavirus. *Virology* **2013**, *446*, 378–388. [CrossRef] [PubMed]
14. Wang, Z.X.; Fang, Y.; Wong, N.S.; Ip, M.; Guo, X.; Wong, S.Y.S. Facilitators and Barriers to Take Up Clinician-Collected and Self-Collected HPV Tests among Chinese Men Who Have Sex with Men. *Viruses* **2021**, *13*, 705. [CrossRef] [PubMed]
15. Dunne, E.F.; Markowitz, L.E.; Chesson, H.; Curtis, C.R.; Saraiya, M.; Gee, J.; Unger, E.R. Recommendations on the Use of Quadrivalent Human Papillomavirus Vaccine in Males-Advisory Committee on Immunization Practices (ACIP). *JAMA J. Am. Med. Assoc.* **2012**, *307*, 557–559.
16. De Vuyst, H.; Clifford, G.M.; Nascimento, M.C.; Madeleine, M.M.; Franceschi, S. Prevalence and type distribution of human papillomavirus in carcinoma and intraepithelial neoplasia of the vulva, vagina and anus: A meta-analysis. *Int. J. Cancer* **2009**, *124*, 1626–1636. [CrossRef] [PubMed]
17. Lin, A.; Ong, K.J.; Hobbelen, P.; King, E.; Mesher, D.; Edmunds, W.J.; Sonnenberg, P.; Gilson, R.; Bains, I.; Choi, Y.H.; et al. Impact and Cost-effectiveness of Selective Human Papillomavirus Vaccination of Men Who Have Sex with Men. *Clin. Infect. Dis.* **2017**, *64*, 580–588. [CrossRef] [PubMed]

18. Hildesheim, A.; Herrero, R.; Wacholder, S.; Rodriguez, A.C.; Solomon, D.; Bratti, M.C.; Schiller, J.T.; Gonzalez, P.; Dubin, G.; Porras, C.; et al. Effect of human papillomavirus 16/18 L1 viruslike particle vaccine among young women with preexisting infection: A randomized trial. *JAMA* **2007**, *298*, 743–755. [CrossRef]
19. Hildesheim, A.; Gonzalez, P.; Kreimer, A.R.; Wacholder, S.; Schussler, J.; Rodriguez, A.C.; Porras, C.; Schiffman, M.; Sidewy, M.; Schiller, J.T.; et al. Impact of human papillomavirus (HPV) 16 and 18 vaccination on prevalent infections and rates of cervical lesions after excisional treatment. *Am. J. Obstet. Gynecol.* **2016**, *215*, 212.e1–212.e5. [CrossRef]
20. National Cancer Institute. Human Papillomavirus (HPV) Vaccines. Available online: https://www.cancer.gov/about-cancer/causes-prevention/risk/infectious-agents/hpv-vaccine-fact-sheet#should-hpv-vaccines-be-given-to-people-who-are-already-infected-with-hpv-or-have-cervical-cell-changes (accessed on 15 October 2021).
21. Centers for Disease Control and Prevention (CDC). HPV Vaccine Recommendations. Available online: https://www.cdc.gov/vaccines/vpd/hpv/hcp/recommendations.html (accessed on 15 May 2021).
22. Centers for Disease Control and Prevention (CDC). Evidence to Recommendations for HPV Vaccination of Adults, Ages 27 through 45 Years. Available online: https://www.cdc.gov/vaccines/acip/recs/grade/HPV-adults-etr.html (accessed on 13 May 2021).
23. Public Health England. HPV Vaccination for Men Who Have Sex with Men (MSM) Programme. Available online: https://www.gov.uk/government/collections/hpv-vaccination-for-men-who-have-sex-with-men-msm-programme (accessed on 14 May 2021).
24. Pollock, K.G.; Wallace, L.A.; Wrigglesworth, S.; McMaster, D.; Steedman, N. HPV vaccine uptake in men who have sex with men in Scotland. *Vaccine* **2019**, *37*, 5513–5514. [CrossRef]
25. McGrath, L.; Fairley, C.K.; Cleere, E.F.; Bradshaw, C.S.; Chen, M.Y.; Chow, E.P.F. Human papillomavirus vaccine uptake among young gay and bisexual men who have sex with men with a time-limited targeted vaccination programme through sexual health clinics in Melbourne in 2017. *Sex. Transm. Infect.* **2019**, *95*, 181–186. [CrossRef]
26. Loretan, C.; Chamberlain, A.T.; Sanchez, T.; Zlotorzynska, M.; Jones, J. Trends and Characteristics Associated with Human Papillomavirus Vaccination Uptake Among Men Who Have Sex with Men in the United States, 2014–2017. *Sex. Transm. Dis.* **2019**, *46*, 465–473. [CrossRef]
27. Checchi, M.; Mesher, D.; McCall, M.; Coukan, F.; Chau, C.; Mohammed, H.; Duffell, S.; Edelstein, M.; Yarwood, J.; Soldan, K. HPV vaccination of gay, bisexual and other men who have sex with men in sexual health and HIV clinics in England: Vaccination uptake and attendances during the pilot phase. *Sex. Transm. Infect.* **2019**, *95*, 608–613. [CrossRef]
28. Wang, Z.X.; Wang, J.; Fang, Y.; Gross, D.L.; Wong, M.C.S.; Wong, E.L.Y.; Lau, J.T.F. Parental acceptability of HPV vaccination for boys and girls aged 9-13years in China—A population-based study. *Vaccine* **2018**, *36*, 2657–2665. [CrossRef]
29. Lau, J.T.F.; Wang, Z.X.; Kim, J.H.; Lau, M.; Lai, C.H.Y.; Mo, P.K.H. Acceptability of HPV Vaccines and Associations with Perceptions Related to HPV and HPV Vaccines Among Men Who Have Sex with Men in Hong Kong. *PLoS ONE* **2013**, *8*, e57204. [CrossRef]
30. Wang, Z.X.; Mo, P.K.H.; Lau, J.T.F.; Lau, M.S.; Lai, C.H.Y. Acceptability of HPV vaccines and perceptions related to genital warts and penile/anal cancers among men who have sex with men in Hong Kong. *Vaccine* **2013**, *31*, 4675–4681. [CrossRef] [PubMed]
31. Wang, Z.X.; Lau, J.T.F.; Ip, T.K.M.; Yu, Y.B.; Fong, F.; Fang, Y.; Mo, P.K.H. Two Web-Based and Theory-Based Interventions With and Without Brief Motivational Interviewing in the Promotion of Human Papillomavirus Vaccination Among Chinese Men Who Have Sex With Men: Randomized Controlled Trial. *J. Med. Internet Res.* **2021**, *23*, e21465. [CrossRef] [PubMed]
32. Janz, N.K.; Becker, M.H. The Health Belief Model—A Decade Later. *Health Educ. Quart.* **1984**, *11*, 1–47. [CrossRef] [PubMed]
33. Wong, H.T.H.; Tam, H.Y.; Chan, D.P.C.; Lee, S.S. Usage and Acceptability of HIV Self-testing in Men who have Sex with Men in Hong Kong. *Aids Behav.* **2015**, *19*, 505–515. [CrossRef] [PubMed]
34. Wang, Z.X.; Yang, X.; Mo, P.K.H.; Fang, Y.; Ip, T.K.M.; Lau, J.T.F. Influence of Social Media on Sexualized Drug Use and Chemsex Among Chinese Men Who Have Sex with Men: Observational Prospective Cohort Study. *J. Med. Internet Res.* **2020**, *22*, e17894. [CrossRef] [PubMed]
35. Wang, Z.X.; Mo, P.K.H.; Ip, M.; Fang, Y.; Lau, J.T.F. Uptake and willingness to use PrEP among Chinese gay, bisexual and other men who have sex with men with experience of sexualized drug use in the past year. *BMC Infect. Dis.* **2020**, *20*, 299. [CrossRef]
36. Reiter, P.L.; Katz, M.L.; Bauermeister, J.A.; Shoben, A.B.; Paskett, E.D.; McRee, A.L. Increasing Human Papillomavirus Vaccination Among Young Gay and Bisexual Men: A Randomized Pilot Trial of the Outsmart HPV Intervention. *LGBT Health* **2018**, *5*, 325–329. [CrossRef]
37. Reiter, P.L.; Gower, A.L.; Kiss, D.E.; Malone, M.A.; Katz, M.L.; Bauermeister, J.A.; Shoben, A.B.; Paskett, E.D.; Mcree, A.L. A Web-Based Human Papillomavirus Vaccination Intervention for Young Gay, Bisexual, and Other Men Who Have Sex with Men: Protocol for a Randomized Controlled Trial. *JMIR Res. Protoc.* **2020**, *9*, e16294. [CrossRef] [PubMed]
38. Fontenot, H.B.; White, B.P.; Rosenberger, J.G.; Lacasse, H.; Rutirasiri, C.; Mayer, K.H.; Zimet, G. Mobile App Strategy to Facilitate Human Papillomavirus Vaccination Among Young Men Who Have Sex with Men: Pilot Intervention Study. *J. Med. Internet Res.* **2020**, *22*, e22878. [CrossRef] [PubMed]
39. Gerend, M.A.; Madkins, K.; Crosby, S.; Korpak, A.K.; Phillips, G.L.; Bass, M.; Houlberg, M.; Mustanski, B. Evaluation of a Text Messaging-Based Human Papillomavirus Vaccination Intervention for Young Sexual Minority Men: Results from a Pilot Randomized Controlled Trial. *Ann. Behav. Med.* **2021**, *55*, 321–332. [CrossRef] [PubMed]

40. Noar, S.M.; Benac, C.N.; Harris, M.S. Does tailoring matter? Meta-analytic review of tailored print health behavior change interventions. *Psychol. Bull.* **2007**, *133*, 673–693. [CrossRef]
41. Redding, C.A.; Brown-Peterside, P.; Noar, S.M.; Rossi, J.S.; Koblin, B.A. One session of TTM-tailored condom use feedback: A pilot study among at-risk women in the Bronx. *Aids Care* **2011**, *23*, 10–15. [CrossRef]
42. Milkman, K.L.; Beshears, J.; Choi, J.J.; Laibson, D.; Madrian, B.C. Using implementation intentions prompts to enhance influenza vaccination rates. *Proc. Natl. Acad. Sci. USA* **2011**, *108*, 10415–10420. [CrossRef]
43. Tucker, J.D.; Fenton, K.A. Innovation challenge contests to enhance HIV responses. *Lancet HIV* **2018**, *5*, e113–e115. [CrossRef]
44. Wang, Z.X.; Lau, J.T.F.; She, R.; Ip, M.; Jiang, H.; Ho, S.P.Y.; Yang, X.Y. Behavioral intention to take up different types of HIV testing among men who have sex with men who were never-testers in Hong Kong. *Aids Care* **2018**, *30*, 95–102. [CrossRef]
45. Suen, Y.T.; Chan, R.C.H.; Wong, E.M.Y. An exploratory study of factors associated with difficulties in accessing HIV services during the COVID-19 pandemic among Chinese gay and bisexual men in Hong Kong. *Int. J. Infect. Dis.* **2021**, *106*, 358–362. [CrossRef]

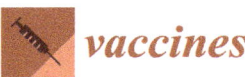

Article

A Long-Term Observation on the Possible Adverse Effects in Japanese Adolescent Girls after Human Papillomavirus Vaccination

Akiyo Hineno [1,2] and Shu-Ichi Ikeda [1,3,*]

1. Intractable Disease Care Center, Shinshu University Hospital, Matsumoto 390-0802, Japan; hineno@shinshu-u.ac.jp
2. Department of Medicine (Neurology and Rheumatology), School of Medicine, Shinshu University, Matsumoto 390-8621, Japan
3. Ikeda Medicine and Neurology Clinic, Azumino 399-8205, Japan
* Correspondence: shu-ichi@ikeda-mnc.jp; Tel.:+81-263-31-6773; Fax:+81-263-31-6783

Abstract: In Japan, a significant number of adolescent females noted unusual symptoms after receiving the human papillomavirus (HPV) vaccination, of which the vast majority of them were initially diagnosed with psychiatric illnesses because of the absence of pathologic radiological images and specific abnormalities in laboratory test results. Later these symptoms were thought to be adverse effects of HPV vaccination. However, a causal link between HPV vaccination and the development of these symptoms has not been demonstrated. Between June 2013 and March 2021, we examined 200 patients who noted various symptoms after HPV vaccination. In total, 87 were diagnosed with HPV vaccination-related symptoms based on our proposed diagnostic criteria. The clinical histories of these 87 patients were analyzed. The age at initial vaccination ranged from 11 to 19 years old (mean ± SD: 13.5 ± 1.5 years old), and the age at the first appearance of symptoms ranged from 12 to 20 years old (mean ± SD: 14.3 ± 1.6 years old). The patients received an initial HPV vaccine injection between May 2010 and May 2013, but the first affected patient developed symptoms in October 2010, and the last affected developed symptoms in October 2015. A cluster of patients with a post-HPV vaccination disorder has not appeared in Japan during the last five years. Our study shows that, in Japan, the period of HPV vaccination considerably overlapped with that of a unique post-HPV vaccination disorder development. This disorder appears as a combination of orthostatic intolerance, chronic regional pain syndrome, and cognitive dysfunction, but its exact pathogenesis remains unclear.

Keywords: human papillomavirus vaccination; adverse effects; orthostatic dysregulation; chronic regional pain syndrome; cognitive dysfunction

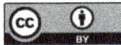

1. Introduction

The human papillomavirus (HPV) infection plays a crucial role in the development of uterine cervical cancers [1]. Therefore, in May 2010, HPV vaccines, Cervarix® (GlaxoSmithKline, Brentford, UK), a papillomavirus recombinant bivalent vaccine, and Gardasil® (Merck & Co, Inc., Kenilworth, NJ, USA), a papillomavirus recombinant quadrivalent vaccine, were widely introduced to Japanese female teenagers [2,3]. Beginning April 2013, female adolescents aged 13–16 years were legally required to receive this vaccination. Soon after this vaccination program began, a significant number of the vaccinated females complained of a unique disorder that was composed of violent tremulous involuntary movement, chronic pain, and weakness in the limbs. The Japanese mass media largely reported that a combination of these symptoms was previously unexperienced, suggesting that this disorder was a possible adverse reaction to HPV vaccination. Repeated presentations of suffering vaccinated females on television had a strong impact on Japanese society, forcing the Japanese Ministry of Public Health, Labour and Welfare to withdraw the recommendation for the use of HPV vaccination at the end of June 2013 [4]. Simultaneously, a special committee was organized to investigate the affected Japanese females, and our institution has been functioning as one of the investigation centers for the past eight years.

In our previous two reports [5,6], we described the clinical features and diagnostic criteria of the involved Japanese females with post HPV vaccination disorder. This disorder seems to include orthostatic dysregulation, chronic regional pain syndrome (CRPS), and cognitive dysfunction [5–7]. Post-vaccination abnormal autoimmune reactions are surmised to be responsible for this disorder [8,9], but a causal link has not been established between HPV vaccination and the appearance of these symptoms. Therefore, in this study, we attempted to clarify the temporal relationship between HPV vaccination and the development of this peculiar disorder on the basis of our single center's long-term observation of the affected Japanese females.

2. Materials and Methods

Between June 2013 and March 2021, we examined the symptoms and objective findings of 200 HPV vaccinated female patients. According to our proposed diagnostic criteria [6], we obtained the necessary patient information, paying special attention to the duration between vaccination and the development of the first symptoms suspected to be related to the vaccine. The patients underwent physical and neurological examinations and routine laboratory tests. Skin temperature and a digital plethysmogram were recorded, and if necessary, the Schellong test was conducted. Moreover, neuropsychological tests and functional brain imaging were performed in patients with cognitive dysfunction. The details of these methods are described in our previous reports [5,6]. The study protocol was approved by the Institutional Review Board (approval nos. 4128 and 4150) of Shinshu University School of Medicine, Matsumoto, Japan.

3. Results

During the past eight years, 200 female patients visited our hospital with the suspicion of HPV vaccine-related adverse effects (33 patients in 2013, 43 in 2014, 38 in 2015, 49 in 2016, 25 in 2017, 8 in 2018, 4 in 2019, 0 in 2020, 0 in 2021). Of these, we excluded 19 patients who had symptoms before vaccination and 5 who received the HPV vaccine after 30 years of age. An additional 28 patients whose symptoms or disorders were explained by known diseases or who had abnormal laboratory data were also excluded, specifically, eight with epilepsy, six with psychiatric or anxiety disorders, three with systemic lupus erythematosus, one with juvenile idiopathic arthritis, one with anti-SGPS antibody-positive polymyositis, and nine with other diseases. For the remaining 148 patients, the clinical manifestations and objective findings were analyzed. The results showed that 32 patients were diagnosed with definite vaccine-related symptoms, and 55 were diagnosed with probable vaccine-related symptoms. The patient's symptoms and signs of the 87 patients diagnosed are summarized in Table 1. The most frequent symptom was prolonged general fatigue, which led to an inability to wake up and subsequently go to school in the morning. Severe headache, widespread pain involving the limbs and trunk, and dysautonomic symptoms including orthostatic fainting and bowel dysfunction were also responsible for markedly decreased daily activity in the patients. Further, widespread pain typically appeared as migratory joint pain without any signs of inflammation, and intermittent neuralgic pain in the chest or abdominal wall was common. Motor dysfunction showed variable patterns, but the distal dominant weakness of the limbs, which was mimicking that of polyneuropathy, was predominant. Abnormal sensations were mainly observed in the thighs or lower legs where dysesthesia or allodynia was frequent. As compared with these symptoms, learning impairment and sleep disorder developed later. The patients complained of a lack of mental clarity. Objective findings that were frequently observed were orthostatic dysregulation, including postural orthostatic tachycardia syndrome (POTS), abnormal digital plethysmogram recordings, and abnormalities on brain SPECT images. The details of these findings have been described in a previous report [6].

Table 1. Frequency of symptoms and signs in the 87 patients studied.

Symptoms	Number of Cases	Frequency (%)
General fatigue	73	83.9
Severe headache	72	82.8
Widespread pain	71	81.6
Dysautonomic symptoms	71	81.6
Motor dysfunction	56	64.4
Abnormal sensation	52	59.8
Learning impairment	52	59.8
Sleep disturbance	44	50.6
Menstrual abnormality	44	50.6
Limb shaking	41	47.1

The temporal distribution of the period of initial vaccination and the appearance of the first symptom in the diagnosed 87 patients is shown in Figure 1. Note that the initial vaccination period ranged from May 2010 to May 2013, and the age at initial vaccination ranged from 11 to 19 years old (mean ± SD: 13.5 ± 1.5 years old). Meanwhile, the first symptom appeared from October 2010 to October 2015, and the age at the appearance of the first symptoms ranged from 12 to 20 years old (mean ± SD: 14.3 ± 1.6 years old). Thus, the time from the first vaccine dose to symptom onset ranged from 0 to 1532 days (median: 199 days). The interval between the onset of symptoms and our initial examination ranged from 0 to 85 months (median: 31 months), indicating the illness duration in the patients before they visited our center.

The temporal relationship between the HPV vaccination and the development of the symptoms was as follows: the first HPV vaccine injection was in May 2010 and the last was in May 2013 (Figure 1a). The first affected vaccinated female developed symptoms in October 2010, and the latest appearance of symptoms occurred in two patients in October 2015; the peak period of the first injection of HPV vaccine seems to be between July 2011 and September 2012, and that of the development of unique post-vaccinated symptoms appeared between September 2011 and August 2013 (Figure 1a,b). Over the previous five years, we did not examine any patients who were newly affected by these unique symptoms (Figure 1b).

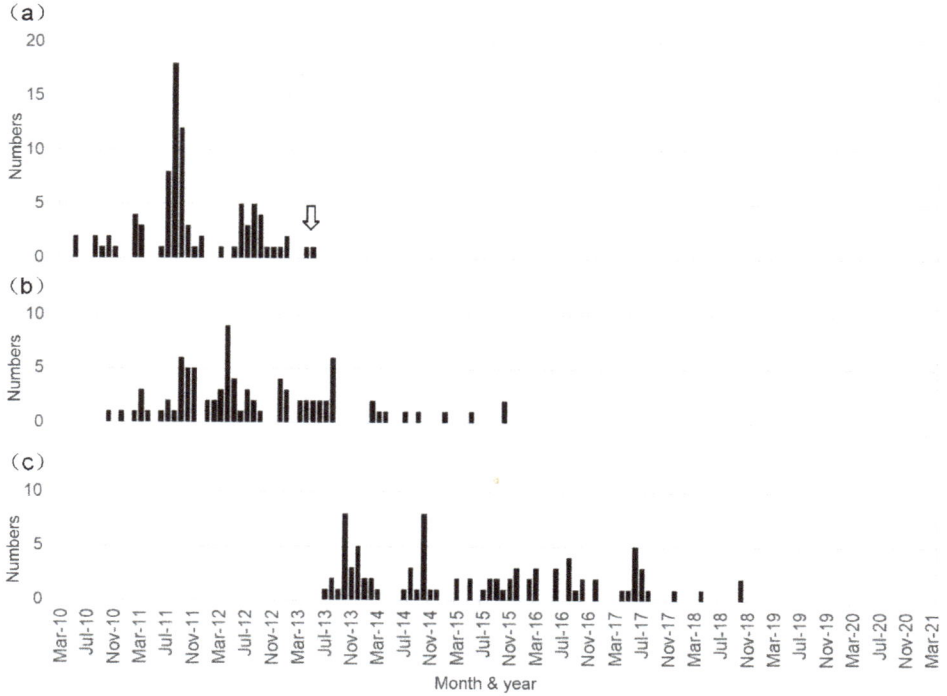

Figure 1. Temporal relationship between HPV vaccination and the development of symptoms in the patients diagnosed as having HPV vaccine-related symptoms. The period presented here ranged from May 2010 to March 2021. (**a**) Number of patients who received the first injection of HPV vaccine each month. The arrow indicates the time when the Japanese Ministry of Public Health, Labour and Welfare stopped the recommendation of HPV vaccination. (**b**) Number of patients who developed symptoms each month. (**c**) Number of patients who visited our institution and were diagnosed as having a post-HPV vaccination disorder each month.

4. Discussion

HPV vaccine safety has been reported in HPV vaccination-predominant countries [10–12]. Especially in Australia, although syncope occasionally occurs after HPV vaccination, the frequency of other serious adverse effects including POTS, CRPS, primary ovarian insufficiency, Guillain-Barré syndrome, autoimmune diseases, and venous thrombosis is very low, suggesting no causal association [13]. However, the potential risk of HPV vaccination and dysautonomia, CRPS, and chronic fatigue syndrome has been identified based on a series of case reports from different countries [14–19]. Thus, safety concerns regarding HPV vaccines remain controversial [20].

According to the reports of a Japanese special committee [21,22], 3.39 million Japanese females received HPV vaccinations between May 2010 and November 2016, and 2024 recipients were reported to have adverse reactions, of which 673 experienced serious symptoms. However, the incidence of adverse reactions in this vaccination period was determined to be low and insignificant, even though similar symptoms were not observed as a result of other vaccines.

Variable clinical manifestations in the post-HPV vaccination disorders can be explained by a combination of orthostatic dysregulation, mainly appearing as POTS, CRPS, and/or cognitive dysfunction [5,6,23]. Recent research has found that among POTS, CRPS, and myalgic encephalomyelitis/chronic fatigue (ME/CFS), some conditions overlap [24–26]; especially for cognitive dysfunction, slow thinking, difficulty in focusing, lack of concentration, forgetfulness, and confusion are commonly observed in all three disorders, and correspond to haziness in thought process, which is currently called "brain fog" [27]. Thus, the cognitive dysfunction observed in patients with post-HPV vaccination disorders may be a secondarily induced pathological condition following the long-lasting POTS and/or CRPS. Furthermore, POTS, CRPS, and ME/CFS seem to share similar autoimmune abnormalities [28], and a few preliminary studies [29–33] and case reports [34–37] have shown that the presence of serum autoantibodies against autonomic nerve receptors may be a critical determinant in the pathogenesis of these three disorders. In relation to this hypothesis, we investigated the autoantibodies against autonomic nerve receptors in the serum of the affected patients and revealed that the serum levels of autoantibodies against the adrenergic receptors and muscarinic acetylcholine receptors were significantly elevated in patients with HPV vaccination, as compared with those in the controls [38]. However, there was no statistically significant association between the clinical symptoms and elevated serum levels of these autoantibodies. Thus, further studies are required to consider the possibility of HPV vaccination-related abnormal autoimmune reactions.

In our previous report [6], we described a close temporal relationship between HPV vaccine administration and the appearance of possible adverse symptoms in 72 Japanese patients on the basis of four years of observation. In this study, we extended this observation period to nearly eight years, and the number of patients diagnosed was increased to 87, reaffirming that the period of HPV vaccination considerably overlapped with that of a unique post-vaccination disorder development in our country. In Japan, HPV vaccine coverage for females aged 12 to 16 years has dropped to less than 1% after the termination of the government's recommendation [39], and during the previous three years, few females visited us for evaluations regarding a suspected post-HPV-vaccination disorder. These observations indicate that intensive injections of HPV vaccines between May 2010 and May 2013 induced a cluster of Japanese patients with a unique post-HPV vaccination disorder. Japan is not the only exceptional country for an extremely lowered rate of HPV vaccination in recent several years; Latin American countries, such as Columbia, followed a similar pattern [40]. Adverse reactions to HPV vaccines seem to be influenced by different genetic backgrounds, cultural, and/or religious conditions. These conditions with no evidence of abnormal radiological images or laboratory data are often difficult to diagnose, easily leading to a pitfall of making the diagnosis of psychiatric illness.

Nevertheless, while there is a possible occurrence of adverse effects after HPV vaccination, these results do not necessarily signal the negation of the usefulness of this vaccine for the prevention of uterine cervical cancer [41]. If the information reported in this study is provided and is widely available at the induction of HPV vaccines, a social distaste for HPV vaccination (All Japan Coordinating Association of HPV Sufferers) would likely not occur in Japan. HPV vaccines are prophylactic and are not therapeutic, and thus, serious adverse effects are not acceptable, even if their incidences are low. Wide monitoring and an open discussion are recommended to ensure the safe announcement of HPV vaccines [42].

Author Contributions: Conceptualization, A.H. and S.-I.I.; designed this study, A.H. and S.-I.I.; analyzed the data, A.H.; writing the manuscript, A.H. and S.-I.I. Both authors have read and agreed to the published version of the manuscript.

Funding: This work was supported by the grant from a Health and Labour Science Research Grant on Emerging and Re-emerging Infectious Diseases (Establishment of Diagnosis and Treatment System on Symptoms after HPV vaccination, grant number 19HA1006) to S.-I.I. from the Ministry of Public Health, Labour and Welfare, Japan.

Institutional Review Board Statement: The study was conducted according to the guidelines of the Declaration of Helsinki and approved by the Institutional Review Board (approval nos. 4128 and 4150) of Shinshu University School of Medicine, Matsumoto, Japan.

Informed Consent Statement: Informed consent was obtained from all subjects involved in the study.

Data Availability Statement: Not applicable.

Conflicts of Interest: The authors declare no conflict of interest directly relevant to the content of this study.

References

1. Walboomers, J.M.; Jacobs, M.V.; Manos, M.M.; Bosch, F.X.; Kummer, J.A.; Shah, K.V.; Snijders, P.J.; Peto, J.; Meijer, C.J.; Muñoz, N. Human papillomavirus is a necessary cause of invasive cervical cancer worldwide. *J. Pathol.* **1999**, *189*, 12–19. [CrossRef]
2. FUTURE II Study Group. Quadrivalent vaccine against human papillomavirus to prevent high-grade cervical lesions. *N. Engl. J. Med.* **2007**, *356*, 1915–1917. [CrossRef] [PubMed]
3. Jeurissen, S.; Makar, A. Epidemiological and economic impact of human papillomavirus vaccines. *Int. J. Gynecol. Cancer* **2009**, *19*, 761–771. [CrossRef] [PubMed]
4. The Ministry of Health, Labour and Welfare. Available online: http://www.mhlw.go.jp/bunya/kenkou/kekkaku-kansenshou2 8/pdf/kankoku_h25_6_01.pdf (accessed on 8 June 2021). (In Japanese)
5. Kinoshita, T.; Abe, R.; Hineno, A.; Tsunekawa, K.; Nakane, S.; Ikeda, S. Peripheral sympathetic nerve dysfunction in adolescent Japanese girls following immunization with the human papillomavirus vaccine. *Intern. Med.* **2014**, *53*, 2185–2200. [CrossRef]
6. Ozawa, K.; Hineno, A.; Kinoshita, T.; Ishihara, S.; Ikeda, S. Suspected adverse effects after human papillomavirus vaccination: A temporal relationship between vaccine administration and the appearance of symptoms in Japan. *Drug Saf.* **2017**, *40*, 1219–1229. [CrossRef] [PubMed]
7. Martínez-Lavín, M.; Amezcua-Guerra, L. Serious adverse events after HPV vaccination: A critical review of randomized trials and post-marketing case series. *Clin. Rheumatol.* **2017**, *36*, 2169–2178. [CrossRef] [PubMed]
8. Blitshetyn, S.; Brinth, L.; Hendrickson, J.E.; Martínez-Lavín, M. Autonomic dysfunction and HPV immunization: An overview. *Immunol. Res.* **2018**, *66*, 744–754. [CrossRef]
9. Hirai, T.; Kuroiwa, Y.; Hayashi, T.; Uchiyama, M.; Nakamura, I.; Yokota, S.; Nakajima, T.; Nishioka, K.; Iguchi, Y. Adverse effects of human papillomavirus virus vaccination on central nervous system: Neuro-endocrinological disorders of hypothalamo-pituitary axis. *Auton. Nerv. Syst.* **2016**, *53*, 49–64. [CrossRef]
10. Larson, H. The world must accept that HPV vaccine is safe. *Nature* **2015**, *528*, 9. [CrossRef]
11. Hviid, A.; Svanström, H.; Schekker, N.M.; Grönlund, O.; Pasternak, B.; Arnheim-Dahlström, L. Human papillomavirus vaccination of adult women and risk of autoimmune and neurological diseases. *J. Intern. Med.* **2017**, *283*, 154–165. [CrossRef]
12. Phillips, A.; Patel, C.; Pillsbury, A.; Brotherton, J.; Macartney, K. Safety of human papillomavirus vaccines: An updated review. *Drug Saf.* **2018**, *41*, 329–346. [CrossRef]
13. Phillips, A.; Hickie, M.; Totterdell, J.; Brotherton, J.; Dey, A.; Hill, R.; Snelling, T.; Macartney, K. Adverse events following HPV vaccination: 11 years of surveillance in Australia. *Vaccine* **2020**, *38*, 6038–6046. [CrossRef]
14. Blitshteyn, S. Postural tachycardia syndrome following human papillomavirus vaccination. *Eur. J. Neurol.* **2014**, *21*, 135–139. [CrossRef]
15. Brinth, L.; Theibel, A.C.; Pors, K.; Mehlsen, J. Suspected side effects to the quadrivalent human papillomavirus vaccine. *Dan. Med. J.* **2015**, *62*, A5064. [PubMed]
16. Brinth, L.S.; Pors, K.; Theibel, A.C.; Mehlsen, J. Orthostatic intolerance and postural tachycardia syndrome as suspected adverse effects of vaccination against human papillomavirus. *Vaccine* **2015**, *33*, 2602–2605. [CrossRef]
17. Palmieri, B.; Poddighe, D.; Vadalà, M.; Laurino, C.; Carnovale, C.; Clementi, E. Severe somatoform and dysautonomic syndromes after HPV vaccination: Case series and review of literature. *Immunol. Res.* **2017**, *65*, 106–116. [CrossRef]
18. Martínez-Lavín, M. Fibromyalgia-like illness in 2 girls after human papillomavirus vaccination. *J. Clin. Rheumatol.* **2014**, *20*, 392–393. [CrossRef] [PubMed]
19. Martinez, P. Motor and Sensory Clinical Findings in Girls Vaccinated against the Human Papillomavirus from Carmen de Bolívar, Colombia. Available online: https://pompiliomartinez.wordpress.com/2016/03/04/motor-and-sensory-clinical-findings-in-girls-vaccinated-against-the-human-papillomavirus-from-carmen-de-bolivar-colombia/ (accessed on 8 June 2021).
20. Chandler, R.E. Safety concerns with HPV vaccines continue to linger: Are current vaccine pharmacovigilance practices sufficient? *Drug Saf.* **2017**, *40*, 1167–1170. [CrossRef] [PubMed]
21. The Ministry of Health, Labour and Welfare. Available online: http://www.mhlw.go.jp/file/05-Shingikai-1060100 0-Daijinkanboukouseikagakuka-Kouseikagakuka/0000161349.pdf (accessed on 8 June 2021). (In Japanese)
22. The Ministry of Health, Labour and Welfare. Available online: http://www.mhlw.go.jp/file/05-Shingikai-10601000-Daijinkanboukouseikagakuka-Kouseikagakuka/0000161329.pdf (accessed on 8 June 2021). (In Japanese)
23. Matsudaira, T.; Takahashi, Y.; Matsuda, K.; Ikeda, H.; Usui, K.; Obi, T.; Inoue, Y. Cognitive dysfunction and regional cerebral blood flow changes in Japanese females after human papillomavirus vaccination. *Neurol. Clin. Neurosci.* **2016**, *4*, 220–227. [CrossRef]
24. Stewart, J.M. Autonomic nervous system dysfunction in adolescents with postural orthostatic tachycardia syndrome and chronic fatigue syndrome is characterized by attenuated vagal baroreflex and potentiated sympathetic vasomotion. *Pediatr. Res.* **2000**, *48*, 218–226. [CrossRef]
25. Karas, B.; Grubb, B.P.; Boeth, K.; Kip, K. The postural orthostatic tachycardia syndrome: A potentially treatable cause of chronic fatigue, exercise intolerance, and cognitive impairment in adolescents. *Pacing Clin. Electrophysiol.* **2000**, *23*, 344–351. [CrossRef] [PubMed]

26. Halicka, M.; Vittersø, A.D.; Proulx, M.J.; Bultitude, J.H. Neuropsychological changes in complex regional pain syndrome (CRPS). *Behav. Neurol.* **2020**, *2020*, 4561831. [CrossRef]
27. Ocon, A.J. Caught in the thickness of brain fog: Exploring the cognitive symptoms of chronic fatigue syndrome. *Front. Physiol.* **2013**, *4*, 63. [CrossRef] [PubMed]
28. Meyer, C.; Heidecke, H. Antibodies against GPCR. *Front Biosci.* **2018**, *23*, 2177–2194.
29. Yub, X.; Stavrakis, S.; Hill, M.A.; Huang, S.; Reim, S.; Lin, H.; Khan, M.; Hamlett, S.; Cunningham, M.W.; Kem, D.C. Autoantibody activation of beta-adrenergic and muscarinic receptors contributes to an "autoimmune" orthostatic hypotension. *J. Am. Soc. Hypertens.* **2012**, *6*, 40–47. [CrossRef]
30. Ruzieh, M.; Batizy, L.; Dasa, O.; Oostra, C.; Grubb, B. The role of autoantibodies in the syndromes of orthostatic intolerance: A systemic review. *Scand. Cardiovasc. J.* **2017**, *51*, 243–247. [CrossRef] [PubMed]
31. Kohr, D.; Singh, P.; Tschernatsch, M.; Kaps, M.; Pouokam, E.; Diener, M.; Kummer, W.; Birklein, F.; Vincent, A.; Goebel, A.; et al. Autoimmunity against the β2 adrenergic receptor and muscarinic-2 receptor in complex regional pain syndrome. *Pain* **2011**, *152*, 2690–2700. [CrossRef]
32. Dubuis, E.; Thompson, V.; Leite, M.I.; Blaes, F.; Maihofner, C.; Greensmith, D.; Vincent, A.; Shenker, N.; Kuttikat, A.; Leuwer, M.; et al. Longstanding complex regional pain syndrome is associated with activating autoantibodies against alpha-1a adrenoreceptors. *Pain* **2014**, *155*, 2408–2417. [CrossRef]
33. Loebel, M.; Grabowski, P.; Heidecke, H.; Bauer, S.; Hanitsch, L.G.; Wittke, K.; Meisel, C.; Reinke, P.; Volk, H.D.; Fluge, Ø.; et al. Antibodies to β adrenergic and muscarinic cholinergic receptors in patients with chronic fatigue syndrome. *Brain Behav. Immun.* **2016**, *52*, 32–39. [CrossRef] [PubMed]
34. Hendrickson, J.E.; Hendrickson, E.T.; Gehrie, E.A.; Sidhe, D.; Wallukat, G.; Schimke, I.; Tormey, C.A. Complex regional pain syndrome and dysautonomia in a 14-year-old girl responsive to therapeutic plasma exchange. *J. Clin. Apher.* **2016**, *31*, 368–374. [CrossRef]
35. Hendrickson, J.E.; Tormey, C.A. Human papilloma virus vaccination and dysautonomia: Consideration for autoantibody evaluation and HLA typing. *Vaccine* **2016**, *34*, 4468. [CrossRef]
36. Blitshteyn, S.; Brook, J. Postural tachycardia syndrome (POTS) with anti-NMDA receptor antibodies after human papillomavirus vaccination. *Immunol. Res.* **2017**, *65*, 282–284. [CrossRef] [PubMed]
37. Schofield, J.R.; Hendrickson, J.E. Autoimmunity, autonomic neuropathy, and the HPV vaccination: A vulnerable subpopulation. *Clin. Pediatr.* **2018**, *57*, 603–606. [CrossRef] [PubMed]
38. Hineno, A.; Ikeda, S.; Scheibenbogen, C.; Heidecke, H.; Schulze-Forster, K.; Junker, J.; Riemekasten, G.; Dechend, R.; Dragun, D.; Shoenfeld, Y. Autoantibodies against autonomic nerve receptors in adolescent Japanese girls after immunization with human papillomavirus vaccine. *Ann. Arthritis Clin. Rheumatol.* **2019**, *2*, 1014.
39. Simms, K.T.; Hanley, S.J.B.; Smith, M.A.; Keane, A.; Canfell, K. Impact of HPV vaccine hesitancy on cervical cancer in Japan: A modelling study. *Lancet Public Health* **2020**, *5*, e223–e234. [CrossRef]
40. Cervantes, J.L.; Doan, A.H. Discrepancies in the evaluation of the safety of the human papillomavirus vaccine. *Mem. Inst. Oswaldo Cruz* **2018**, *113*, e180063. [CrossRef] [PubMed]
41. Chambuso, R.S.; Rebello, G.; Kaambo, E. Personalized human papillomavirus vaccination for persistence of immunity for cervical cancer prevention: A critical review with experts' opinions. *Front. Oncol.* **2020**, *10*, 548. [CrossRef] [PubMed]
42. Wick, G. Allowing an Open Discussion of the Side Effects of Vaccines. Available online: https://science.sciencemag.org/content/allowing-open-discussion-side-effects-vaccines (accessed on 8 June 2021).

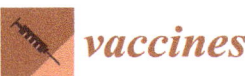

Review

A Systematic Review of Interventions to Improve HPV Vaccination Coverage

Edison J. Mavundza [1,*], Chinwe J. Iwu-Jaja [2], Alison B. Wiyeh [3], Blessings Gausi [4], Leila H. Abdullahi [5], Gregory Halle-Ekane [6] and Charles S. Wiysonge [1,4,7]

1. Cochrane South Africa, South African Medical Research Council, Francie van Zijl Drive, Parow Valley, Cape Town 7501, South Africa; Charles.Wiysonge@mrc.ac.za
2. Department of Nursing and Midwifery, Stellenbosch University, Francie van Zijl Drive, Tygerberg, Cape Town 7505, South Africa; chinwelolo@gmail.com
3. Department of Epidemiology, University of Washington, Seattle, WA 98145, USA; wberiliy@yahoo.co.uk
4. Division of Epidemiology and Biostatistics, School of Public Health and Family Medicine, University of Cape Town, Anzio Road, Observatory, Cape Town 7925, South Africa; sibusiso.gausi@alumni.uct.ac.za
5. African Institute for Development Policy, Nairobi P.O. Box 14688-00800, Kenya; leylaz@live.co.za
6. Faculty of Health Sciences, University of Buea, Buea P.O. Box 63, Cameroon; halle-ekane.edie@ubuea.cm
7. Division of Epidemiology and Biostatistics, Department of Global Health, Stellenbosch University, Francie van Zijl Drive, Tygerberg, Cape Town 7505, South Africa
* Correspondence: Edison.mavundza@mrc.ac.za

Citation: Mavundza, E.J.; Iwu-Jaja, C.J.; Wiyeh, A.B.; Gausi, B.; Abdullahi, L.H.; Halle-Ekane, G.; Wiysonge, C.S. A Systematic Review of Interventions to Improve HPV Vaccination Coverage. *Vaccines* **2021**, *9*, 687. https://doi.org/10.3390/vaccines9070687

Academic Editor: Gloria Calagna

Received: 6 April 2021
Accepted: 24 May 2021
Published: 23 June 2021

Publisher's Note: MDPI stays neutral with regard to jurisdictional claims in published maps and institutional affiliations.

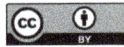

Copyright: © 2021 by the authors. Licensee MDPI, Basel, Switzerland. This article is an open access article distributed under the terms and conditions of the Creative Commons Attribution (CC BY) license (https://creativecommons.org/licenses/by/4.0/).

Abstract: Human papillomavirus (HPV) infection is the most common sexually transmitted infection worldwide. Although most HPV infections are transient and asymptomatic, persistent infection with high-risk HPV types may results in diseases. Although there are currently three effective and safe prophylactic HPV vaccines that are used across the world, HPV vaccination coverage remains low. This review evaluates the effects of the interventions to improve HPV vaccination coverage. We searched the Cochrane Central Register of Controlled Trials, PubMed, Web of Science, Scopus, and the World Health Organization International Clinical Trials Registry Platform and checked the reference lists of relevant articles for eligible studies. Thirty-five studies met inclusion criteria. Our review found that various evaluated interventions have improved HPV vaccination coverage, including narrative education, outreach plus reminders, reminders, financial incentives plus reminders, brief motivational behavioral interventions, provider prompts, training, training plus assessment and feedback, consultation, funding, and multicomponent interventions. However, the evaluation of these intervention was conducted in high-income countries, mainly the United States of America. There is, therefore, a need for studies to evaluate the effect of these interventions in low-and middle-income countries, where there is a high burden of HPV and limited HPV vaccination programs.

Keywords: human papillomavirus; vaccination coverage; recipient-oriented interventions; provider-oriented interventions; systematic review

1. Introduction

Human papillomavirus (HPV) infection is the most common sexually transmitted infection worldwide [1]. It is estimated that 75% of sexually active men and women will acquire HPV infection in their lifetime. HPV infections are most prevalent in young adults, as sexual risk behaviors are greatest in this age group. Sexually active young women, in particular, carry the highest risk of infection, with studies documenting rates as high as 68–71% [2]. To date, more than 200 HPV types have been identified and classified into two groups: high-risk and low-risk types [3]. Although most HPV infections are transient and asymptomatic, persistent infection with high-risk HPV types may result in cancers, including cervical, anal, vulvar, vaginal, penile, and oropharyngeal cancers [4–6], and genital warts [6]. High-risk HPV types, including HPV-16, -18, -31, -33, -35, -39, -45, -51,

-52, -56, -58, and -59 are associated with cancers in humans, whereas low-risk HPV types, including HPV-6, -11, -40, -42, -43, -44, -54, -61, and -72 cause benign diseases such as genital warts [7]. Among these HPV types, the majority of HPV-related clinical diseases are associated with HPV-16, -18, -6, and -11. HPV types 16 and 18 cause approximately 70% of cervical cancer, and HPV-6 and HPV-11 are responsible for approximately 90% of genital warts. Most HPV-associated morbidity and mortality is due to cervical cancer, the fourth most common cancer in women worldwide, with an estimated 604,127 cases and 341,831 deaths in 2020 [8]. HPV vaccination is an important tool to prevent and control HPV infection and its complications [5]. There are currently three prophylactic HPV vaccines that are used across the world: Cervarix, a bivalent HPV vaccine that targets HPV-16 and -18; Gardasil, a quadrivalent HPV vaccine that targets HPV-6, -11, -16, and -18; and Gardasil 9, a nonavalent HPV vaccine that targets HPV-6, -11, -16, -18, -31, -33, -45, -52, and -58 [9]. All three vaccines have proven to be highly efficacious against persistent infection of their vaccine genotypes. However, HPV vaccines are most effective when administered before debut and exposure to HPV [10]. HPV vaccination is currently recommended for adolescent males and females aged 9–14 years in a two-dose series and as a three-dose series for young men and women aged 15–26 years [11].

Despite its effectiveness, safety, and recommendations, HPV vaccination coverage remains low. Numerous barriers to HPV vaccination have been identified, including lack of health care provider recommendations, concerns about safety, concerns about side effects, and a general lack of awareness and knowledge about HPV vaccination [12]. There is, therefore, an urgent need for effective interventions to improve HPV vaccination coverage and reduce the burden of HPV-associated infections and cancers. Several reviews have assessed interventions to improve HPV vaccination coverage. However, the reviews assessed the effectiveness of interventions among adolescents [13], young adults [14], adolescents and young adults [15], the effectiveness of practice- and community-based interventions [6], and communication technology interventions [16]. A comprehensive systematic review on interventions to increase HPV vaccination coverage was published in 2016 [17]. However, the review included only studies conducted in the United States of America. Therefore, this review's findings may not be applicable to low- and middle-income countries, where the burden of HPV is high, and vaccination coverage is very low. In addition, the review included only studies up to 2015, while there have been numerous potentially eligible studies published since then. To the best of our knowledge, there is no comprehensive systematic review that has assessed interventions to improve HPV vaccination coverage across all country income categories. These limitations justify the need for a comprehensive systematic review on the interventions to improve HPV vaccination coverage.

2. Materials and Methods

The protocol for this review was registered in the International Prospective Register of Systematic Reviews (PROSPERO) (CRD42019138971) [18], and the review was prepared according to the Preferred Reporting Items for Systematic Reviews and Meta-Analyses (PRISMA) guideline [19].

2.1. Criteria for Considering Studies for This Review

We included randomized trials, non-randomized trials, interrupted time-series studies, and controlled before–after studies that met the quality criteria used by the Cochrane Effective Practice and Organization of Care (EPOC) [20]. We only included cluster-randomized controlled trials with at least two intervention and two control clusters. Interrupted time-series studies were only included if their outcomes were measured during at least three points before and after the intervention. We also included controlled before–after studies only if they had at least two intervention groups and at least two comparable control groups. We included studies conducted among all individuals eligible for HPV vaccines and their parents/legal guardians or healthcare providers. Included studies evaluated recipient-oriented, provider-oriented, legislative, health system, and multi-component interventions. Eligible studies compared the interventions to standard HPV vaccination practices, alternative interventions, or similar interventions implemented with different degrees of intensity. Our primary outcome of interest was HPV vaccination coverage, while our secondary outcomes were adverse effects and the cost of the intervention.

2.2. Search Methods for Identification of Studies

We developed a comprehensive search strategy with the help of an information specialist. We searched the following databases: the Cochrane Central Register of Controlled Trials (CENTRAL), PubMed, Web of Science, and Scopus. We searched databases from inception until the day of the search. We searched for published articles with no language restriction. We provided the search strategies for databases searched (Appendix A, Table A1). We also searched the WHO International Clinical Trials Registry Platform for ongoing trials and the reference lists of included studies and related reviews for other relevant studies. In addition, we searched the abstracts of the latest conferences of relevant scientific societies related to vaccination and HPV virology for new or pending information not yet published in peer-reviewed journals.

2.3. Selection of Studies

Two review authors (Edison Mavundza [EM] and Chinwe Iwu-Jaja [CI]) independently screened the titles and abstracts to identify potentially eligible studies. Disagreements between the two authors were resolved by discussion and consensus. We obtained the full texts of all potentially eligible studies. Two authors independently screened the full texts and identified included studies, resolving discrepancies through discussion and consensus. Excluded studies are described in the table of excluded studies alongside their reasons for exclusion.

2.4. Data Extraction and Management

Two review authors (EM and CI) independently extracted data from each included study using a structured and standardized data extraction form. Extracted data included study setting, type of study, type of participants, type of intervention, type of comparator, and type of outcomes measured. Differences between the two review authors were resolved by discussion and consensus.

2.5. Assessment of Risk of Bias in Included Studies

Two review authors (EM and CI) independently assessed the risk of bias within each included study by addressing seven specific domains, namely, random sequence generation, allocation concealment, blinding of participants and personnel, blinding of outcome assessment, incomplete outcome data, selective outcome reporting, and "other issues" [21]. For each included study, the two review authors independently described what the study authors reported that they did for each domain and then made a decision relating to the risk of bias for that domain by assigning a judgement of "low risk" of bias, "high risk" of bias, or "unclear risk" of bias. The review authors compared the results of their independent assessments of risk of bias and resolved any discrepancies by discussion and consensus.

3. Results

3.1. Results of the Search

The search yielded 3936 records. After removing 1078 duplicates, 2858 titles and abstracts were screened, and 2764 were not relevant. We reviewed the remaining 94 potentially eligible full-text articles for inclusion; 49 met our inclusion criteria, and we excluded 45 articles. The 49 included publications reported data on 35 studies. The 45 excluded articles reported data on 38 studies. The process used for the search and selection of studies for this review is described in Figure 1.

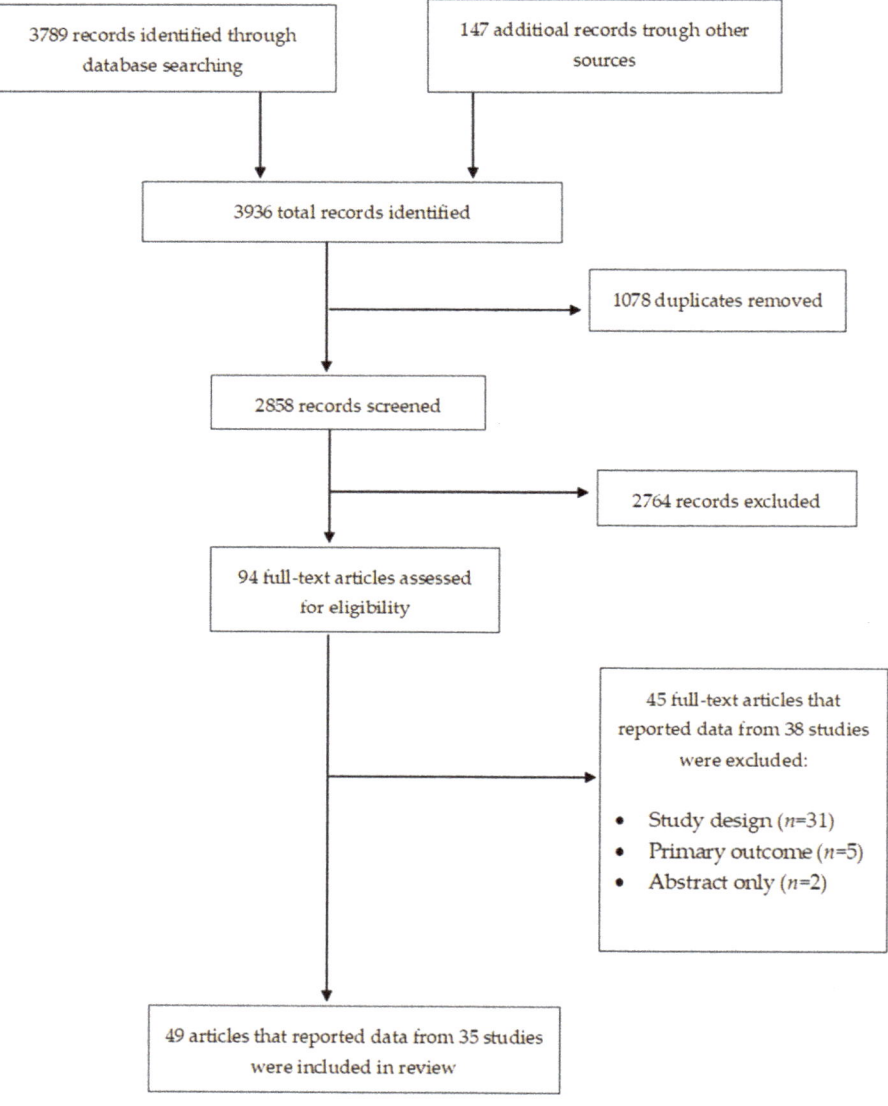

Figure 1. PRISMA flow diagram showing the study search and selection process.

3.2. Description of Studies

The characteristics of the included studies are summarized in Appendix A, Table A2.

3.2.1. Study Design and Setting

Thirty-two studies were randomized trials [22–53], two studies were controlled before–after studies [54,55], and one study was a non-randomized trial [56]. Thirty-two studies were conducted in the USA [22–35,37,39–48,50–56]. The remaining three studies were carried out in the UK [36], the Netherlands [38], and Australia [49].

3.2.2. Participants

Seven studies were conducted among females only [22,24,27,33,36,37,51]; one study was conducted among males only [41]; one study was conducted among males and females [43]; thirteen studies were conducted among parents/ guardians [25,31,32,34,38–40,42,44,45,47,49,56]; nine studies were conducted among providers [23,28–30,46,52–55]. The remaining four studies were conducted among mixed participants: adolescents and parents/guardians [35,48,50] and young adults and parents/guardians [26].

3.2.3. Interventions and Comparators

Twenty-six studies assessed recipient-oriented interventions [22,24–27,31–45,47–51,56]. The remaining nine studies assessed provider-oriented interventions [23,28–30,46,52–55]. Comparators ranged from the standard of care in each setting to alternative interventions.

3.2.4. Outcome Measures

All included studies reported data on our primary outcome, HPV vaccination coverage. Twenty-two studies reported data on the initiation of the HPV vaccine series [22,23,25,27–37,39,41,44,48,53–56]. Nineteen studies reported data on the completion of HPV vaccine series [22,24,25,27,30,34,36,40–44,46,48,51,52,54–56]. Four studies reported data on the receipt of any HPV vaccine dose [26,38,49,50].

Only four studies reported data on our pre-specified secondary outcomes. Three studies reported data on the cost of the intervention strategies [25,45,47], and one study reported data on adverse effects of the intervention [44].

3.2.5. Excluded Studies

Thirty-eight studies were excluded for reasons described in the characteristics of excluded studies (Appendix A, Table A3).

3.2.6. Risk of Bias in Included Studies

The risk of bias in the included studies is summarized in Appendix A, Table A4. Below, we briefly describe the risk related to sequence generation, allocation concealment, blinding, completeness of outcome data, selective reporting, and other potential biases.

The risk of bias linked to the adequacy of the generation of the randomization sequence was low for twenty-two studies [22,23,25–28,32–34,36,37,39–41,44–49,51,52], unclear for ten studies [24,29–31,35,38,42,43,50,53], and high for two studies [55,56].

The risk of bias resulting from the adequacy of allocation concealment was low for five studies [22,27,37,46,47], unclear for fourteen studies [23,24,26,28–31,35,38,41–43,50,53], and high for fifteen studies [25,32–34,36,39,40,44,45,48,49,51,52,55,56].

The risk of bias linked to the adequacy of blinding of participants and research personnel was low for thirteen studies [22,26,32,39,42,43,45,47–49,51–53], unclear for thirteen studies [24,25,30,31,33,35–37,40,46,50,55,56], and high for eight studies [23,27–29,34,38,41,44].

The risk of bias related to the blinding of outcome assessors was low for four studies [24,26,32,40], unclear for twenty-six studies [22,25,27–31,33,36,37,39,42–53,55,56], and high for four studies [23,34,38,41].

The risk of bias linked to the completeness of outcome data was low for twenty-five studies [23,24,27–37,40,41,43–46,48–53], unclear for three studies [25,47,55], and high for six studies [22,26,38,39,42,56].

We did not find evidence of reporting bias or other biases beyond the ones reported above.

3.3. Effects of Interventions

3.3.1. Recipient-Oriented Interventions

Comparison 1: Tailored Education Compared to Standard of Care

Three studies assessed the effect of HPV-tailored education compared to the standard of care on the initiation of the HPV vaccine series. The studies showed that HPV-tailored education had no effect on the initiation of the HPV vaccine series (RR 1.00, 95% CI 0.86

to 1.17; 1350 participants) [22,27,48]. We judged the certainty of the evidence as very low because of concerns regarding the risk of bias in the included studies and serious imprecision in the findings.

Three studies assessed the effect of HPV-tailored education compared to the standard of care on the completion of the HPV vaccine series. Meta-analysis of data from these three studies showed that tailored education improved the completion of HPV vaccination series (RR 1.35, 95% CI 1.03 to 1.77; I^2 = 27%; 880 participants) [22,27,51]. We downgraded the certainty of the evidence to low because of study limitations (i.e., a high risk of bias in all studies).

Two studies assessed the impact of tailored education compared to the standard of care on receipt of any dose of the HPV vaccine. The study showed that tailored education had no effect on uptake of HPV vaccine (RR 1.01, 95% CI 0.98 to 1.04; 8931 participants) [26,35]. We judged the certainty of the evidence as very low because of concerns regarding the risk of bias in the included studies and serious imprecision in the findings.

The studies reported no relevant secondary outcomes.

Comparison 2: Tailored Education Compared to Untailored Education

One study assessed the effect of tailored education compared to untailored education on receipt of any dose of HPV vaccine. The study showed untailored education had a slight effect on uptake of HPV vaccine compared to the tailored education intervention (RR 0.97, 95% CI 0.80 to 1.19; 855 participants) [26]. We downgraded the certainty of the evidence to very low because of concerns regarding the risk of bias in the included study and serious imprecision in the findings.

The study reported no relevant secondary outcomes.

Comparison 3: Narrative Education Compared to Non-Narrative Education

Two studies showed that narrative education improved the initiation of the HPV vaccination series compared to non-narrative education (RR 1.38, 95% CI 0.95 to 2.00; I^2 = 24%; 728 participants) [33,35]. We judged the certainty of the evidence as very low because of concerns regarding the risk of bias in the included studies and very serious imprecision in the findings.

The studies reported no relevant secondary outcomes.

Comparison 4: Multicomponent Education Compared to Standard of Care

A study showed that a multicomponent HPV education led to a very small decrease in the uptake of HPV vaccine compared to the standard of care (RR 0.98, 95% CI 0.87 to 1.11; 2912 participants) [50]. We downgraded the certainty of the evidence to low because of concerns regarding the risk of bias in the included study and serious imprecision in the findings.

The study reported no relevant secondary outcomes.

Comparison 5: Outreach Plus Reminders Compared to Standard of Care

One study assessed the impact of outreach plus reminders compared to the standard of care on the initiation of the HPV vaccine series. The study showed that the intervention improved the initiation of the HPV vaccine series (RR 1.28, 95% CI 1.02 to 1.60; 1624 participants) [31]. We judged the certainty of the evidence as moderate because of an unclear risk of bias in the included study.

The study reported no relevant secondary outcomes.

Comparison 6: Outreach Plus Education Compared to Standard of Care

A study assessed the impact of education and outreach compared to the standard of care on the initiation of the HPV vaccine series. The study reported that 84% of participants in both groups (Brochure only and *Entre Madre e Hija* (EMH)) initiated HPV vaccination, and no differences were observed between EMH program and brochure-only participants [56].

We downgraded the certainty of the evidence to moderate because of study limitations (i.e., non-randomized study).

One study assessed the impact of education and outreach compared to standard of care on the completion of the HPV vaccine series. The study showed that the intervention improved the completion of the HPV vaccine series (RR 1.70, 95% CI 1.30 to 2.22; 288 participants) [56]. We downgraded the certainty of the evidence to moderate because of study limitations (i.e., non-randomized study).

The study reported no relevant secondary outcomes.

Comparison 7: Education Plus Reminders Compared to Standard of Care

A study assessed the effect of education plus reminders compared to the standard of care on the initiation of the HPV vaccine series. The study showed that the intervention improved the initiation of the HPV vaccine series (RR 1.74, 95% CI 1.10 to 2.76; 150 participants) [41]. We downgraded the certainty of the evidence to low because of study limitations, as the included study had a high risk of bias.

Another study assessed the impact of HPV education plus reminders compared to the standard of care on the initiation of the HPV vaccine series. The study showed that the intervention was significantly associated with HPV vaccine uptake (RR: 0.84; 95% CI: 0.31–2.28) [37]. We judged the certainty of the evidence as very low because of concerns regarding the risk of bias in the included study and serious imprecision in the findings.

Three studies assessed the impact of HPV education plus reminders compared to the standard of care on the completion of the HPV vaccine series. A meta-analysis of data from these three studies showed that the intervention improved the completion of the HPV vaccine series (RR 1.18, 95% CI 0.92 to 1.51; I^2 = 28%; 6711 participants) [41–43]. We downgraded the certainty of the evidence to very low because of concerns regarding the risk of bias in the included studies and serious imprecision in the findings.

The studies reported no relevant secondary outcomes.

Comparison 8: Reminders vs. Standard of Care

Three studies assessed the effect of a reminder compared to the standard of care on the initiation of the HPV vaccine series. Two studies showed that the intervention improved the initiation of the HPV vaccine series (RR 1.16, 95% CI 1.13 to 1.18; I^2 = 40%; 166,264 participants) [25,39]. We judged the certainty of the evidence as low because of study limitations, as the included studies had a high risk of bias.

Suh (2012) [45] reported that 26.5% of female adolescents initiated HPV vaccine series in the intervention group compared to 15.3% in the control group. We judged the certainty of the evidence as low because of study limitations, as the included studies had a high risk of bias.

Four studies assessed the effect of reminders compared to the standard of care on the completion of the HPV vaccine series. The study showed that intervention improved the completion of the HPV vaccination series (RR 1.23, 95% CI 1.18 to 1.29; I^2 = 63%; 175,743 participants) [24,25,40,48]. We downgraded the certainty of the evidence to very low because of concerns regarding the risk of bias and serious inconsistency in the included studies.

Tull (2019) [49] assessed the effect of reminders compared to the standard of care on the uptake of any HPV dose. The study found that the intervention had no effect on the uptake of HPV vaccine (RR 1.03, 95% CI 1.01 to 1.05; 5912 participants). We judged the certainty of the evidence as moderate because of a high risk of bias in the included study.

Three studies measured the costs of the intervention [25,45,47]. Coley (2018) [25] calculated the reminder mailing and vaccination costs. The mailing costs were $13,698 for address verification, $44,312 for printing, and $57,991 for postage. The vaccination cost was $30.95 per adolescent who initiated the HPV vaccine series. Szilagyi (2013) [47] measured the cost of the intervention on pertussis, meningococcal, and HPV vaccination among adolescents. The delivery cost of the intervention was $18.78 for mailed and $16.68 for phone reminders per adolescent per year, respectively. The cost per additional fully vaccinated adolescent was $463.99 for mailed and $714.98 for telephone reminders. Suh (2012) [45] calculated the total operating cost of reminder/recall intervention per additional adolescent who received tetanus-diphtheria-acellular pertussis, meningococcal conjugate, or a first dose of human papillomavirus vaccine in four practices. The total operating cost, which included personnel and supply costs, ranged between $1087 and $1349.

Comparison 9: Educational Reminders Compared to Plain Reminders

Hofstetter (2017) [32] showed that educational reminders improve the initiation of the HPV vaccination series compared to plain reminders (RR 0.53, 95% CI 0.27 to 1.06; 90 participants). We downgraded the certainty of the evidence to very low because of concerns regarding the risk of bias in the included study and serious imprecision in the findings.

The study reported no relevant secondary outcomes.

Comparison 10: Financial Incentives Plus Reminders Compared to Standard of Care

One study assessed the impact of financial incentives plus reminders compared to the standard of care on the initiation of the HPV vaccine series. The study showed that intervention improved the initiation of the HPV vaccine series (RR 1.73, 95% CI 1.34 to 2.24; I^2 = 64%; 1000 participants) [36]. We judged the certainty of the evidence as very low because of concerns regarding the risk of bias in the included study and serious inconsistency.

A study assessed the impact of financial incentives plus reminders compared to the standard of care on the completion of the HPV vaccine series. The study showed that intervention improved the initiation of the HPV vaccine series (RR 1.82, 95% CI 1.26 to 2.63; I^2 = 0%; 1000 participants) [36]. We downgraded the certainty of the evidence to low because of a high risk of bias in the included study.

The study reported no relevant secondary outcomes.

Comparison 11: Brief Motivational Behavioral Intervention Compared to Standard of Care

One study assessed the impact of the brief motivational behavioral intervention compared to the standard of care on the initiation of the HPV vaccine series. The study showed that intervention improved initiation of the HPV vaccine series (RR 1.10, 95% CI 0.85 to 1.43; 200 participants) [34]. We downgraded the certainty of the evidence to very low because of concerns regarding the risk of bias in the included study and serious imprecision in the findings.

A study assessed the impact of the brief motivational behavioral intervention compared to the standard of care on the completion of the HPV vaccine series. The study showed that intervention improved the completion of HPV vaccine series (RR 1.73, 95% CI 0.66 to 4.59; 200 participants) [34]. We judged the certainty of the evidence as very low, because of concerns regarding the risk of bias in the included studies and serious imprecision in the findings.

The study reported no relevant secondary outcomes.

Comparison 12: Brief Health Messaging Using Different Formats

One study assessed the effect of brief health messaging on the initiation of the HPV vaccine series. The study reported that rhetorical questions did not increase the initiation of the HPV vaccine series (RR = 1.15, CI 0.89, 1.50). One-sided and two-sided messages also had no effect on the initiation of the HPV vaccine series [44]. We downgraded the certainty of the evidence to very low because of concerns regarding the risk of bias in the included study and serious imprecision in the findings.

A study assessed the effect of brief health messaging on the completion of the HPV vaccine series. The study reported that rhetorical questions and message sidedness had no significant effect on the completion of the HPV vaccine series [44]. We judged the certainty of the evidence as very low because of concerns regarding the risk of bias in the included studies and serious imprecision in the findings.

Rickert (2015) evaluated the adverse events of the intervention, but none occurred.

3.3.2. Provider-Oriented Intervention

Comparison 13: Prompts Compared to Standard of Car

One study assessed the impact of provider prompts compared to the standard of care on the initiation of the HPV vaccine series. The study showed that provider prompts improved the initiation of the HPV vaccine series (RR 1.36, 95% CI 1.20 to 1.54; 925 participants) [53]. We downgraded the certainty of the evidence to moderate because of study limitations, as the included study had an unclear risk of bias.

Two studies assessed the effect of provider prompts compared to the standard of care on the completion of the HPV vaccine series. The study showed that intervention improved the completion of the HPV vaccine series (RR 1.12, 95% CI 1.06 to 1.19; $I^2 = 72\%$; 3056 participants) [46,52]. We downgraded the certainty of the evidence to very low because of concerns regarding the risk of bias in the included studies and serious inconsistency.

The studies reported no relevant secondary outcomes.

Comparison 14: Provider Training Compared to Standard of Care

A study assessed the effect of provider announcement and conversation training compared to the standard of care on the initiation of the HPV vaccine series. The study reported that clinics that received announcement training had increases in HPV vaccine initiation coverage that exceeded control clinics' increases (5.4% difference, 95% CI 1.1 to 9.7). Clinics that received conversation training did not differ from the control arm on uptake for HPV vaccine initiation (all $Ps > 0.05$) [23]. We judged the certainty of the evidence as very low because of concerns regarding the risk of bias in the included studies and serious imprecision in the findings.

The study reported no relevant secondary outcomes.

Comparison 15: Provider Training Plus Assessment and Feedback Compared to Wait List Control

One study assessed the impact of provider training plus assessment and feedback intervention compared to wait list control on the initiation of the HPV vaccine series. The study showed that initiation of the HPV vaccine series rates increased by 10.2 percentage points in the intervention arm and 6.9 percentage points in the control arm [29]. We downgraded the certainty of the evidence to very low because of concerns regarding the risk of bias in the included studies and very serious imprecision in the findings.

The study reported no relevant secondary outcomes.

Comparison 16: Assessment and Feedback Compared to Standard of Care Series

Irving (2018) [54] evaluated the effect of assessment and feedback intervention compared to the standard of care on the initiation of the HPV vaccine series among adolescent boys and girls aged 11–17 years. The study reported that there was no significant difference in the initiation of the HPV vaccine series between intervention and control clinics. We downgraded the certainty of the evidence to very low because of study limitations (i.e., before–after study).

One study evaluated the effect of assessment and feedback intervention compared to the standard of care on the initiation of the HPV vaccine series among adolescent boys and girls aged 11–17 years [54]. The study found that the completion of the HPV vaccine series between the intervention and control clinics was not significantly different. We downgraded the certainty of the evidence to very low because of study limitations (i.e., before–after study).

The study reported no relevant secondary outcomes.

Comparison 17: Provider Consultation Compared to Standard of Care

A study assessed the effect of in-person and webinar-delivered Assessment, Feedback, Incentives, and eXchange (AFIX) consultations compared to standard of care on the initiation of the HPV vaccine series. The study reported that participants served by clinics in the in-person arm had uptake that exceed those in the control arm for HPV vaccine initiation (1.5% (95% CI: 0.3 to 2.7)). Participants served by clinics in the webinar versus control arms also had larger coverage increases for HPV vaccine initiation (1.9 (95% CI: 0.7 to 3.1)) [26]. We downgraded the certainty of the evidence to very low because of concerns regarding the risk of bias in the included study and very serious imprecision in the findings.

The study reported no relevant secondary outcomes.

Comparison 18: Funding Compared to Training and Technical Assistance

One study compared the effect of $90,000 (2-year grant fund), $10,000 (3-month grant fund), and training and technical assistance on the initiation of the HPV vaccine series among patients aged 11–12 years. The study found that initiation of the HPV vaccine series rates increased by 18.4, 14.6, and 11.1 percentage points in the $90,000 grant fund, training and technical assistance, and $10,000 grant fund, respectively [30]. We judged the certainty of the evidence as low because of concerns regarding the risk of bias in the included study and serious imprecision in the findings.

A study compared the effect of $90,000 (2-year grant fund), $10,000 (3-month grant fund), and training and technical assistance on the completion of the HPV vaccine series among patients aged 11–12 years. The study reported that completion of HPV vaccine series rates increased only in the $90,000 grant fund by 5 percentage points and decreased by 4.5 and 1.7 percentage points in the $10,000 grant fund and training and technical assistance arm, respectively [30]. We judged the certainty of the evidence as low because of concerns regarding the risk of bias in the included study and serious imprecision in the findings.

The study reported no relevant secondary outcomes.

Comparison 19: Multicomponent Intervention Compared Standard of Care

One study assessed the impact of a multicomponent intervention compared to the standard of care on the initiation of the HPV vaccine series among adolescents aged 11–12 and 13–17 years. Among adolescents aged 11–12 years, HPV vaccine series initiation rates increased by 18.7 percentage points in the intervention arm and 12.6 percentage points in the control arm, whereas, among adolescents aged 13–17 years, the rates increased by 8.7 percentage points in the intervention arm and 7 percentage points in the control arm [55]. We downgraded the certainty of the evidence to very low because of study limitations (i.e., before–after study).

A study assessed the impact of a multicomponent intervention compared to the standard of care on the completion of the HPV vaccine series among adolescents aged 11–12 and 13–17 years. HPV vaccine series completion rates among adolescents aged 11–12 years increased by the same 20.7 percentage points both in the intervention and control arms, whereas, among adolescents aged 13–17 years, the completion rates increased by 12.5 percentage points in the intervention and 11.9 percentage points in the control arms [55]. We downgraded the certainty of the evidence to very low because of study limitations (i.e., before–after study).

The study reported no relevant secondary outcomes.

4. Discussion

Our study found that recipient-oriented interventions that improved the initiation of the HPV vaccine series were narrative education, reminders, outreach plus reminders, education plus reminders, financial incentives plus reminders, and brief motivational behavioral interventions. We also found that the recipient-oriented interventions that improved the completion of the HPV vaccine series were tailored education, outreach and education, education plus reminders, reminders in general, financial incentives plus reminders, and brief motivational behavioral interventions. Tailored education, outreach and education, and brief health messaging were recipient-oriented interventions that had no effect on the initiation of the HPV vaccine series. Brief health messaging was also found to be a recipient-oriented intervention that had no effect on the completion of the HPV vaccine series. The provider-oriented interventions that improved the initiation of the HPV vaccine series were prompts, training, training plus assessment and feedback, consultation, funding, and multicomponent interventions. Prompts, funding and multicomponent were also found to be provider-oriented interventions that improved the completion of HPV vaccine series. Assessment and feedback were provider-oriented interventions that had no effect on both the initiation and the completion of the HPV vaccine series. With regards to the improvement of uptake of any HPV vaccine dose, all assessed recipient-oriented interventions, tailored education, untailored education, multicomponent education, and reminders did not have any effect.

Our systematic review was comprehensive. We included all known types of interventions, including recipient- and provider-oriented interventions, and all country settings. Our comprehensive search resulted in 35 studies that met our inclusion criteria. However, all studies were conducted in high-income countries, mainly the USA, where the burden of HPV is relatively low. None of the included studies were conducted in low-income countries, where the burden of HPV is very high. Therefore, the findings of these studies may be applicable only in the settings of the high-income countries. Another limitation is that there is very small number of studies that reported data on our secondary outcomes. Among the included studies, there were only one and three studies that reported data on the adverse effects and the cost of the interventions, respectively. However, because of variations in the measures of costs between the three studies, we were unable to conduct a meta-analysis. One study that reported on the adverse effects of the intervention stated that there were no effects documented in the study. Given that there is insufficient data on adverse effects and costs of the interventions, there is an urgent need for more studies to address these gaps. In addition, these studies should be well-designed and should evaluate outcomes and report results in ways that will allow the clear assessment of the cost and adverse effects of the interventions.

Thirty-five studies were excluded in this review mainly based on the methods used to conduct them. In addition, most of these studies were published after 2015, the period in which a previous similar review by Smulian (2016) [17] included studies up to. We may therefore have missed important findings from these studies. Well-designed studies that assess the effect of the interventions on HPV vaccination coverage are needed.

We used the Grading of Recommendations, Assessment, Development and Evaluations (GRADE)approach to assess the certainty of the evidence on the effects of the included interventions on HPV vaccination coverage. Among the recipient-oriented interventions that improved HPV vaccination coverage, we judged the certainty of the evidence as moderate for outreach plus reminders, low for reminders, and very low for education, financial incentives plus reminders, and brief motivational behavioral interventions. Regarding provider-oriented interventions that improved HPV vaccination coverage, we judged the certainty of the evidence as moderate for provider prompts, low for funding, and very low for training, consultation, training plus assessment and feedback, consultation, and multicomponent interventions. Overall, the certainty of evidence of interventions that improved HPV vaccination coverage was very low to moderate. Our main concerns with the evidence related to study limitations: risk of bias, indirectness, and imprecision in the studies. There is, therefore, an urgent need for well-designed, well-implemented, and well-reported studies to increase the certainty of the current evidence. We minimized potential biases in the review process by adhering to the Cochrane guidelines for conducting a systematic review [21]. We conducted comprehensive searches of both peer-reviewed and grey literature, without limiting the searches to a specific language. Two review authors independently assessed study eligibility, extracted data, and assessed the risk of bias in each included study. We are not aware of any biases in the review process.

Several systematic reviews have assessed the effectiveness of interventions for improving HPV vaccination coverage [6,13–17,57]. Smulian (2016) [17] evaluated the effectiveness of the interventions for improving HPV vaccination coverage in USA. The review found that many types of intervention strategies (targeting recipients, providers, and the health system) increased HPV vaccination coverage in different settings. Contrary to our review, which included 35 studies, this similar comprehensive review, which searched five databases for studies published between 2006 to 2015, resulted in 34 eligible studies. Like their review, all the studies included in our review were conducted in high-income countries. Of the 35 studies included in our review, 32 were conducted in the USA and the remaining three were from Australia, the Netherlands, and the UK. Acampora (2020) [13] and colleagues evaluated the effectiveness of interventions for improving HPV vaccination coverage among adolescents. The authors found that reminder-based interventions, either alone or in combination with other interventions, had a positive effect on vaccination coverage [13]. In another review, the effectiveness of intervention for improving HPV coverage among college students was assessed. The authors reported that the educational intervention that utilized a joint peer and medical provider message was the only intervention in their review that significantly increased HPV vaccine uptake [14]. The effectiveness of communication technology interventions on HPV vaccination coverage was assessed by Francis (2017) [16] and found that usage of computer, mobile, or internet technologies as the sole or primary mode for intervention delivery increased vaccination coverage. Niccolai (2015) [6] conducted a systematic review to assess the effectiveness of practice- and community-based interventions on improving HPV vaccination coverage. The review reported that several interventions including reminder and recall systems, physician-focused strategies (e.g., audit and feedback), school-located programs, and social marketing have improved vaccination coverage. The effectiveness of the interventions that applied new media to improve vaccination coverage was assessed by Odone and colleagues. The authors reported that text messaging, accessing immunization campaign websites, using patient-held web-based portals and computerized reminders, and standing orders increased vaccination coverage rates [57]. Walling and colleagues compared the effectiveness of the informational-, behavioral-, and environmental-based interventions on improving HPV vaccination coverage among adolescents and young adults aged 11 to 26 years. The authors found that environmental interventions, particularly school-based vaccination programs were most effective in increasing vaccination coverage [15].

5. Conclusions

Although several interventions improved HPV vaccination coverage, the certainty of the evidence varied from moderate to low. Although many studies were included in our review, all of them were conducted in high-income countries. There is, therefore, a need for further high-quality studies in low- and middle-income countries. At the same time, many studies assessing the effect of different interventions on improving HPV vaccination coverage were excluded because of the way they were conducted. As a result, well-designed, well-implemented, and well-reported studies are needed. In addition, given that there is limited information from existing studies on the cost of the tested interventions, further studies are needed to address this challenge.

Author Contributions: Conceptualization, E.J.M., C.J.I.-J. and C.S.W.; methodology and analysis, E.J.M. and C.S.W.; writing—original draft preparation, E.J.M.; writing—review and editing, E.J.M., C.J.I.-J., A.B.W., B.G., L.H.A., G.H.-E. and C.S.W. All authors have read and agreed to the published version of the manuscript.

Funding: This research was funded by the South African Medical Research Council.

Institutional Review Board Statement: Not applicable.

Informed Consent Statement: Not applicable.

Data Availability Statement: Not applicable.

Acknowledgments: The authors would like to thank Elizabeth Pienaar at Cochrane South Africa for assisting with the search strategy.

Conflicts of Interest: The authors declare no conflict of interest.

Appendix A

Table A1. Search strategies (search date: 9 July 2019).

Search	Query	Results
	PubMed	
#1	Search ("papillomavirus vaccines"(MeSH Terms) OR ("papillomavirus"[All Fields] AND "vaccines"[All Fields]) OR "papillomavirus vaccines"(All Fields) OR ("hpv"[All Fields] AND "vaccine"[All Fields]) OR "hpv vaccine"(All Fields)) AND (VACCINATE[All Fields] OR ["vaccination"[MeSH Terms] OR "vaccination"[All Fields]])	6876
#2	Search (randomized controlled trial(pt) OR controlled clinical trial(pt) OR randomized(tiab) OR placebo(tiab) OR "drug therapy"(Subheading) OR randomly(tiab) OR trial(tiab) OR groups(tiab)) NOT ("animals"(MeSH Terms) NOT "humans"(MeSH Terms))	3,933,624
#3	Search ("case-control studies"(MeSH Terms) OR ("case-control"[All Fields] AND "studies"[All Fields]) OR "case-control studies"(All Fields) OR ("case"[All Fields] AND "control"[All Fields] AND "studies"[All Fields]) OR "case control studies"(All Fields)) OR ("cohort studies"[MeSH Terms] OR ["cohort"[All Fields] AND "studies"[All Fields]] OR "cohort studies"(All Fields))	2,188,056
#4	Search (#2 OR #3)	5,407,771
#5	Search (#1 AND #4)	1815
	Web of Science	
#1	Search ((("papillomavirus vaccines" OR ["papillomavirus" AND "vaccines"] OR "papillomavirus vaccines" OR ["hpv" AND "vaccine"] OR "hpv vaccine") AND (VACCINATE OR ["vaccination" OR "vaccination"]))	5810
#2	Search ((([randomized controlled trial] OR [controlled clinical trial]) OR (["case-control studies" OR ["case-control" AND "studies"] OR ["case"AND "control" AND "studies"] OR "case control studies"] OR ["cohort studies" OR ["cohort" AND "studies"]]))	652,297
#3	Search (#2 AND #1)	669
	Scopus	
#1	Search ("papillomavirus vaccines" OR "papillomavirus vaccine" OR "hpv vaccine" OR "HPV vaccines")	9447
#2	Search ("Randomized controlled trial" OR "controlled clinical trial" OR "Randomized Controlled trials" OR "Controlled Clinical trials" OR "case-control studies" OR "Case control studies")	1,175,572
#3	Search (#1 AND #2)	738

Table A2. Characteristics of included studies.

No.	Study Id	Country	Study Type	Sample Size	Participants	Intervention	Comparator	Outcome Measure
1	Bennett (2015) [22] Bennett (2014) [58] NCT01769560 [59]	USA	RCT	661	Female students aged 18–26 years	330 participants were randomized to individually tailored educational website.	331 participants were randomized to the website of the standard CDC information factsheet on the HPV vaccine.	Initiation and completion of HPV vaccine series
2	Brewer (2017) [23] NCT02377843 [60]	USA	RCT	30	Providers	10 clinics were randomized to announcement training. Participating clinicians received 1 h of training on announcement to recommend HPV vaccination. 10 clinics were randomized to conservation training. Participating clinicians received 1 h of training on conservation to recommend HPV vaccination.	10 clinics were randomized to the waitlist control condition. Participating clinics received a video recording of the announcement training, which was sent 1 month after the 6-month assessment of vaccination outcomes.	Initiation of HPV vaccine series
3	Chao (2015) [24]	USA	RCT	12,225	Females aged 9–26 years	9804 participants were randomized to reminder letter. Participants received a letter reminding them of the HPV vaccination.	2451 participants were randomized to the standard of care. Participants received no reminder letters.	Completion of HPV vaccine series
4	Coley (2018) [25]	USA	RCT	303,965	Parents of adolescents aged 11–13 years	151,982 participants were randomized to reminder letter. Parents received letters reminding them to vaccinate their adolescents.	151,983 participants were randomized to control letters. Participants received letters six months after the observation period was completed.	Initiation and completion of HPV vaccine series Cost of intervention
5	Dempsey (2019) [26] NCT02145156 [61]	USA	RCT	1294	Young adults aged 18–26 years and their parents	430 participants were randomized to web-based tailored messaging called CHICOs (Combatting HPV Infections and Cancers). Participants received an iPad with the CHICOS intervention programmed onto it. 425 participants were randomized to web-based untailored messaging. Participants received an iPad-based version of the Vaccine Information Sheet from the Centers for Disease Control and Prevention.	439 participants were randomized to usual care. Participants received care routinely provided by the clinician and did not interact with or have access to the iPad	Receipt of any HPV vaccine dose

Table A2. *Cont.*

No.	Study Id	Country	Study Type	Sample Size	Participants	Intervention	Comparator	Outcome Measure
6	DiClemente (2015) [27] NCT00813319 [62]	USA	RCT	216	Female adolescents aged 14–18 years	108 participants were randomized to theory-based, multi-component computer-delivered media-based intervention called Girls OnGuard. Participants viewed a 12-min interactive computer-delivered media presentation on HPV vaccination.	108 participants were randomized to placebo. Participants viewed a time-equivalent health promotion media presentation on physical activity and nutrition.	Initiation and completion of HPV vaccine series
7	Fisher-Borne (2018) [30]	USA	RCT	30	Providers	10 participants were randomized to $90,000 2-year grant. 10 participants were randomized to $10,000 3-month grant.	10 participants were randomized to no funding. Participants received training and technical assistance.	Initiation and completion of HPV vaccine series
8	Gilkey (2014) [28]	USA	RCT	91	Providers Primary care clinics (pediatric and family practice clinics) serving adolescents 11–18 years old.	30 clinics were randomized to in-person delivered Assessment, Feedback, Incentives, and eXchange (AFIX) consultation. 30 clinics were randomized to webinar-delivered AFIX consultation.	30 clinics were randomized to no consultation	Initiation of HPV vaccine series
9	Gilkey (2019) [29]	USA	RCT	78	Pediatricians	43 participants were randomized to quality improvement plus assessment and feedback.	35 participants were randomized to wait-list control arm. Participants received QI program after 6 months of follow-up.	Initiation of the HPV vaccine series
10	Henrikson (2018) [31] Henrikson (2017) [63]	USA	RCT	1805	Parents of adolescents aged 10–12 years	1354 participants were randomized to outreach letter, brochure, and reminder. Participants received outreach letter and brochure recommending HPV vaccination followed by automated HPV vaccine reminder call for dose 1.	451 participants were randomized to usual care. Participants received no outreach letter or reminder call.	Initiation of the HPV vaccine series
11	Hofstetter (2017) [32]	USA	RCT	295	Parents of adolescents with chronic medical conditions	154 participants were randomized to educational text message reminders. Participants received educational text message reminders on receipt of HPV.	141 participants were randomized to plaint text message reminders.	Initiation of the HPV vaccine series

175

Table A2. Cont.

No.	Study Id	Country	Study Type	Sample Size	Participants	Intervention	Comparator	Outcome Measure
12	Hopfer (2012) [33]	USA	RCT	404	College women aged 18–26 years	252 participants were randomized to narrative messages Participants viewed one of three videos: (1) a video of vaccine decision narratives delivered by peers (101), (2) a video of narratives delivered by medical experts (50), or (3) a video of narratives delivered by a combination of peers and experts (101)	152 participants were randomized to no narrative messages Participants viewed one of three controls: (1) an informational video without narratives, (2) the campus website providing information about HPV and the vaccine, or (3) no message.	Initiation of the HPV vaccine series
13	Irving (2018) [54]	USA	BA	12	Providers (clinics)	9 clinics were enrolled in the provider-focused assessment and feedback intervention.	3 clinics were enrolled in the standard of care.	Initiation and completion of HPV vaccine series
14	Joseph (2016) [34] NCT01254669 [64]	USA	RCT	200	Mothers of daughters aged 11–15 years	100 participants were randomized to brief negotiated interviewing (BNI). Participants received the BNI intervention, which addressed mothers' beliefs, values, and concerns about HPV prevention and accounting for their priorities for health and well-being.	100 participants were randomized to no BNI. Participants received the low literacy, standard-practice HPV vaccine information sheet given to all patients prior to vaccination	Initiation and completion of HPV vaccine series
15	Lee (2018) [35]	USA	RC	19	Mothers and daughters aged 14–17 years dyads	10 participants were randomized to storytelling narrative videos. The participants watched a 26-min storytelling narrative DVD on HPV vaccine, entitled "Save My Daughter from Cervical Cancer."	9 participants were randomized to written non-narrative education materials. Participants received CDC flyers on the HPV vaccine.	Initiation of the HPV vaccine series
16	Mantzari (2015) [36]	UK	RCT	1000	Girls aged 16–18 years	500 participants were randomized to financial incentives. Participants received the offer of "Love2Shop" vouchers worth £45 for receiving the three vaccinations.	500 participants were randomized to no financial incentives. Participants received no incentives.	Initiation and completion of HPV vaccine series
17	Mclean (2017) [55]	USA	BA	43	Providers (clinics)	9 participants were enrolled in the multi-component interventions. Participants received education on HPV vaccination, assessment and feedback, and patient reminder and recall notifications.	34 participants were enrolled in the standard of care.	Initiation and completion of HPV vaccine series

Table A2. *Cont.*

No.	Study Id	Country	Study Type	Sample Size	Participants	Intervention	Comparator	Outcome Measure
18	Parra Medina (2015) [56]	USA	N-RCT	372	Hispanic mothers with a daughter aged 11–17 years	257 participants were enrolled in the outreach and education program called Entre Madre e Hija (EMH), a culturally relevant cervical cancer prevention program. Participants received health education, referral, and navigation support for HPV vaccination. They also received an HPV vaccine educational brochure.	115 participants were enrolled in the HPV vaccine educational brochure only.	Initiation and completion of HPV vaccine series
19	Patel (2012) [37]	USA	RCT	256	Female college students aged 18–26 years	128 were randomized to HPV-specific patient education and reminder letter. Participants received HPV and Vaccination" fact sheet plus reminder letter for HPV vaccination.	128 were randomized to standard of care. Participants did not receive "HPV and Vaccination" fact sheet and reminder letter.	Initiation of the HPV vaccine series
20	Pot (2017) [38]	The Netherlands	RCT	806	Mothers of girls aged 12 years	3995 participants were randomized to web-based tailored intervention with virtual assistants. Participants received tailored information on HPV and HPV vaccination.	4067 participants were randomized to standard of care. Participants received universal information about the HPV vaccination	Receipt of any HPV vaccine dose
21	Rand (2015) [39]	USA	RCT	3812	Parents of adolescents aged 11–16 years	1893 participants were randomized to text message reminders. Parents received text message reminding them that their adolescents were due for HPV vaccine doses.	1919 participants were randomized to general adolescent health text message. Parents received general adolescent health text message each time their adolescents were due for HPV vaccine dose.	Initiation of the HPV vaccine series
22	Rand (2017) [40] NCT01731496 [65]	USA	RCT	749	Parents of adolescents aged 11–17 years	178 participants were randomized to telephone message reminder. Parents received telephone call reminding them that their adolescents were due for an HPV vaccine dose. 191 participants were randomized to text message reminders. Parents received text message reminding them that their adolescents were due for HPV vaccine dose.	180 participants were randomized to standard of care (telephone reminder control). 200 participants were randomized to standard of care (text reminder control).	Completion of HPV vaccine series

Table A2. Cont.

No.	Study Id	Country	Study Type	Sample Size	Participants	Intervention	Comparator	Outcome Measure
23	Reiter (2018) [41] Mcree (2018) [66], NCT01769560 [59]	USA	RCT	150	Young gay and bisexual men aged 18-25 years	76 participants were randomized to outsmart HPV intervention. Participants received population-targeted, individually tailored content about HPV and the HPV vaccine, and monthly HPV vaccination reminders sent via email and/or text message.	74 participants were randomized to standard HPV information. Participants received standard information about HPV and the HPV vaccine.	Completion of HPV vaccine series
24	Richman (2019) [42]	USA	RCT	257	Parents of adolescences aged 9-17 years.	129 participants were randomized to electronic messaging (text or email).Participants received appointment reminders and education messages about HPV and the HPV vaccine.	128 participants were randomized to standard of care. Participants received a paper card with the date of their next appointment written on it.	Completion of HPV vaccine series
25	Richman (2016) [43]	US	RCT	264	College students aged 18-26 years	130 participants were randomized to electronic messaging (text or email). Participants received appointment reminders and education messages about HPV and the HPV vaccine. In addition, participants received a paper card with the date of their nextappointment written on it.	134 participants were randomized to standard of care. Participants received a paper card with the date of their next appointment written on it.	Completion of HPV vaccine series
26	Rickert (2015) [44]	USA	RCT	445	Parents of male and female adolescents aged 11-15 years	109 participants were randomized to rhetorical questions (RQ) plus one-sided message. 114 participants were randomized to RQ plus two-sided message.	116 participants were randomized to no RQ plus one-sided message. 106 participants were randomized to no RQ plus two-sided message.	Initiation and completion of HPV vaccine series
27	Suh (2012) [45]	USA	RCT	1600	Parents of adolescents aged 11 to 18 years	800 participants were randomized to letter and telephone reminders. Parents received letter and autodialed telephone call informing them that their adolescents were due for an HPV vaccination.	800 participants were randomized to usual care. Parents received no reminder/recall	Initiation and completion of HPV vaccine series Cost of intervention

Table A2. Cont.

No.	Study Id	Country	Study Type	Sample Size	Participants	Intervention	Comparator	Outcome Measure
28	Szilagyi (2015) [46]	USA	RCT	22	Providers / Primary care practices attendant by adolescents aged 11–17 years	11 practices were randomized to provider prompts on HPV vaccination (electronic health record (EHR) or nurse- or staff-initiated prompts). Participants received prompts indicating the specific HPV vaccine doses that the adolescents were due for during their practice visits.	11 practices were randomized to standard of care. Participants did not receive any prompts.	Completion of HPV vaccine series
29	Szilagyi (2013) [47]	USA	RCT	7404	Parents of adolescents aged 11–17 years	2494 participants were randomized to letter reminder. Parents received reminder letters advising them to call their adolescent's primary care practice to schedule an appointment for HPV vaccination. 2504 participants were randomized to telephone reminder. Parents received autodialed reminder calls advising them to call their adolescent's primary care practice to schedule an appointment for HPV vaccination.	2406 participants were randomized to standard of care. Parents received no reminder.	Initiation and completion of HPV vaccine series Costs of the intervention
30	Tiro (2015) [48]	USA	RCT	814	Parents and girls /daughters aged 11–18 years dyads	410 participants were randomized to HPV-vaccine-specific brochure and recalls. Participants received HPV-vaccine-specific brochures and telephone recalls for vaccination.	404 participants were randomized to general adolescent vaccine brochure. Participants received a CDC brochure about all Advisory Committee on Immunization Practices' recommended vaccines.	Initiation and completion of HPV vaccine series

Table A2. Cont.

No.	Study Id	Country	Study Type	Sample Size	Participants	Intervention	Comparator	Outcome Measure
31	Tull (2019) [49]	Australia	RCT	4386	Parents of Year 7 students	1442 participants were randomized to motivational short message service (SMS) Reminders. Participants received a motivational SMS: "Vaccine preventable diseases are still a problem in the community and children most at risk are those that have not been immunized." 1418 participants were randomized to self-regulatory SMS reminders. Participants received an SMS: "make a plan now for how your child will get to school on-time on immunization day."	1526 participants were randomized to no SMS reminders. Participants received no SMS reminders.	Receipt of any HPV vaccine dose
32	Underwood (2019) [50] Herbert (2014) [67]	USA	RCT	2135	Parents and adolescents	668 participants (parents only) were randomized to educational intervention. Participants received an educational brochure about adolescent vaccines. 690 participants (parents and adolescents) were randomized to multicomponent educational intervention. Participants (parents) received educational brochures about vaccines recommended during adolescence. Participants (adolescents) received a vaccine-focused curriculum delivered by science teachers.	777 participants were randomized to no intervention. Parents received no information.	Receipt of any HPV vaccine dose
33	Vanderpool (2013) [51]	USA	RCT	344	Young women aged 18–26 years	178 participants were randomized to an educational DVD, entitled "1-2-3 Pap." Participants watched a 13-min educational DVD on HPV, HPV vaccines, and pap tests	166 participants were randomized to Standard of care.	Completion of HPV vaccine series

Table A2. *Cont.*

No.	Study Id	Country	Study Type	Sample Size	Participants	Intervention	Comparator	Outcome Measure
34	Wilkinson (2019) [52] Zimet (2016) [68] NCT02555803 [69]	USA	RCT	29	Providers (pediatric clinicians)	15 participants were randomized to automated reminder. Participants received automated reminders via Child Health Improvement through Computer Automation (CHICA) to recommend the 2nd and 3rd doses of HPV vaccine to adolescents aged 11–17 years who had already initiated the vaccine series.	14 participants were randomized to usual practice. Participants received reminders to recommend the 2nd and 3rd doses of HPV vaccine manually from the nurses who looked them up in the Children and Hoosier Immunization Registry Program (CHIRP).	Completion of HPV vaccine series
35	Zimet (2018) [53]	USA	RCT	29	Providers (health care providers)	8 participants were randomized to simple reminder prompt. Participants received computer-generated messages reminding them of HPV vaccination eligibility. 11 participants were randomized to elaborated reminder prompt. Participants received computer-generated reminders with a suggested script for recommending the three adolescent platform vaccines.	10 participants were randomized to usual practice. Participants did not receive any reminder prompt. They made HPV vaccination recommendations their existing methods for determining eligibility.	Initiation of the HPV vaccine series

Table A3. Characteristics of excluded studies.

Study No.	Study Id.	Reason
1	Chigbu (2017) [70]	A before–after study evaluating the impact of trained community health educators on the uptake of cervical and breast cancer screening and HPV vaccination. The study was excluded because it had one intervention and control group.
2	Cory (2019) [71]	A randomized study assessing the effects of educational interventions on human papillomavirus vaccine acceptability. Reported outcome was intention to vaccinate.
3	Daley (2014) [72]	A cluster-randomized controlled study assessing the program costs, the proportion of costs reimbursed, and the likelihood of vaccination in a school-located adolescent vaccination program that billed health insurance. One intervention and control cluster.
4	Davies (2017) [73] Skinner (2015) [74]	A cluster-randomized controlled study evaluating the effect of educational intervention on HPV vaccination uptake. One intervention and control cluster.
5	Dempsey (2018) [75] O'Leary (2017) [76] NCT02456077 [77]	A cluster-randomized controlled study evaluating the effect of a health care professional communication training intervention on adolescent human papillomavirus vaccination. One intervention and control cluster.
6	Deshmukh (2018) [78]	A before–after study evaluating the impact of a clinical intervention bundle on the rate of missed opportunities and uptake of the vaccine among young adult women. One intervention and control group.
7	Dixon (2019) [79] Dixon (2016) [80] NCT02546752 [81]	A cluster-randomized controlled study assessing the effects an educational intervention in improving HPV vaccination. One intervention and control cluster.
8	Fiks (2013) [82]	A cluster-randomized controlled study evaluating the effectiveness of decision support for families, clinicians, or both on HPV vaccine receipt. One intervention and control cluster.
9	Fiks (2016) [83]	A before–after study evaluating the impact of Maintenance-of-Certification program on improving HPV vaccination rates. One intervention and control group.
10	Forster (2017) [84]	A cluster-randomized controlled study evaluating the effect of an adolescent incentive intervention on improving HPV vaccination uptake. One intervention and control cluster.
11	Grandahl (2016) [85]	A cluster-randomized controlled study assessing the effect of the educational intervention on increasing HPV vaccination among adolescents. One intervention and control cluster.
12	Jacobs-Wingo (2017) [86]	A cross-sectional study assessing the impact of multi-component interventions on increasing HPV vaccine coverage.
13	Jiménez-Quiñones (2017) [87]	A descriptive study assessing the impact of a pharmacist administered educational program on the vaccination rates of HPV. A descriptive study.
14	Keeshin (2017) [88]	A prospective cohort study evaluating the impact of text message reminder recall on increasing HPV vaccination in young HIV-1-infected patients. A prospective study.
15	Kempe (2012) [89]	A demonstration study assessing the effectiveness and cost of immunization recall at school-based health centers. A demonstration study.
16	Kim (2018) [90]	Conference abstract only
17	Lee (2016) [91]	A before–after study evaluating the effect of the text messaging intervention on HPV vaccination among Korean-American women. One intervention group.
18	Mayne (2014) [92]	A cluster-randomized controlled study evaluating the effect of decision support on HPV vaccination. One intervention and control cluster
19	Mehta (2013) [93]	A randomized-controlled study evaluating a health-belief-model-based intervention to increase vaccination rates in college men. The reported outcome was intention to vaccinate.
10	O'Leary (2019) [94]	A cluster-randomized controlled study assessing the effectiveness of a multimodal intervention in obstetrics/gynecology clinics in increasing vaccination uptake. One intervention and control cluster.

Table A3. Cont.

Study No.	Study Id.	Reason
21	Patel (2014) [95] NCT01343485 [96]	A cluster-randomized control study evaluating the impact of an automated reminders in increasing on-time completion of the three-dose HPV vaccine series. One intervention and control cluster.
22	Perez (2016) [2]	A randomized controlled study evaluating the effect of an information–motivation–behavioral skills (IMB) intervention in increasing HPV vaccination knowledge, motivation, and intentions among college-aged women. Reported outcome was intentions to vaccinate
23	Perkins (2015) [97]	A before–after study assessing the effectiveness of a provider-focused intervention in improving HPV vaccination rates in boys and girls. One intervention group and control group.
24	Rahman (2013) [98]	A cross-sectional study evaluating the impact of attending a well-woman clinic on HPV vaccine intent and uptake among both their sons and daughters. A cross-sectional study.
25	Rickert (2014) [99]	A before–after study assessing the impact of health beliefs on intent and first dose uptake of HPV vaccine among young adolescent males. One intervention and control cluster.
26	Roblin (2014) [100]	An observational study evaluating the influence of deductible health plans on receipt of the human papillomavirus vaccine series. An observational study.
27	Ruffin (2015) [101]	A retrospective study assessing the impact of electronic health record reminder on HPV vaccine initiation and timely completion among female patients. A retrospective study.
28	Russel (2012) [102]	A randomized controlled study assessing the effectiveness of text message reminders in improving vaccination appointment attendance and series completion among adolescents and adults. Abstract only.
29	Sanderson (2017) [103] NCT02808832 [104]	A cluster-randomized controlled study evaluating the effectiveness of provider-focused and patient-focused intervention strategies in increasing HPV vaccination. One intervention and control cluster.
30	Spleen (2012) [105]	A before–after study evaluating the impact of theory and community-based educational intervention on increasing parents' HPV-related knowledge and parental intent to vaccinate their daughters against HPV. One intervention and control group.
31	Valdez (2015) [106]	A randomized controlled trial evaluating the effects of HPV vaccine education intervention on promoting informed decision-making about HPV vaccination among parents. Reported outcome were intentions to vaccinate
32	Whadera (2015) [107]	A prospective study assessing the effect of HPV educational intervention on HPV knowledge, vaccine acceptance, and vaccine series completion among female entertainment and sex workers. A prospective study.
33	Wedel (2016) [108]	A before–after study evaluating the effect of HPV educational intervention on increasing HPV vaccinations among military women. Not a controlled before and after study.
34	Wegwart (2014) [109]	A before–after study evaluating the effect of evidence-based HPV vaccination leaflets on understanding, intention, and actual vaccination decision. One intervention and control group
35	Whelan (2014) [110]	A retrospective study examining the relationship between school-based strategies and uptake of HPV vaccine. A retrospective study.
36	Winer (2016) [111]	A cluster-randomized controlled study evaluating the impact of an educational intervention on increasing HPV vaccination coverage in American Indian girls. One intervention and control cluster.
37	Zimmerman (2017) [112]	A before–after study evaluating the effect of the 4 Pillars™ Practice Transformation Program on improving adolescent HPV vaccination. One intervention and control group.
38	Zimmerman (2017) [113]	A cluster-randomized controlled study evaluating the effect of the 4 Pillars™ Practice Transformation Program on improving adolescent HPV vaccination. One intervention and control cluster.

Table A4. Risk of bias summary.

Study	Random Sequence Generation (Selection Bias)	Allocation Concealment (Selection Bias)	Blinding of Participants and Personnel (Performance Bias)	Blinding of Outcome Assessment (Detection Bias)	Incomplete Outcome Data (Attrition Bias)	Selective Reporting (Reporting Bias)	Other Bias
Bennett (2015) [22]	+	+	+	?	−	+	+
Brewer (2017) [23]	+	?	−	−	+	+	+
Chao (2015) [24]	?	?	?	?	+	+	+
Coley (2018) [25]	+	−	?	?	?	+	+
Dempsey (2019b) [26]	+	?	+	+	−	+	+
DiClemente (2015) [27]	+	+	−	?	+	+	+
Fisher-Borne (2018) [30]	?	?	?	?	−	+	+
Gilkey (2014) [28]	+	?	−	?	+	+	+
Gilkey (2019) [29]	?	?	−	?	+	+	+
Henrikson (2018) [31]	?	?	?	?	+	+	+
Hofstetter (2017) [32]	+	−	+	+	+	+	+
Hopfer (2012) [33]	+	−	?	?	+	+	+
Irving (2018) [54]	−	−	?	?	+	+	+
Joseph (2016) [34]	+	−	−	−	+	+	+
Lee (2018) [35]	?	?	?	?	+	+	+
Mantzari (2015) [36]	+	−	?	?	+	+	+
Mclean (2017) [55]	−	−	?	?	?	+	+
Parra-Medina (2015) [56]	−	−	?	?	−	?	+
Patel (2012) [37]	+	+	?	?	+	+	+

Table A4. *Cont.*

Study	Random Sequence Generation (Selection Bias)	Allocation Concealment (Selection Bias)	Blinding of Participants and Personnel (Performance Bias)	Blinding of Outcome Assessment (Detection Bias)	Incomplete Outcome Data (Attrition Bias)	Selective Reporting (Reporting Bias)	Other Bias
Pot (2017) [38]	?	?	−	−	−	+	+
Rand (2015) [39]	+	−	+	?	−	+	+
Rand (2017) [40]	+	−	?	+	+	+	+
Reiter (2018) [41]	+	?	−	−	+	+	+
Richman (2019) [42]	?	?	+	?	−	+	+
Richman (2016) [43]	?	?	+	?	+	+	+
Rickert (2015) [44]	+	−	−	?	+	+	+
Suh (2012) [45]	+	−	+	?	+	+	+
Szilagyi (2015) [46]	+	+	?	?	+	+	+
Szilagyi (2013) [47]	+	+	+	?	?	+	+
Tiro (2015) [48]	+	−	+	?	+	+	+
Tull (2019) [49]	+	−	+	?	+	+	+
Underwood (2019) [50]	?	?	?	?	+	+	+
Vanderpool (2013) [51]	+	−	+	?	+	+	+
Wilkinson (2019) [52]	+	−	+	?	+	+	+
Zimet (2018) [53]	?	?	?	?	+	+	+

References

1. Loke, A.Y.; Kwan, M.L.; Wong, Y.-T.; Wong, A.K.Y. The Uptake of Human Papillomavirus Vaccination and Its Associated Factors Among Adolescents: A Systematic Review. *J. Prim. Care Community Health* **2017**, *8*, 349–362. [CrossRef]
2. Perez, G.K.; Cruess, D.G.; Strauss, N.M. A brief information–motivation–behavioral skills intervention to promote human papillomavirus vaccination among college-aged women. *Psychol. Res. Behav. Manag.* **2016**, *9*, 285–296. [CrossRef]
3. Fontes, A.; Andreoli, M.A.; Villa, L.L.; Assone, T.; Gaester, K.; Fonseca, L.A.; Duarte, A.J.; Casseb, J. High specific immune response to a bivalent anti-HPV vaccine in HIV-1-infected men in São Paulo, Brazil. *Papillomavirus Res.* **2016**, *2*, 17–20. [CrossRef]
4. Holman, D.M.; Benard, V.; Roland, K.; Watson, M.; Liddon, N.; Stockley, S. Barriers to human papillomavirus vaccination among US adolescents: A systematic review of the literature. *JAMA Pediatr.* **2014**, *168*, 76–82. [CrossRef]

5. Lu, P.-J.; Yankey, D.; Jeyarajah, J.; O'Halloran, A.; Elam-Evans, L.D.; Smith, P.J.; Stokley, S.; Singleton, J.A.; Dunne, E.F. HPV Vaccination Coverage of Male Adolescents in the United States. *Pediatrics* **2015**, *136*, 839–849. [CrossRef]
6. Niccolai, M.L.; Hansen, C.E. Practice- and Community-Based Interventions to Increase Human Papillomavirus Vaccine Coverage: A Systematic Review. *JAMA Pediatr.* **2015**, *169*, 686–692. [CrossRef]
7. Egawa, N.; Doorbar, J. The low-risk papillomaviruses. *Virus Res.* **2017**, *231*, 119–127. [CrossRef]
8. Globocan. Available online: https://gco.iarc.fr (accessed on 30 March 2021).
9. Chabeda, A.; Yanez, R.J.; Lamprecht, R.; Meyers, A.E.; Rybicki, E.P.; Hitzeroth, I.I. Therapeutic vaccines for high-risk HPV-associated diseases. *Papillomavirus Res.* **2018**, *5*, 46–58. [CrossRef]
10. Gallagher, K.E.; Howard, N.; Kabakama, S.; Mounier-Jack, S.; Burchett, H.E.D.; Lamontagne, D.S.; Watson-Jones, D. Human papillomavirus (HPV) vaccine coverage achievements in low and middle-income countries 2007–2016. *Papillomavirus Res.* **2017**, *4*, 72–78. [CrossRef]
11. Carney, P.A.; Hatch, B.; Stock, I.; Dickinson, C.; Davis, M.; Larsen, R.; Valenzuela, S.; Marino, M.; Darden, P.M.; Gunn, R.; et al. A stepped-wedge cluster randomized trial designed to improve completion of HPV vaccine series and reduce missed opportunities to vaccinate in rural primary care practices. *Implement. Sci.* **2019**, *14*, 30. [CrossRef]
12. Brandt, H.M.; Pierce, J.Y.; Crary, A. Increasing HPV vaccination through policy for public health benefit. *Hum. Vaccines Immunother.* **2015**, *12*, 1623–1625. [CrossRef] [PubMed]
13. Acampora, A.; Grossi, A.; Barbara, A.; Colamesta, V.; Causio, F.A.; Calabrò, G.E.; Boccia, S.; De Waure, C. Increasing HPV Vaccination Uptake among Adolescents: A Systematic Review. *Int. J. Environ. Res. Public Health* **2020**, *17*, 7997. [CrossRef] [PubMed]
14. Barnard, M.; Cole, A.C.; Ward, L.; Gravlee, E.; Cole, M.L.; Compretta, C. Interventions to increase uptake of the human papillomavirus vaccine in unvaccinated college students: A systematic literature review. *Prev. Med. Rep.* **2019**, *14*, 100884. [CrossRef] [PubMed]
15. Walling, E.B.; Benzoni, N.; Dornfeld, J.; Bhandari, R.; Sisk, B.A.; Garbutt, J.; Colditz, G. Interventions to Improve HPV Vaccine Uptake: A Systematic Review. *Pediatrics* **2016**, *138*. [CrossRef] [PubMed]
16. Francis, D.B.; Cates, J.R.; Wagner, K.P.G.; Zola, T.; Fitter, J.E.; Coyne-Beasley, T. Communication technologies to improve HPV vaccination initiation and completion: A systematic review. *Patient Educ. Couns.* **2017**, *100*, 1280–1286. [CrossRef]
17. Smulian, E.A.; Mitchell, K.R.; Stokley, S. Interventions to increase HPV vaccination coverage: A systematic review. *Hum. Vaccines Immunother.* **2016**, *12*, 1566–1588. [CrossRef]
18. PROSPERO. Available online: https://www.crd.york.ac.uk/prospero/ (accessed on 30 March 2021).
19. Liberati, A.; Altman, D.G.; Tetzlaff, J.; Mulrow, C.; Gøtzsche, P.C.; Ioannidis, J.P.A.; Clarke, M.; Devereaux, P.J.; Kleijnen, J.; Moher, D. The PRISMA statement for reporting systematic reviews and meta-analyses of studies that evaluate health care interventions: Explanation and elaboration. *J. Clin. Epidemiol.* **2009**, *62*, e1–e34. [CrossRef]
20. Cochrane Effective Practice and Organisation of Care. EPOC Resources for Review Authors. Available online: https://epoc.cochrane.org/resources/epoc-resources-review-authors/ (accessed on 20 March 2021).
21. Higgins, J.; Altman, D.; Sterne, J. Assessing Risk of Bias in Included Studies. In *Cochrane Handbook for Systematic Reviews of Interventions*; Version 5.1.0 Updated March, 2011; Higgins, J.P.T., Green, S., Eds.; The Cochrane Collaboration: London, UK, 2011.
22. Bennett, A.T.; Patel, D.A.; Carlos, R.C.; Zochowski, M.K.; Pennewell, S.M.; Chi, A.M.; Dalton, V.K. Human Papillomavirus Vaccine Uptake after a Tailored, Online Educational Intervention for Female University Students: A Randomized Controlled Trial. *J. Women Health* **2015**, *24*, 950–957. [CrossRef]
23. Brewer, N.T.; Hall, M.E.; Malo, T.L.; Gilkey, M.B.; Quinn, B.; Lathren, C. Announcements Versus Conversations to Improve HPV Vaccination Coverage: A Randomized Trial. *Pediatrics* **2016**, *139*, e20161764. [CrossRef]
24. Chao, C.; Preciado, M.; Slezak, J.; Xu, L. A Randomized Intervention of Reminder Letter for Human Papillomavirus Vaccine Series Completion. *J. Adolesc. Health* **2015**, *56*, 85–90. [CrossRef]
25. Coley, S.; Hoefer, D.; Rausch-Phung, E. A population-based reminder intervention to improve human papillomavirus vaccination rates among adolescents at routine vaccination age. *Vaccine* **2018**, *36*, 4904–4909. [CrossRef] [PubMed]
26. Dempsey, A.F.; Maertens, J.; Sevick, C.; Jimenez-Zambrano, A.; Juarez-Colunga, E. A randomized, controlled, pragmatic trial of an iPad-based, tailored messaging intervention to increase human papillomavirus vaccination among Latinos. *Hum. Vaccines Immunother.* **2019**, *15*, 1577–1584. [CrossRef] [PubMed]
27. DiClemente, R.J.; Murray, C.C.; Graham, T.; Still, J. Overcoming barriers to HPV vaccination: A randomized clinical trial of a culturally-tailored, media intervention among African American girls. *Hum. Vaccines Immunother.* **2015**, *11*, 2883–2894. [CrossRef]
28. Gilkey, M.B.; Dayton, A.M.; Moss, J.L.; Sparks, A.C.; Grimshaw, A.H.; Bowling, J.M.; Brewer, N.T. Increasing Provision of Adolescent Vaccines in Primary Care: A Randomized Controlled Trial. *Pediatrics* **2014**, *134*, e346–e353. [CrossRef]
29. Gilkey, M.B.; Parks, M.J.; Margolis, M.A.; McRee, A.-L.; Terk, J.V. Implementing Evidence-Based Strategies to Improve HPV Vaccine Delivery. *Pediatrics* **2019**, *144*, e20182500. [CrossRef] [PubMed]
30. Fisher-Borne, M.; Preiss, A.J.; Black, M.; Roberts, K.; Saslow, D. Early Outcomes of a Multilevel Human Papillomavirus Pilot Intervention in Federally Qualified Health Centers. *Acad. Pediatr.* **2018**, *18*, S79–S84. [CrossRef]
31. Henrikson, N.B.; Zhu, W.; Baba, L.; Nguyen, M.; Berthoud, H.; Gundersen, G.; Hofstetter, A.M. Outreach and Reminders to Improve Human Papillomavirus Vaccination in an Integrated Primary Care System. *Clin. Pediatr.* **2018**, *57*, 1523–1531. [CrossRef]

32. Hofstetter, A.M.; Barrett, A.; Camargo, S.; Rosenthal, S.L.; Stockwell, M.S. Text message reminders for vaccination of adolescents with chronic medical conditions: A randomized clinical trial. *Vaccine* **2017**, *35*, 4554–4560. [CrossRef]
33. Hopfer, S. Effects of a Narrative HPV Vaccination Intervention Aimed at Reaching College Women: A Randomized Controlled Trial. *Prev. Sci.* **2011**, *13*, 173–182. [CrossRef]
34. Joseph, N.P.; Bernstein, J.; Pelton, S.; Goff, G.; Horanieh, N.; Freund, K.M. Brief Client-Centered Motivational and Behavioral Intervention to Promote HPV Vaccination in a Hard-to-Reach Population: A Pilot Randomized Controlled Trial. *Clin. Pediatr.* **2016**, *55*, 851–859. [CrossRef]
35. Lee, H.; Kim, M.; Cooley, M.E.; Kiang, P.N.-C.; Kim, D.; Tang, S.; Shi, L.; Thiem, L.; Kan, P.; Peou, S.; et al. Using narrative intervention for HPV vaccine behavior change among Khmer mothers and daughters: A pilot RCT to examine feasibility, acceptability, and preliminary effectiveness. *Appl. Nurs. Res.* **2018**, *40*, 51–60. [CrossRef]
36. Mantzari, E.; Vogt, F.; Marteau, T.M. Financial incentives for increasing uptake of HPV vaccinations: A randomized controlled trial. *Health Psychol.* **2015**, *34*, 160–171. [CrossRef]
37. Patel, D.A.; Zochowski, M.; Peterman, S.; Dempsey, A.F.; Ernst, S.; Dalton, V.K. Human Papillomavirus Vaccine Intent and Uptake Among Female College Students. *J. Am. Coll. Health* **2012**, *60*, 151–161. [CrossRef]
38. Pot, M.; Paulussen, T.G.; Ruiter, R.A.; Eekhout, I.; De Melker, H.E.; Spoelstra, M.E.; Van Keulen, H.M.; Grandahl, M.; Glanz, J.; Bragazzi, N. Effectiveness of a Web-Based Tailored Intervention With Virtual Assistants Promoting the Acceptability of HPV Vaccination Among Mothers of Invited Girls: Randomized Controlled Trial. *J. Med. Internet Res.* **2017**, *19*, e312. [CrossRef]
39. Rand, C.M.; Brill, H.; Albertin, C.; Humiston, S.G.; Schaffer, S.; Shone, L.P.; Blumkin, A.K.; Szilagyi, P.G. Effectiveness of Centralized Text Message Reminders on Human Papillomavirus Immunization Coverage for Publicly Insured Adolescents. *J. Adolesc. Health* **2015**, *56*, S17–S20. [CrossRef] [PubMed]
40. Rand, C.M.; Vincelli, P.; Goldstein, N.P.; Blumkin, A.; Szilagyi, P.G. Effects of Phone and Text Message Reminders on Completion of the Human Papillomavirus Vaccine Series. *J. Adolesc. Health* **2017**, *60*, 113–119. [CrossRef]
41. Reiter, P.L.; Katz, M.L.; Bauermeister, J.A.; Shoben, A.B.; Paskett, E.D.; McRee, A.-L. Increasing Human Papillomavirus Vaccination Among Young Gay and Bisexual Men: A Randomized Pilot Trial of the Outsmart HPV Intervention. *LGBT Health* **2018**, *5*, 325–329. [CrossRef]
42. Richman, A.R.; Torres, E.; Wu, Q.; Carlston, L.; O'Rorke, S.; Moreno, C.; Olsson, J. Text and Email Messaging for Increasing Human Papillomavirus Vaccine Completion among Uninsured or Medicaid-insured Adolescents in Rural Eastern North Carolina. *J. Health Care Poor Underserved* **2019**, *30*, 1499–1517. [CrossRef] [PubMed]
43. Richman, A.R.; Maddy, L.; Torres, E.; Goldberg, E.J. A randomized intervention study to evaluate whether electronic messaging can increase human papillomavirus vaccine completion and knowledge among college students. *J. Am. Coll. Health* **2016**, *64*, 269–278. [CrossRef] [PubMed]
44. Rickert, V.I.; Auslander, B.; Cox, D.S.; Rosenthal, S.L.; Rupp, R.E.; Zimet, G.D. School-based HPV immunization of young adolescents: Effects of two brief health interventions. *Hum. Vaccines Immunother.* **2015**, *11*, 315–321. [CrossRef]
45. Suh, C.A.; Saville, A.; Daley, M.F.; Glazner, J.E.; Barrow, J.; Stokley, S.; Dong, F.; Beaty, B.; Dickinson, L.M.; Kempe, A. Effectiveness and Net Cost of Reminder/Recall for Adolescent Immunizations. *Pediatrics* **2012**, *129*, e1437–e1445. [CrossRef]
46. Szilagyi, P.G.; Serwint, J.R.; Humiston, S.G.; Rand, C.M.; Schaffer, S.; Vincelli, P.; Dhepyasuwan, N.; Blumkin, A.; Albertin, C.; Curtis, C.R. Effect of Provider Prompts on Adolescent Immunization Rates: A Randomized Trial. *Acad. Pediatr.* **2015**, *15*, 149–157. [CrossRef] [PubMed]
47. Szilagyi, P.G.; Albertin, C.; Humiston, S.G.; Rand, C.M.; Schaffer, S.; Brill, H.; Stankaitis, J.; Yoo, B.-K.; Blumkin, A.; Stokley, S. A Randomized Trial of the Effect of Centralized Reminder/Recall on Immunizations and Preventive Care Visits for Adolescents. *Acad. Pediatr.* **2013**, *13*, 204–213. [CrossRef] [PubMed]
48. Tiro, J.A.; Sanders, J.M.; Pruitt, S.L.; Stevens, C.F.; Skinner, C.S.; Bishop, W.P.; Fuller, S.; Persaud, D. Promoting HPV Vaccination in Safety-Net Clinics: A Randomized Trial. *Pediatrics* **2015**, *136*, 850–859. [CrossRef] [PubMed]
49. Tull, F.; Borg, K.; Knott, C.; Beasley, M.; Halliday, J.; Faulkner, N.; Sutton, K.; Bragge, P. Short Message Service Reminders to Parents for Increasing Adolescent Human Papillomavirus Vaccination Rates in a Secondary School Vaccine Program: A Randomized Control Trial. *J. Adolesc. Health* **2019**, *65*, 116–123. [CrossRef] [PubMed]
50. Underwood, N.L.; Gargano, L.M.; Sales, J.; Vogt, T.M.; Seib, K.; Hughes, J.M. Evaluation of Educational Interventions to Enhance Adolescent Specific Vaccination Coverage. *J. Sch. Health* **2019**, *89*, 603–611. [CrossRef]
51. Vanderpool, R.C.; Cohen, E.L.; Crosby, R.A.; Jones, M.G.; Bates, W.; Casey, B.R.; Collins, T. "1-2-3 Pap" Intervention Improves HPV Vaccine Series Completion Among Appalachian Women. *J. Commun.* **2013**, *63*, 95–115. [CrossRef] [PubMed]
52. Wilkinson, T.A.; Dixon, B.E.; Xiao, S.; Tu, W.; Lindsay, B.; Sheley, M.; Dugan, T.; Church, A.; Downs, S.M.; Zimet, G. Physician clinical decision support system prompts and administration of subsequent doses of HPV vaccine: A randomized clinical trial. *Vaccine* **2019**, *37*, 4414–4418. [CrossRef]
53. Zimet, G.; Dixon, B.E.; Xiao, S.; Tu, W.; Kulkarni, A.; Dugan, T.; Sheley, M.; Downs, S.M. Simple and Elaborated Clinician Reminder Prompts for Human Papillomavirus Vaccination: A Randomized Clinical Trial. *Acad. Pediatr.* **2018**, *18*, S66–S71. [CrossRef]
54. Irving, S.A.; Groom, H.C.; Stokley, S.; McNeil, M.M.; Gee, J.; Smith, N.; Naleway, A.L. Human Papillomavirus Vaccine Coverage and Prevalence of Missed Opportunities for Vaccination in an Integrated Healthcare System. *Acad. Pediatr.* **2018**, *18*, S85–S92. [CrossRef]

55. McLean, H.Q.; VanWormer, J.J.; Chow, B.D.W.; Birchmeier, B.; Vickers, E.; Devries, E.; Meyer, J.; Moore, J.; McNeil, M.M.; Stokley, S.; et al. Improving Human Papillomavirus Vaccine Use in an Integrated Health System: Impact of a Provider and Staff Intervention. *J. Adolesc. Health* **2017**, *61*, 252–258. [CrossRef] [PubMed]
56. Parra-Medina, D.; Morales-Campos, D.Y.; Mojica, C.; Ramirez, A.G. Promotora Outreach, Education and Navigation Support for HPV Vaccination to Hispanic Women with Unvaccinated Daughters. *J. Cancer Educ.* **2015**, *30*, 353–359. [CrossRef]
57. Odone, A.; Ferrari, A.; Spagnoli, F.; Visciarelli, S.; Shefer, A.; Pasquarella, C.; Signorelli, C. Effectiveness of interventions that apply new media to improve vaccine uptake and vaccine coverage: A systematic review. *Hum. Vaccines Immunother.* **2015**, *11*, 72–82. [CrossRef]
58. Bennett, A. Use of "mefirst," a tailored, online educational intervention to promote HPV vaccination among female university students. *J. Women Health* **2014**, *23*, 22.
59. MeFirst: A Tailored Intervention to HPV Vaccine Decision Making. Available online: https://clinicaltrials.gov/ct2/show/NCT01769560/ (accessed on 30 March 2021).
60. Making Effective Human Papillomavirus (HPV) Vaccine Recommendations. Available online: https://clinicaltrials.gov/ct2/show/NCT02377843/ (accessed on 30 March 2021).
61. Educational Intervention to Minimize Disparities in Humanpapillomavirus Vaccination (HPV). Available online: https://clinicaltrials.gov/ct2/show/NCT02145156/ (accessed on 30 March 2021).
62. Girls OnGuard: HPV Vaccination Uptake Among African American Adolescent Females (Girls OnGuard). Available online: https://www.clinicaltrials.gov/ct2/show/study/NCT00813319/ (accessed on 30 March 2021).
63. Henrikson, N.; Zhu, W.; Nguyen, M.; Baba, L.; Berthoud, H.; Hofstetter, A. Health System-Based HPV Vaccine Reminders: Randomized Trial Results. *Cancer Epidemiol. Biomark. Prev.* **2017**, *26*, 435. [CrossRef]
64. An Intervention Study To Improve Human PapillomaVirus (HPV) Immunization in Haitian and African American Girls (HPV). Available online: https://clinicaltrials.gov/ct2/show/NCT01254669/ (accessed on 30 March 2021).
65. The Efficacy of Reminders to Complete HPV Series (ICHAT). Available online: https://clinicaltrials.gov/ct2/show/NCT01731496/ (accessed on 30 March 2021).
66. McRee, A.-L.; Shoben, A.; Bauermeister, J.A.; Katz, M.L.; Paskett, E.D.; Reiter, P.L. Outsmart HPV: Acceptability and short-term effects of a web-based HPV vaccination intervention for young adult gay and bisexual men. *Vaccine* **2018**, *36*, 8158–8164. [CrossRef]
67. Herbert, N. Parental Attitudes and Beliefs About Human Papillomavirus (HPV) Vaccination and Vaccine Receipt Among Adolescents in Richmond County, Georgia. *J. Adolesc. Health* **2014**, *54*, S82. [CrossRef]
68. Zimet, G.; Dixon, B.; Xiao, S.; Tu, W.; Lindsay, B.; Sheley, M.; Downs, S.; Dugan, T.; Church, A. Can automated physician reminders increase 2nd and 3rd dose administration of HPV vaccine? *Sex. Transm. Dis.* **2016**, *43*, S158.
69. HPV Vaccination: Evaluation of Reminder Prompts for Doses 2 & 3. Available online: https://clinicaltrials.gov/ct2/show/NCT02558803/ (accessed on 30 March 2021).
70. Chigbu, C.O.; Onyebuchi, A.K.; Onyeka, T.C.; Odugu, B.U.; Dim, C.C. The impact of community health educators on uptake of cervical and breast cancer prevention services in Nigeria. *Int. J. Gynecol. Obstet.* **2017**, *137*, 319–324. [CrossRef] [PubMed]
71. Cory, L.; Cha, B.; Ellenberg, S.; Borger, H.; Hwuang, W.-T.; Smith, J.; Haggerty, A.; Morgan, M.; Burger, R.; Chu, C.; et al. Effects of Educational Interventions on Human Papillomavirus Vaccine Acceptability: A Randomized Controlled Trial. *Obstet. Gynecol.* **2019**, *134*, 376–384. [CrossRef] [PubMed]
72. Daley, M.F.; Kempe, A.; Pyrzanowski, J.; Vogt, T.M.; Dickinson, L.M.; Kile, D.; Fang, H.; Rinehart, D.J.; Shlay, J.C. School-Located Vaccination of Adolescents With Insurance Billing: Cost, Reimbursement, and Vaccination Outcomes. *J. Adolesc. Health* **2014**, *54*, 282–288. [CrossRef]
73. Davies, C.; Skinner, S.R.; Stoney, T.; Marshall, H.S.; Collins, J.; Jones, J.; Hutton, H.; Parrella, A.; Cooper, S.; McGeechan, K.; et al. 'Is it like one of those infectious kind of things?' The importance of educating young people about HPV and HPV vaccination at school. *Sex Educ.* **2017**, *17*, 256–275. [CrossRef]
74. Skinner, S.R.; Davies, C.; Cooper, S.; Stoney, T.; Marshall, H.; Jones, J.; Collins, J.; Hutton, H.; Parrella, A.; Zimet, G.; et al. HPV.edu study protocol: A cluster randomised controlled evaluation of education, decisional support and logistical strategies in school-based human papillomavirus (HPV) vaccination of adolescents. *BMC Public Health* **2015**, *15*, 896. [CrossRef] [PubMed]
75. Dempsey, A.F.; Pyrznawoski, J.; Lockhart, S.; Barnard, J.; Campagna, E.J.; Garret, K.; Fisher, A.; Dickinson, L.M.; O'Leary, S.T. Effect of a Health Care Professional Communication Training Intervention on Adolescent Human Papillomavirus Vaccination. A Cluster Randomized Clinical Trial. *JAMA Pediatr.* **2018**, *172*, e180016. [CrossRef]
76. O'Leary, S.; Pyrzanowski, M.J.; Lockhart, B.S.; Barnard, M.J.; Campagna, M.E.; Garrett, M.K.; Fisher, M.A.; Dickinson, M.; Dempsey, A. Impact of a Provider Communication Training Intervention on Adolescent Human Papillomavirus Vaccination: A Cluster Randomized, Clinical Trial. *Open Forum Infect. Dis.* **2017**, *4*, S61. [CrossRef]
77. Strengthening Physician Communication About HPV Vaccines. Available online: https://clinicaltrials.gov/ct2/show/NCT02456077/ (accessed on 30 March 2021).
78. Deshmukh, U.; Oliveira, C.R.; Griggs, S.; Coleman, E.; Avni-Singer, L.; Pathy, S.; Shapiro, E.D.; Sheth, S.S. Impact of a clinical interventions bundle on uptake of HPV vaccine at an OB/GYN clinic. *Vaccine* **2018**, *36*, 3599–3605. [CrossRef]
79. Dixon, B.E.; Zimet, G.D.; Xiao, S.; Tu, W.; Lindsay, B.; Church, A.; Downs, S.M. An Educational Intervention to Improve HPV Vaccination: A Cluster Randomized Trial. *Pediatrics* **2019**, *143*, e20181457. [CrossRef]

80. Dixon, B.; Downs, S.; Zhang, Z.; Tu, W.; Lindsay, B.; Dugan, T.; Zimet, G. A mhealth intervention trial to improve HPV vaccination rates in urban primary care clinics. *Sex. Transm. Dis.* **2016**, *43*, S199.
81. Use of a Patient Education/Messaging Platform to Increase Uptake and Series Completion of the HPV Vaccine. Available online: https://clinicaltrials.gov/ct2/show/NCT02546752/ (accessed on 30 March 2021).
82. Fiks, A.G.; Grundmeier, R.W.; Mayne, S.; Song, L.; Feemster, K.; Karavite, D.; Hughes, C.C.; Massey, J.; Keren, R.; Bell, L.M.; et al. Effectiveness of Decision Support for Families, Clinicians, or Both on HPV Vaccine Receipt. *Pediatrics* **2013**, *131*, 1114–1124. [CrossRef] [PubMed]
83. Fiks, A.G.; Luan, X.; Mayne, S.L. Improving HPV Vaccination Rates Using Maintenance-of-Certification Requirements. *Pediatrics* **2016**, *137*, e20150675. [CrossRef] [PubMed]
84. Forster, A.S.; Cornelius, V.; Rockliffe, L.; Marlow, L.A.; Bedford, H.; Waller, J. A cluster randomised feasibility study of an adolescent incentive intervention to increase uptake of HPV vaccination. *Br. J. Cancer* **2017**, *117*, 1121–1127. [CrossRef]
85. Grandahl, M.; Rosenblad, A.; Stenhammar, C.; Tydén, T.; Westerling, R.; Larsson, M.; Oscarsson, M.; Andrae, B.; Dalianis, T.; Nevéus, T. School-based intervention for the prevention of HPV among adolescents: A cluster randomised controlled study. *BMJ Open* **2016**, *6*, e009875. [CrossRef]
86. Jacobs-Wingo, J.L.; Jim, C.C.; Groom, A.V. Human Papillomavirus Vaccine Uptake: Increase for American Indian Adolescents, 2013–2015. *Am. J. Prev. Med.* **2017**. [CrossRef]
87. Jiménez-Quiñones, E.M.; Melin, K.; Jiménez-Ramírez, F.J. Impact of a Pharmacist Conducted Educational Program on Human Papilloma Virus Vaccination Rates in a Low Socioeconomic Population in the City of Lares, PR. *P. R. Health Sci. J.* **2017**, *36*, 67–70. [PubMed]
88. Keeshin, S.W.; Feinberg, J. Text Message Reminder–Recall to Increase HPV Immunization in Young HIV-1-Infected Patients. *J. Int. Assoc. Provid. AIDS Care* **2017**, *16*, 110–113. [CrossRef] [PubMed]
89. Kempe, A.; Barrow, J.; Stokley, S.; Saville, A.; Glazner, J.E.; Suh, C.; Federico, S.; Abrams, L.; Seewald, L.; Beaty, B.; et al. Effectiveness and Cost of Immunization Recall at School-Based Health Centers. *Pediatrics* **2012**, *129*, e1446–e1452. [CrossRef]
90. Kim, M.; Lee, H.; Aronowitz, T.; Sheldon, L.K.; Kiang, P.; Allison, J.; Shi, L. Abstract C56: An online-based storytelling video intervention on promoting Korean American female college students' HPV vaccine uptake. *Cancer Epidemiol. Biomark. Prev.* **2018**, *27*, C56. [CrossRef]
91. Lee, H.Y.; Koopmeiners, J.S.; McHugh, J.; Raveis, V.H.; Ahluwalia, J.S. mHealth Pilot Study: Text Messaging Intervention to Promote HPV Vaccination. *Am. J. Health Behav.* **2016**, *40*, 67–76. [CrossRef]
92. Mayne, S.L.; Durivage, N.E.; Feemster, K.A.; Localio, A.R.; Grundmeier, R.W.; Fiks, A.G. Effect of Decision Support on Missed Opportunities for Human Papillomavirus Vaccination. *Am. J. Prev. Med.* **2014**, *47*, 734–744. [CrossRef]
93. Mehta, P.; Lee, R.C.; Sharma, M. Designing and Evaluating a Health Belief Model-Based Intervention to Increase Intent of HPV Vaccination among College Males. *Int. Q. Community Health Educ.* **2013**, *34*, 101–117. [CrossRef]
94. O'Leary, S.T.; Pyrzanowski, J.; Brewer, S.E.; Sevick, C.; Dickinson, L.M.; Dempsey, A.F. Effectiveness of a multimodal intervention to increase vaccination in obstetrics/gynecology settings. *Vaccine* **2019**, *37*, 3409–3418. [CrossRef]
95. Patel, A.; Stern, L.; Unger, Z.; Debevec, E.; Roston, A.; Hanover, R.; Morfesis, J. Staying on track: A cluster randomized controlled trial of automated reminders aimed at increasing human papillomavirus vaccine completion. *Vaccine* **2014**, *32*, 2428–2433. [CrossRef]
96. Innovative Tool to Increase Completion of Human Papillomavirus (HPV) Vaccine Series. Available online: https://clinicaltrials.gov/ct2/show/NCT01343485 (accessed on 18 May 2021).
97. Perkins, R.B.; Zisblatt, L.; Legler, A.; Trucks, E.; Hanchate, A.; Gorin, S.S. Effectiveness of a provider-focused intervention to improve HPV vaccination rates in boys and girls. *Vaccine* **2015**, *33*, 1223–1229. [CrossRef] [PubMed]
98. Rahman, M.; Elam, L.B.; Balat, M.I.; Berenson, A.B. Well-woman visit of mothers and human papillomavirus vaccine intent and uptake among their 9–17 year old children. *Vaccine* **2013**, *31*, 5544–5548. [CrossRef] [PubMed]
99. Rickert, V.I.; Auslander, B.A.; Cox, D.S.; Rosenthal, S.L.; Rickert, J.A.; Rupp, R.; Zimet, G.D. School-based vaccination of young US males: Impact of health beliefs on intent and first dose acceptance. *Vaccine* **2014**, *32*, 1982–1987. [CrossRef] [PubMed]
100. Roblin, D.W.; Ritzwoller, D.P.; Rees, D.I.; Carroll, N.M.; Chang, A.; Daley, M.F. The influence of deductible health plans on receipt of the human papillomavirus vaccine series. *J. Adolesc. Health* **2014**, *54*, 275–281. [CrossRef]
101. Ruffin, M.T.; Plegue, M.A.; Rockwell, P.G.; Young, A.P.; Patel, D.A.; Yeazel, M.W. Impact of an Electronic Health Record (EHR) Reminder on Human Papillomavirus (HPV) Vaccine Initiation and Timely Completion. *J. Am. Board Fam. Med.* **2015**, *28*, 324–333. [CrossRef] [PubMed]
102. Russell, S. PIN62 Effectiveness of Text Message Reminders for Improving Vaccination Appointment Attendance and Series Completion Among Adolescents and Adults. *Value Health* **2012**, *15*, A248. [CrossRef]
103. Sanderson, M.; Canedo, J.R.; Khabele, D.; Fadden, M.K.; Harris, C.; Beard, K.; Burress, M.; Pinkerton, H.; Jackson, C.; Mayo-Gamble, T.; et al. Pragmatic trial of an intervention to increase human papillomavirus vaccination in safety-net clinics. *BMC Public Health* **2017**, *17*, 158. [CrossRef]
104. An HPV Vaccine Provider Intervention in Safety Net Clinics. Available online: https://clinicaltrials.gov/ct2/show/NCT02808832/ (accessed on 30 March 2021).

105. Spleen, A.M.; Kluhsman, B.C.; Clark, A.D.; Dignan, M.B.; Lengerich, E.J.; The ACTION Health Cancer Task Force. An Increase in HPV-Related Knowledge and Vaccination Intent Among Parental and Non-parental Caregivers of Adolescent Girls, Age 9–17 Years, in Appalachian Pennsylvania. *J. Cancer Educ.* **2011**, *27*, 312–319. [CrossRef]
106. Valdez, A.; Stewart, S.L.; Tanjasari, S.P.; Levy, V.; Garza, A. Design and efficacy of a multilingual, multicultural HPV vaccine education intervention. *J. Commun. Health* **2015**, *8*, 106–118. [CrossRef]
107. Wadhera, P.; Evans, J.L.; Stein, E.; Gandhi, M.; Couture, M.-C.; Sansothy, N.; Sichan, K.; Maher, L.; Kaldor, J.; Page, K.; et al. Human papillomavirus knowledge, vaccine acceptance, and vaccine series completion among female entertainment and sex workers in Phnom Penh, Cambodia: The Young Women's Health Study. *Int. J. STD AIDS* **2015**, *26*, 893–902. [CrossRef]
108. Wedel, S.; Navarrete, C.R.; Burkard, C.J.F.; Clark, M.J. Improving Human Papillomavirus Vaccinations in Military Women. *Mil. Med.* **2016**, *181*, 1224–1227. [CrossRef]
109. Wegwarth, O.; Kurzenhäuser-Carstens, S.; Gigerenzer, G. Overcoming the knowledge–behavior gap: The effect of evidence-based HPV vaccination leaflets on understanding, intention, and actual vaccination decision. *Vaccine* **2014**, *32*, 1388–1393. [CrossRef] [PubMed]
110. Whelan, N.W.; Steenbeek, A.; Martin-Misener, R.; Scott, J.; Smith, B.; D'Angelo-Scott, H. Engaging parents and schools improves uptake of the human papillomavirus (HPV) vaccine: Examining the role of the public health nurse. *Vaccine* **2014**, *32*, 4665–4671. [CrossRef] [PubMed]
111. Winer, R.L.; Gonzales, A.A.; Noonan, C.J.; Buchwald, D.S. A Cluster-Randomized Trial to Evaluate a Mother–Daughter Dyadic Educational Intervention for Increasing HPV Vaccination Coverage in American Indian Girls. *J. Community Health* **2016**, *41*, 274–281. [CrossRef] [PubMed]
112. Zimmerman, R.K.; Raviotta, J.M.; Nowalk, M.P.; Moehling, K.K.; Reis, E.C.; Humiston, S.G.; Lin, C.J. Using the 4 Pillars™ Practice Transformation Program to increase adolescent human papillomavirus, meningococcal, tetanus-diphtheria-pertussis and influenza vaccination. *Vaccine* **2017**, *35*, 6180–6186. [CrossRef] [PubMed]
113. Zimmerman, R.K.; Moehling, K.K.; Lin, C.J.; Zhang, S.; Raviotta, J.M.; Reis, E.C.; Humiston, S.G.; Nowalk, M.P. Improving adolescent HPV vaccination in a randomized controlled cluster trial using the 4 Pillars™ practice Transformation Program. *Vaccine* **2017**, *35*, 109–117. [CrossRef]

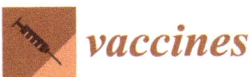

Review

Internal and External Validity of Social Media and Mobile Technology-Driven HPV Vaccination Interventions: Systematic Review Using the Reach, Effectiveness, Adoption, Implementation, Maintenance (RE-AIM) Framework

Matthew Asare [1,*], Braden Popelsky [1], Emmanuel Akowuah [1], Beth A. Lanning [1] and Jane R. Montealegre [2]

1. Department of Public Health, Baylor University, Waco, TX 76708, USA; braden_popelsky@baylor.edu (B.P.); emmanuel_akowuah@baylor.edu (E.A.); Beth_Lanning@baylor.edu (B.A.L.)
2. Dan L Duncan Comprehensive Cancer Center, Baylor College of Medicine, Houston, TX 77030, USA; jrmontea@bcm.edu
* Correspondence: matt_asare@baylor.edu

Abstract: Social media human papillomavirus (HPV) vaccination interventions show promise for increasing HPV vaccination rates. An important consideration for the implementation of effective interventions into real-world practice is the translation potential, or external validity, of the intervention. To this end, we conducted a systematic literature review to describe the current body of evidence regarding the external validity of social media HPV vaccination-related interventions. Constructs related to external validity were based on the reach, effectiveness, adoption, implementation, maintenance (RE-AIM) framework. Seventeen articles published between 2006 and 2020 met the inclusion criteria. Three researchers independently coded each article using a validated RE-AIM framework. Discrepant codes were discussed with a fourth reviewer to gain consensus. Of these 17 studies, 3 were pilot efficacy studies, 10 were randomized controlled trials (RCTs) to evaluate effectiveness, 1 was a population-based study, and 3 did not explicitly state which type of study was conducted. Reflecting this distribution of study types, across all studies the mean level of reporting RE-AIM dimensions varied with reach recording 90.8%, effectiveness (72.1%), adoption (40.3%), implementation (45.6%), and maintenance (26.5%). This review suggests that while the current HPV vaccination social media-driven interventions provide sufficient information on internal validity (reach and effectiveness), few have aimed to gather data on external validity needed to translate the interventions into real world implementation. Our data suggest that implementation research is needed to move HPV vaccination-related interventions into practice. Included in this review are recommendations for enhancing the design and reporting of these HPV vaccination social media-related interventions.

Keywords: HPV; HPV vaccine; social media; mobile phone; HPV vaccine intervention; RE-AIM Framework

---

1. Introduction

The human papillomavirus (HPV) vaccine protects against HPV-associated cancers, including most cervical cancer, as well as vulvar, vaginal, anal, penile, and oropharyngeal cancer. Cervical cancer is the fourth most common cancer among women worldwide, with approximately 570,000 new cervical cancer cases reported in 2018, representing 6.6% of female cancers [1]. The incidence of oral and anal cancers is increasing [2,3]. The HPV vaccine is recommended for adolescents aged 11–12 years, with catch-up vaccination through age 26 and FDA approval for adults up to age 45 years [4]. As part of the Global Strategy for the Elimination of Cervical Cancer as a Public Health Problem, the World Health Organization's (WHO) goal is for 90% vaccination of girls age 15 by 2030. The Healthy People 2030 goal is to increase the proportion of adolescents who receive recommended doses of the HPV vaccine with a target goal of 80% [5]. Although integrated programs and efforts to increase the HPV vaccination have occurred in many countries over the last 14 years, HPV vaccine rates remain low [6]. For instance, in 2019, only 54.2% of adolescents in the US [7] and 15% of adolescents globally [8] were current on HPV vaccinations.

Multiple factors including lack of opportunity for vaccination, parental attitudes or perceptions towards vaccination, lack of recommendations from healthcare providers, concerns about the vaccine's effect on sexual behavior, religious objection, low perceived risk of HPV infection, social influences, irregular preventive care, and vaccine cost have contributed to the low vaccination rates [9–11]. In efforts to address these barriers, researchers have included mobile technology-related media including text-message, e-mail, phone calls, and private Facebook messages, in their interventions to increase vaccination awareness, uptakes, and dose completion [12,13]. These interventions have been efficacious in increasing HPV vaccination uptake and completion [12–15]. However, the prospect of translating these efficacious interventions into regular clinical practice is unknown due in part to the lack of reported external validity [16]. External validity is the ability to generalize an evidence-based study to different measures, persons, settings, and times [17]. Several translational researchers have argued that reporting detailed components and processes of evidence-based studies would increase studies' generalizability (external validity) and the ability to translate those interventions into practice [18–20].

To address the research-practice issue, Glasgow and colleagues developed the Reach, Effectiveness, Adoption, Implementation, and Maintenance (RE-AIM) framework [21] with a set of metrics critical for evaluating the generalizability of an evidence-based intervention into routine practice. They proposed that the translatability of an intervention is best evaluated through the five dimensions (RE-AIM). The reach dimension is designed to assess the proportion of potentially eligible individuals who participate in the intervention study. Efficacy/effectiveness is the function of the intended positive impact of the intervention. Adoption reflects the potential settings and intervention agents that participate in a study. Implementation refers to the quantity and quality of delivery of the intervention's various components. Finally, the maintenance dimension is the longer-term efficacy/effectiveness of an intervention on an individual (see Table 1 for the definitions and indicators for each RE-AIM dimension). This framework can be used to organize and evaluate threats to the transferability of research to practice. Further, by evaluating a study through the five-dimension lens of the framework, researchers are able to assess internal and external validity equally [16,21].

The RE-AIM framework has been used recently in several systematic reviews to evaluate the internal and external validities of health intervention studies such as weight management intervention [18], physical activity intervention [22,23], worksite health behavior interventions [24], community settings [20], school-based health promotion [25,26], childhood obesity prevention [27–29], children dietary interventions with parents [30], injury prevention strategies [31], faith-based intervention [32], mobile phone-based intervention for diabetes self-management [33], and HIV prevention intervention [34]. While encouraging, there is little reporting on its potential use for translating HPV vaccination social media-driven intervention methods into regular practice settings, specifically at the population level. The two most recent comprehensive literature reviews on HPV vaccination mobile technology-related interventions evaluated the effectiveness of interventions in increasing the HPV vaccine [35], and the effectiveness of communication technology interventions on HPV vaccine [36]. However, the scope of these two previous literature reviews was narrow, focusing primarily on internal validity with limited information on the external validity of the HPV vaccination intervention studies [18,19].

Table 1. Average scores for the RE-AIM dimensions and the scores for each 33-item indicator as used in the current study.

Dimension	Definition	Indicator	Percentage (%)
Reach (R)	The proportion and representativeness of individuals willing to participate in a given intervention.	1. Described Target Population	100
		2. Demographic & behavioral information	100
		3. Recruitment Strategies	94.1
		4. Inclusion & exclusion criteria	94.1
		5. Method to identify the target population	76.5
		6. Sample size	88.2
		7. Participation rate	82.4
			Average: 90.8
Efficacy/Effectiveness (E)	The influence of an intervention on important outcomes, including potential negative effects, quality of life, and economic outcomes	1. Design/Conditions	100
		2. Efficacy, Effectiveness, Translational?	100
		3. Measure of the primary outcome	100
		4. Results (shortest assessment)	94.1
		5. Intent-to-treat or present at FU	35.3
		6. Imputation procedure	76.5
		7. Measure of robustness across subgroups	47.1
		8. Measure of short-term attrition	23.5
			Average: 72.1
Adoption (A)	The proportion and representativeness of locations and intervention staff willing to initiate and adopt an intervention	1. Description of intervention location	88.2
		2. Description of delivery staff	64.7
		3. Method to identify target delivery agent	47.1
		4. Level of expertise of delivery agent	58.8
		5. Delivery staff participation rate	11.8
		6. Organizational spread	5.9
		7. Measures of cost of adoption	5.9
			Average: 40.3

Table 1. Cont.

Dimension	Definition	Indicator	Percentage (%)
Implementation (I)	How consistently various elements of an intervention are delivered as intended by staff, and the time and cost of the intervention	1. Intervention frequency	88.2
		2. Extent protocol delivered as intended (%)	11.8
		3. Participant attendance/completion rates	82.4
		4. Measures of cost	0
			Average: 45.6
Maintenance (M)	The extent to which participants make and maintain a behavior change and the sustainability of a program or policy in the setting in which it was intervened	1. Follow-up assessment (3- or 6-months)	70.6
		2. Attrition	35.3
		3. Is the program still in place?	0
		4. Was the program institutionalized?	0
			Average: 26.5

Our study aimed to use the RE-AIM framework to evaluate HPV vaccination intervention studies that included mobile technology to increase HPV vaccination completion (i.e., receiving all the recommended doses: two doses for 9–14 years old and three doses for those between 15 and 45 years old) and/or vaccination uptake (defined as receiving at least one dose of vaccine). To our knowledge, this is the first review using the RE-AIM framework to evaluate the HPV vaccination mobile technology-related (Facebook, text messaging, and mobile health (miHealth)) interventions. Unlike the two previous reviews on HPV vaccine interventions [35,36], our current systematic review was structured to determine the translation potential or external validity of published HPV vaccination intervention studies by determining the extent to which those studies reported information across all five of the RE-AIM framework dimensions. We further provide recommendations for future research based on these findings.

2. Materials and Methods

2.1. Search Strategy and Selection Criteria

We conducted an extensive literature search to identify research articles related to HPV vaccination technology-based interventions. We searched nine databases (PubMed, EMBASE, Medline, ERIC, CINAHL, Academic Search Complete, Web of Science, PsycINFO, Cochrane Library) using the following terms: human papillomavirus OR human papillomavirus* OR HPV and social media OR social medium OR Web 2.0 OR twitter messaging OR Instagram OR Facebook OR WhatsApp OR Tito OR text message OR mobile technology AND intervention OR RCT. An article was included in the review if it met the following inclusion criteria: published in English, between 2006 and 2020, and in peer-reviewed journals; outcome variables included HPV vaccination completion and/or vaccination uptake; intervention study; the intervention's mode of delivery included social media (WhatsApp, Facebook) and text messages. Articles were excluded if they were cross-sectional studies and included assessment of only participants' knowledge, attitude, and intention (see Figure 1).

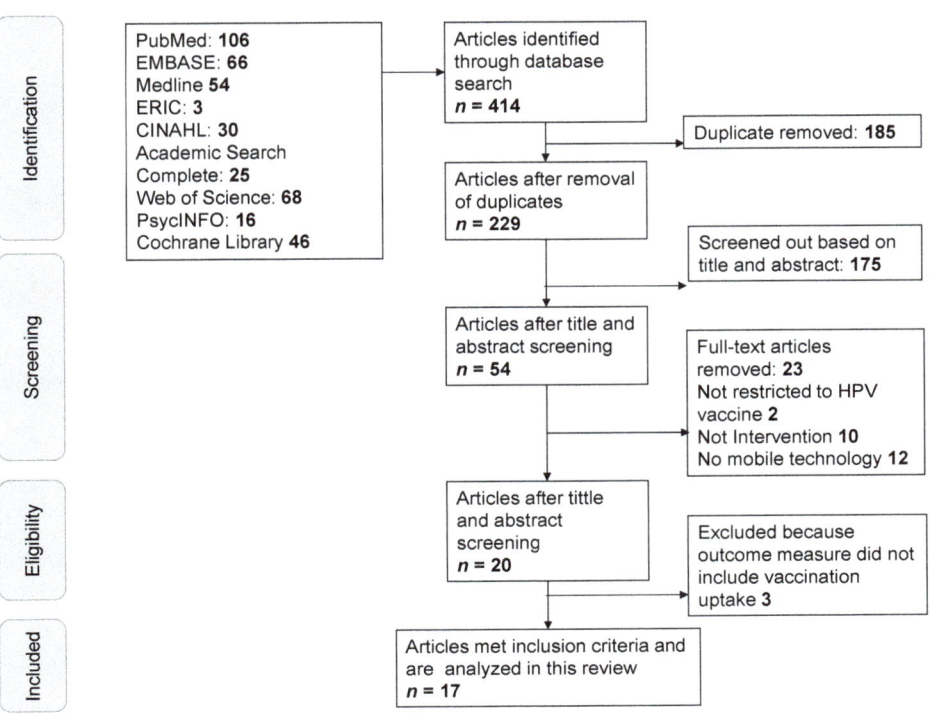

Figure 1. Flowchart of the search strategy.

2.2. RE-AIM Criteria

A modified version of the RE-AIM 30-item data extraction tool (https://www.re-aim.org, accessed on 10 February 2021) was used to code eligible articles on the degree to which internal and external validity indicators were reported. The RE-AIM dimensions and corresponding indicators are listed in Table 1.

2.2.1. Reach Dimension

Seven indicators were used to evaluate the reach dimension of the study. They included the description of the target population, description of the participants' HPV vaccination behavior, recruitment strategies, inclusion and exclusion criteria, description of the sample size determination, and participation rate.

2.2.2. Effectiveness Dimension

Eight metrics for effectiveness included the efficacy of the intervention in changing vaccination behavior, measurement of primary and/or secondary outcome (i.e., vaccination completion, or uptake), a short-term assessment, intent-to-treat assessment, description of imputation procedure, the measure of robustness across subgroups, and short-term attrition assessment.

2.2.3. Adoption Dimension

The seven indicators used for adoption were a description of intervention location, intervention delivery staff, the method used to identify delivery staff, inclusion and exclusion criteria for the staff, and rate of staff participation.

2.2.4. Implementation Dimension

The four metrics used for the implementation dimension were intention frequency, duration, the extent to which the intervention was implemented as planned, completion rates, and measurement of cost of implementing the intervention.

2.2.5. Maintenance Dimension

The four metrics for maintenance included follow-up (3 and 6 months) assessments, attrition rates, continuation, and institutionalization of the program.

2.3. Coding and Analysis

Articles that met the inclusion criteria for this review were independently coded by three graduate research assistants (B.P., N.T., and C.M.) and supervised by the principal investigator (PI) of the research team (M.A.). Each reviewer coded a "yes" indicating the presence or "no," indicating the absence of the RE-AIM indicators outlined above. Following the individual coding, the PI and the three research assistants met to discuss articles and coding results, resolve uncertainty, and gain consensus in coding. The articles that had "yes" for any indicator were scored as 1 and "no" was scored as 0. Each of the 17 articles was tabulated and scored with a column totaling individual dimension scores for each article. Analyses included providing count and percentage data across RE-AIM indicators. Row percentages were calculated to display the proportion of articles addressing each of the dimension indicators. Finally, column totals, averages, and average percentages were computed to summarize the number of articles reporting each of the five dimensions. To determine the overall quality of RE-AIM reporting, we also examined the number of articles that included the 33 indicators from the data extraction tool (see Table 1). Based on the 33-item RE-AIM indicators, articles that scored between 0 and 11 indicated fewer reporting of RE-AIM indicators, between 12 and 22 indicated moderate reporting, and between 23 and 33 indicated high reporting of RE-AIM indicators.

3. Results

The literature search yielded 414 total articles. After removing duplicate articles and conducting a preliminary screening process based on title and abstract, a total of 53 eligible articles remained. The secondary screenings restricted articles to HPV vaccine interventions and social media-driven interventions. The complete article identification strategy produced 17 articles that met the inclusion criteria and were analyzed in this review [15,37–52]. Of these 17 studies, 3 were pilot efficacy studies [39,44,51], 10 were randomized controlled trials (RCTs) to evaluate effectiveness [15,38,43,45–50,52], 1 was a population-based study [41], and 3 did not explicitly state which type of study was conducted [37,40,42]. The target population for the reviewed articles includes parents with adolescents (boys and girls) [15,45,46,50], Young Sexual Minority Men [51,52], college students [37,38,44,47–49], adolescents (boy and girls) [40–42], young women (19–26 years) [39,43]. The vaccination uptake rates in the review ranged from 6.6% to 89% and the completion rates range from 17% to 88%, indicating successful implementation of many of the interventions. A total number of 189,877 participants were reached in the reviewed HPV vaccine interventions. Out of 189,769, (we excluded 108 participants in Ortiz et al.'s study because they did not provide absolute numbers for vaccination uptake) participants enrolled in the re-viewed articles, pooled estimate of 19,294 participants in studies received at least one dose of HPV vaccine representing a 10.2% vaccination rate among the participants in those reviewed articles. Mohanty et al. [41] and Chodick [50] used Facebook to deliver the intervention and they reached the largest target population or had highest penetrations (155,110 and 21,592 participants, respectively) and text messaging interventions. The most common social media used were mobile phone text messaging [39,46,49,52], combination of text messaging and email systems [15,43,47,48], Facebook [41,42,50], and mobile web technology [38,40]. Other studies mentioned that they used social media but did not mention specific social media [37,44,51]. Supplementary Table S1 shows the details on study design, outcome, demographic characteristics, social media used, and RE-AIM indicators used.

3.1. RE-AIM Reporting Scores

Using RE-AIM rating procedures, we found that 14 (82.35%) articles moderately reported RE-AIM indicators [15,37,39–46,48,50–52], and three articles (17.65%) had high reporting of RE-AIM indicators [38,45,47,49]. The three studies that were rated as high quality addressed between 69.70% (23 out of 33) and 72.73% (24 out of 33) of the indicators. The 14 medium reporting quality articles addressed between 42.42% (14 out of 33) and 66.67% (22 out of 33) of the indicators. The reach and effectiveness dimensions were the most addressed domains with an average score of 90.8% and 85.8%, respectively. The adoption, implementation, and maintenance domains were the least addressed domains with average scores of 38.2%, 45.6%, and 26.48%, respectively (see Table 1).

3.1.1. Reach Dimension

The indicators with the greatest reporting scores under the reach dimension were description of the target population, including race/ethnicity and other demographic information (100%), behavioral information (100%), inclusion/exclusion criteria (94.1%), and recruitment strategies (94.1%). The least reported reach indicator was the method to identify the target population with an average score of 76.5% (see Table 1). Overall, ten articles [15,38,41,42,46–49,51,52] reported all seven indicators under the reach dimension, four studies [37,40,44,45] reported the least (5 out of 7) of the indicators in the reach dimension (see Figure 2).

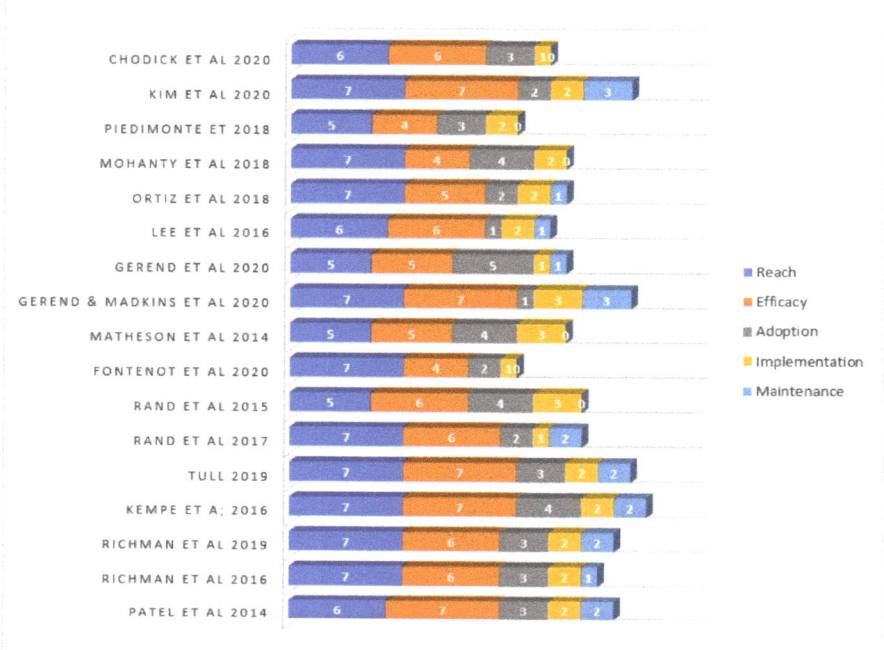

Figure 2. The scores for the reviewed articles on the RE-AIM Dimensions (*n* = 17). Note: Reach scale 0–7; Efficacy scale 0–10; Adoption scale 0–8; Implementation and Maintenance scales 0–4.

3.1.2. Efficacy/Effectiveness Dimension

The most common efficacy/effectiveness dimension indicators reported by the reviewed articles include intervention effectiveness in changing behavior (100%), measurement of the primary outcome (100%), short-term assessment (94.1%), and description of intervention design/conditions (100%). Indicators such as intent-to-treat, imputation procedure, quality of life, unintended consequence measurement, a measure of robustness across subgroups, and measures of short-term attrition were scarcely reported in the articles (see Table 1). Three articles reported eight out of 10 effectiveness dimension indicators [38,43,47]. Fontenot et al. [51] and Mohanty et al. [41] reported the least amount, 4 out of 10 indicators (see Figure 2).

3.1.3. Adoption Dimension

For the adoption dimension, the most reported indicators were the description of intervention location (88.2%) and the staff who delivered intervention (64.7%). Organizational spread and measures of the cost of adoption were two adoption indicators that received the lowest reporting score of 5.9% (see Table 1). Only Gerend et al.'s [37] article reported six out of the eight adoption dimension indicators. The remaining articles reported a few of the adoption dimension indicators with scores ranging from 1 to 5 (out of 8 indicators) (see Figure 2).

3.1.4. Implementation

Per our inclusion criteria for this review, all 17 articles included in the review used some form of technology including social media (Facebook), mobile phone (text messages), and emails to deliver the intervention. The most addressed implementation dimension indicators were intervention frequency and duration (88.2%) and participation/completion rates (82.4%)

(see Table 1). The extent to which the protocol was delivered as intended was the least reported indicator (11.8%) and none of the studies reported the total cost of implementing the intervention. However, eight reported incentives given to each participant, and one reported that vaccines were given to participants at no cost (see Figure 2).

3.1.5. Maintenance

The most common maintenance dimension indicator addressed in the reviewed articles was the 3-month and 6-month follow-up assessment (70.6%). The long-term attrition rate was addressed in 35.3% of articles. None of the articles addressed whether the programs were institutionalized or were still in place (see Table 1).

4. Discussion

4.1. Summary

This systematic review utilized the RE-AIM framework to evaluate the impact of HPV vaccine intervention studies that incorporated mobile technology to increase vaccine uptake and recommended dose completion. Eleven articles' outcome of measure included vaccination uptake [37–39,41,44,46,47,49–52], and six articles' outcome measure was vaccination completion [15,40,42,43,45,48]. The vaccination uptake rates in the review ranged from 6.6% to 89% and the completion rates range from 17% to 88%, indicating successful implementation of many of the interventions.

Our review of 17 articles showed the emphasis on reporting internal validity (i.e., reach and efficacy), and the collective absence of reporting external validity per Glasgow et al.'s (1999) reporting criteria. This finding is consistent with other RE-AIM literature reviews that found that the most common indicators reported in studies are reach and efficacy/effectiveness [23,25–28,32,53]. On the other hand, the external validity dimensions which include adoption, implementation, and maintenance were underreported. Therefore, making the translation of those intervention studies into the practice setting difficult.

4.1.1. Reach Dimension

A total number of 189,877 participants were reached in the reviewed HPV vaccine interventions. Lee et al.'s [39] article reached the lowest number of participants ($n = 30$) while Mahanty et al.'s [41] Facebook intervention reached the highest number of participants ($n = 155,110$). The reporting for the reach dimension indicators ranges from 77% to 100%. Many of the articles included in this review provided detailed descriptions of the target population which is consistent with the literature [25,27–30,34,54,55]. Several articles targeted college students [37,38,43,44,48] which is not surprising given that the majority of those within the college-age groups are social media consumers. A few of the articles reviewed reached or targeted parents with adolescents (boys and girls) [15,45,46,50]. Parents are critical target audience for any HPV vaccination interventions because parental knowledge, positive attitude, affordability, and willingness are precursor to successful HPV vaccination programs [56–59]. The reach dimension indicator rarely discussed is the target population denominator. While reporting of this indicator tends to be challenging [55], by not reporting the target population denominator, there is no context given to help determine the sample sizes. In the efficacy studies the concern is recruiting enough participants to provide the necessary power to detect effect size; therefore, understanding the target population that was exposed to recruitment materials can provide an estimate of the likely reach the program will achieve [18].

4.1.2. Efficacy/Effectiveness

Out of 189,769 participants enrolled in the reviewed articles, a pooled estimate of 19,294 received at least one dose of HPV vaccine, representing a 10.2% vaccination rate among the participants in those reviewed articles. Tull et al.'s [49] study reported the highest vaccination rates (motivational arm 88%, self-regulatory arm 89%, and control arm 86%). Our systematic review showed that four indicators in the Efficacy/Effectiveness dimension including design/conditions, efficacy or effectiveness, the measure of the outcome with or without comparison to the vaccination goal, and short-term assessments, were regularly reported which is consistent with the literature [25,27–30,34,54,55]. Across all 17 articles, less than half the authors described their chosen method of analysis for missing variables and/or attrition whether to use intent-to-treat or per-protocol analysis (analysis by treatment administered) approach. The intention-to-treat principle states that all randomized participants are included in the statistical analysis and analyzed according to the group they were originally assigned, regardless of what treatment (if any) they received [60]. Whenever treatment groups are not analyzed according to the group to which they were originally assigned, the risk of bias increases [61]. Similar to the conclusion drawn by Hollis and Campbell [58] the intention to treat approach is often insufficiently described and inadequately applied. This lack of reporting can diminish the accurate (unbiased) conclusions regarding the effectiveness of an intervention [61]. Authors should explicitly describe the handling of any deviations from randomized allocation and discuss missing responses and their potential effect on the studies' outcomes [62]. However, the use of randomization in some of the studies [15,38,40,42,43,45,52] may attenuate the possible confounding bias. Although most of the articles reported short-term pre-post assessments, only four articles [38,43,45,53] calculated short-term attrition rates. Attrition prevents a full intention to treat analysis and it can occur when participants have missing data and/or loss to follow-up. We argue that researchers need to be more explicit about the loss to follow-up, especially if rates are high [63].

4.1.3. Adoption Dimension

The average score of the adoption dimension was 38% with observed scores for the adoption indicators ranging from 6% to 88%. The description of the location of the intervention score (88%) for our reviewed articles is higher than the previous reviews scores of 48% to 60% [18,54], but lower when compared with the scores in Allen et al.'s [16] review findings. The description of the delivery staff received the second-highest in reporting (65%). The skill sets of the intervention staff, the description of the setting of the intervention staff, and information about the staff can help determine the translating potentials of the study in another setting. Less than half of the articles discussed the methods used to identify target delivery agents and the level of expertise. Crucial to the implementation of an intervention is the selection of the target delivery agents but indicators such as inclusion and exclusion criteria for selecting delivery staff, delivery staff participation rate, organizational spread, and measure of the cost of adoption were underreported. The underreporting of selection criteria of delivery agents has been debated by other reviews [16,27]. By not reporting a level of expertise or a method to select the interventionists, it becomes difficult not only to measure the intervention effectiveness but also to translate those studies to other settings to achieve the same level of success. Rarely reported is the organizational spread dimension indicator, which measures if the intervention used a multi-level approach. This is an important indicator because of the focus on collaboration and communication between multiple levels of an organization which can increase the overall impact of the intervention and the probability of the behavior being adopted and/or maintained. The full support of adopting agents directly influences implementation fidelity and program sustainability [64].

4.1.4. Implementation

In the implementation dimension, we were interested in intervention studies that incorporated social media technology to deliver the intervention. Although the authors did not evaluate whether using a specific social media type was effective in delivering the intervention, based on our review we found that interventions that utilized Facebook [41,50] and text messages [15,45,49] reported significant improvements in HPV vaccination. The most frequent technology used was text messaging [15,37,39,43,45–49]. Additionally, only eight articles reported the underlying theoretical framework used in intervention development [38,39,41,42,49–52]. Theories provide a systematic view of phenomena by specifying the relationship between program inputs (resources), program activities (how the program is implemented), and their outputs or outcomes [65,66]. Reporting the theoretical framework used in intervention could facilitate replication and implementation of HPV intervention studies in several different settings.

The HPV vaccine intervention studies included in this review required multiple visits and multiple contacts (reminders) with the study population. Omitting information about the number of contacts or the exact reminder messages introduces a bias. The types of reminders and the difficulty in reaching vaccination sites can greatly influence vaccination uptake. Additionally, the impact of the intervention is weakened by the lack of reporting on the extent to which the protocol was delivered as intended, including sending reminders to participants. Furthermore, none of the articles included the costs incurred during the implementation phase of the interventions, which once again eliminates a monetary reference point to consider when designing future interventions. While many researchers incorporated incentives for participation and offered vaccines at reduced or no costs, there is minimal discussion of the cost incurred in implementing the interventions. Reporting cost is essential in understanding how resources are utilized in both effective and non-effective interventions. Cost is a critical aspect of interventions designed for low resource areas, as the success of those interventions is partly dependent on study participants' ability to pay for the cost of the vaccination.

4.1.5. Maintenance

Our review showed the maintenance dimension was by far the most underreported indicator, with only 68.75% of articles reported conducting follow-up assessments. The lack of reporting could be due to researchers' financial and time limitations [20]. For HPV vaccines, it requires 12 months or more to complete the recommended dosing. HPV intervention studies should include a measurement of long-term effects and address the issue of maintenance. Without such measures, it is difficult to determine if the intervention strategies affect vaccination completion rates.

4.2. Limitations

There were several limitations to our study. First, this review focused on increasing the uptake of the HPV vaccine series. Because the vaccine comprises two to three doses administered at varying intervals in large catchment periods and populations, follow-up and series completion can be inherently difficult to ensure. Second, the RE-AIM framework served as the guide for evaluating the effectiveness of public health interventions. However, we utilized a modified or shortened version of the RE-AIM criteria in each dimension. Third, it is possible that our scope for article selection was significantly narrowed because we concentrated on reviewing recent articles involving a mobile technology and social media component through electronic messages/reminders, and/or social media campaigns. Fourth, while the interventions targeted several different populations, (e.g., college students, Appalachian women, adolescents, urban, rural, etc.) three of the articles in the review took place outside the United States with different contextual factors. Public health attitudes, perceptions, resources, and procedures may differ across cultures. Finally, researchers of the reviewed articles may argue that their studies were intended to demonstrate the efficacy of the intervention and that the scope of reporting might preclude effectiveness or generalizability information [20,67]. Further, researchers may collect data on external validity, but due to article length restriction may not report the date. However, even in efficacy trials, it would be beneficial to document and report adoption and implementation dimensions so that future researchers can replicate the study [20,67].

4.3. Strengths

Despite the above limitations, this review has several strengths. First, the use of the RE-AIM framework as a guiding metric for evaluating HPV vaccination interventions.

The RE-AIM framework allows for the inclusion of the internal and external validity criteria that are important for evaluating the possibilities of translating interventions to other settings instead of evaluating just the efficacy of the interventions. Second, RE-AIM offers a systematic and structured examination of system-level considerations to the adoption of efficacious interventions. The RE-AIM framework has shown utility in assessing multiple criteria related to prevention research, namely, elements of efficacy, effectiveness, efficiency, and other implications for public health decision making such as quality of life and safety [64].

4.4. Implications and Recommendations

4.4.1. Implication for Future Publication

The application of the RE-AIM framework to evaluate the effectiveness of HPV vaccine social mobile interventions is limited, yet our review demonstrates the utility of RE-AIM to evaluate HPV interventions and highlights the potential transferability of selected HPV intervention programs to a broader audience. To increase the potential to translate social media related HPV vaccine research findings to practice, researchers should place a greater emphasis on obtaining and reporting external validity information, such as adoption, implementation, and maintenance dimensions. Providing external validity information enhances other researchers' and practitioners' ability to judge the generalizability of effects and the comparative utility of interventions [20,67]. All stakeholders, including researchers, reviewers, editorial board, and funders, should emphasize the need for external validity information [20].

4.4.2. Implications for Future HPV Vaccine Intervention

I. While a few reviewed studies included parents of adolescents [15,45,46,50], there is a need to consider social media strategies as a potential method to reach parents. Parents either make decisions to vaccinate their teenagers or influence their children's decisions so not including them in the target population is a missed opportunity to influence behavior [68].

II. The overall penetration or reach of the studies was high, especially in studies that used Facebook to reach a large population [41,50]. However, the impact of social media on the vaccine uptake was rarely measured in the reviewed studies. Future studies should compare the effectiveness of different social media platforms (e.g., Facebook vs. text messaging) on HPV vaccine uptake.

5. Conclusions

In conclusion, our findings show that social media-related HPV vaccination intervention studies demonstrated some effect on vaccination uptake (at least one dose of vaccination rate of 10.2% of the study population), reached larger study participants, and demonstrated that college students and college-aged groups are the targets of most social media intervention studies. While most articles in our review met the Consolidated Standards of Reporting Trials (CONSORT) metrics for reporting, specifically for internal validity reporting, the adoption, implementation, and maintenance dimensions for the RE-AIM framework were underreported. To ensure that these successful community-based interventions can be translated into practices, stakeholders should not only embrace the reporting of all the RE-AIM dimensions but should encourage researchers to adhere to external validity reporting standards similar to CONSORT internal validity reporting.

Supplementary Materials: The following are available online at https://www.mdpi.com/2075-393X/9/3/197/s1, Table S1: RE-AIM Dimensions and selected indicators reported by the reviewed articles ($n = 17$).

Author Contributions: Conceptualization, M.A. and B.P.; methodology, M.A. and J.R.M.; validation, B.P., M.A., E.A., and B.A.L.; formal analysis, M.A. and B.P.; data curation, M.A. and B.P.; writing—original draft preparation, B.P. and M.A.; writing—review and editing, M.A., B.P., E.A., B.A.L., and J.R.M.; supervision, M.A.; All authors have read and agreed to the published version of the manuscript.

Funding: This research received no external funding.

Institutional Review Board Statement: Not applicable.

Informed Consent Statement: Not applicable.

Acknowledgments: We are thankful to Vedana Vaidhyanathan at the Baylor library for helping in the databases search during the literature review.

Conflicts of Interest: The authors declare no conflict of interest.

References

1. WHO. Cervical Cancer. Available online: https://www.who.int/cancer/prevention/diagnosis-screening/cervical-cancer/en/ (accessed on 16 November 2020).
2. Deshmukh, A.A.; Suk, R.; Shiels, M.S.; Sonawane, K.; Nyitray, A.G.; Liu, Y.; Gaisa, M.M.; Palefsky, J.M.; Sigel, K. Recent Trends in Squamous Cell Carcinoma of the Anus Incidence and Mortality in the United States, 2001–2015. *J. Natl. Cancer Inst.* **2020**, *112*, 829–838. [CrossRef] [PubMed]
3. Ellington, T.D.; Henley, S.J.; Senkomago, V.; O'Neil, M.E.; Wilson, R.J.; Singh, S.; Richardson, L.C. Trends in Incidence of Cancers of the Oral Cavity and Pharynx—United States 2007–2016. *MMWR Morb. Mortal Wkly. Rep.* **2020**, *69*, 433. [CrossRef]
4. U.S. Food and Drug Administration. FDA Approves Expanded Use of Gardasil 9 to Include Individuals 27 through 45 Years Old. Available online: https://www.fda.gov/news-events/press-announcements/fda-approves-expanded-use-gardasil-9-include-individuals-27-through-45-years-old (accessed on 14 November 2020).
5. Healthy People 2030. Increase the Proportion of Adolescents Who Get Recommended Doses of the HPV Vaccine—IID 08. Available online: https://health.gov/healthypeople/objectives-and-data/browse-objectives/vaccination/increase-proportion-adolescents-who-get-recommended-doses-hpv-vaccine-iid-08 (accessed on 2 December 2020).
6. Peterson, C.E.; Dykens, J.A.; Brewer, N.T.; Buscemi, J.; Watson, K.; Comer-Hagans, D.; Ramamonjiarivelo, Z.; Fitzgibbon, M. Society of Behavioral Medicine Supports Increasing HPV Vaccination Uptake: An Urgent Opportunity for Cancer Prevention. *Transl. Behav. Med.* **2016**, *6*, 672–675. [CrossRef] [PubMed]
7. Elam-Evans, L.D.; Yankey, D.; Singleton, J.A.; Sterrett, N.; Markowitz, L.E.; Williams, C.L.; Stokley, S. National, Regional, State, and Selected Local Area Vaccination Coverage among Adolescents Aged 13–17 Years—United States, 2019. *MMWR Morb. Mortal Wkly. Rep.* **2020**, *69*, 1109. [CrossRef] [PubMed]
8. Immunization Coverage. Available online: https://www.who.int/news-room/fact-sheets/detail/immunization-coverage (accessed on 6 November 2020).
9. Holman, D.M.; Benard, V.; Roland, K.B.; Watson, M.; Liddon, N.; Stokley, S. Barriers to Human Papillomavirus Vaccination among US Adolescents: A Systematic Review of the Literature. *JAMA Pediatr.* **2014**, *168*, 76–82. [CrossRef] [PubMed]
10. Leung, S.O.A.; Akinwunmi, B.; Elias, K.M.; Feldman, S. Educating Healthcare Providers to Increase Human Papillomavirus (HPV) Vaccination Rates: A Qualitative Systematic Review. *Vaccine X* **2019**, *3*, 100037. [CrossRef] [PubMed]
11. Palmer, J.; Carrico, C.; Costanzo, C. Identifying and Overcoming Perceived Barriers of Providers towards HPV Vaccination: A Literature Review. *J. Vaccines* **2015**, *2015*, 869468. [CrossRef]
12. Wilson, A.R.; Hashibe, M.; Bodson, J.; Gren, L.H.; Taylor, B.A.; Greenwood, J.; Jackson, B.R.; She, R.; Egger, M.J.; Kepka, D. Factors Related to HPV Vaccine Uptake and 3-Dose Completion among Women in a Low Vaccination Region of the USA: An Observational Study. *BMC Womens Health* **2016**, *16*. [CrossRef] [PubMed]
13. Fishman, J.; Taylor, L.; Frank, I. Awareness of HPV and Uptake of Vaccination in a High-Risk Population. *Pediatrics* **2016**, *138*, e20152048. [CrossRef]
14. Chao, C.; Preciado, M.; Slezak, J.; Xu, L. A Randomized Intervention of Reminder Letter for Human Papillomavirus Vaccine Series Completion. *J. Adolesc. Health* **2015**, *56*, 85–90. [CrossRef]
15. Kempe, A.; O'Leary, S.T.; Shoup, J.A.; Stokley, S.; Lockhart, S.; Furniss, A.; Dickinson, L.M.; Barnard, J.; Daley, M.F. Parental Choice of Recall Method for HPV Vaccination: A Pragmatic Trial. *Pediatrics* **2016**, *137*, e20152857. [CrossRef] [PubMed]
16. Allen, K.; Zoellner, J.; Motley, M.; Estabrooks, P.A. Understanding the Internal and External Validity of Health Literacy Interventions: A Systematic Literature Review Using the RE-AIM Framework. *J. Health Commun.* **2011**, *16*, 55–72. [CrossRef]
17. Steckler, A.; McLeroy, K.R. The Importance of External Validity. *Am. J. Public Health* **2008**, *98*, 9–10. [CrossRef]
18. Akers, J.D.; Estabrooks, P.A.; Davy, B.M. Translational Research: Bridging the Gap between Long-Term Weight Loss Maintenance Research and Practice. *J. Am. Diet. Assoc.* **2010**, *110*, 1511–1522. [CrossRef] [PubMed]
19. Glasgow, R.E.; Klesges, L.M.; Dzewaltowski, D.A.; Bull, S.S.; Estabrooks, P. The Future of Health Behavior Change Research: What Is Needed to Improve Translation of Research into Health Promotion Practice? *Ann. Behav. Med.* **2004**, *27*, 3–12. [CrossRef] [PubMed]
20. Dzewaltowski, D.A.; Estabrooks, P.A.; Klesges, L.M.; Bull, S.; Glasgow, R.E. Behavior Change Intervention Research in Community Settings: How Generalizable Are the Results? *Health Promot. Int.* **2004**, *19*, 235–245. [CrossRef]

21. Glasgow, R.E.; Vogt, T.M.; Boles, S.M. Evaluating the Public Health Impact of Health Promotion Interventions: The RE-AIM Framework. *Am. J. Public Health* **1999**, *89*, 1322–1327. [CrossRef]
22. McGoey, T.; Root, Z.; Bruner, M.W.; Law, B. Evaluation of Physical Activity Interventions in Children via the Reach, Efficacy/Effectiveness, Adoption, Implementation, and Maintenance (RE-AIM) Framework: A Systematic Review of Randomized and Non-Randomized Trials. *Prev. Med.* **2016**, *82*, 8–19. [CrossRef]
23. Craike, M.; Hill, B.; Gaskin, C.J.; Skouteris, H. Interventions to Improve Physical Activity during Pregnancy: A Systematic Review on Issues of Internal and External Validity Using the RE-AIM Framework. *BJOG* **2017**, *124*, 573–583. [CrossRef]
24. Bull, S.S.; Gillette, C.; Glasgow, R.E.; Estabrooks, P. Work Site Health Promotion Research: To What Extent Can We Generalize the Results and What Is Needed to Translate Research to Practice? *Health Educ. Behav.* **2003**, *30*, 537–549. [CrossRef]
25. Estabrooks, P.; Dzewaltowski, D.A.; Glasgow, R.E.; Klesges, L.M. School-Based Health Promotion: Issues Related to Translating Research into Practice. *J. Sch. Health* **2002**, *73*, 21–28. [CrossRef]
26. Bastos, P.d.O.; Cavalcante, A.S.P.; Pereira, W.M.G.; de Castro, V.H.S.; Ferreira Júnior, A.R.; Guerra, P.H.; da Silva, K.S.; da Silva, M.R.F.; Barbosa Filho, V.C. Health Promoting School Interventions in Latin America: A Systematic Review Protocol on the Dimensions of the RE-AIM Framework. *Int. J. Environ. Res. Public Health* **2020**, *17*, 5558. [CrossRef]
27. Klesges, L.M.; Dzewaltowski, D.A.; Glasgow, R.E. Review of External Validity Reporting in Childhood Obesity Prevention Research. *Am. J. Prev. Med.* **2008**, *34*, 216–223. [CrossRef] [PubMed]
28. Economos, C.D.; Anzman-Frasca, S.; Koomas, A.H.; Bakun, P.J.; Brown, C.M.; Brown, D.; Folta, S.C.; Fullerton, K.J.; Sacheck, J.M.; Sharma, S.; et al. Dissemination of Healthy Kids out of School Principles for Obesity Prevention: A RE-AIM Analysis. *Prev. Med.* **2019**, *119*, 37–43. [CrossRef] [PubMed]
29. Sanchez-Flack, J.C.; Herman, A.; Buscemi, J.; Kong, A.; Bains, A.; Fitzgibbon, M.L. A Systematic Review of the Implementation of Obesity Prevention Interventions in Early Childcare and Education Settings Using the RE-AIM Framework. *Transl. Behav. Med.* **2020**, *10*, 1168–1176. [CrossRef] [PubMed]
30. Schlechter, C.R.; Rosenkranz, R.R.; Guagliano, J.M.; Dzewaltowski, D.A. A Systematic Review of Children's Dietary Interventions with Parents as Change Agents: Application of the RE-AIM Framework. *Prev. Med.* **2016**, *91*, 233–243. [CrossRef]
31. Barden, C.; Bekker, S.; Brown, J.C.; Stokes, K.A.; McKay, C.D. Evaluating the Implementation of Injury Prevention Strategies in Rugby Union and League: A Systematic Review Using the RE-AIM Framework. *Int. J. Sports Med.* **2021**, *42*, 112–121.
32. Isaacs, S.A.; Roman, N.V.; Savahl, S.; Sui, X.-C. Using the RE-AIM Framework to Identify and Describe Best Practice Models in Family-Based Intervention Development: A Systematic Review. *Child Fam. Soc. Work* **2018**, *23*, 122–136. [CrossRef]
33. Yoshida, Y.; Patil, S.J.; Brownson, R.C.; Boren, S.A.; Kim, M.; Dobson, R.; Waki, K.; Greenwood, D.A.; Torbjørnsen, A.; Ramachandran, A.; et al. Using the RE-AIM Framework to Evaluate Internal and External Validity of Mobile Phone-Based Interventions in Diabetes Self-Management Education and Support. *J. Am. Med. Inform. Assoc.* **2020**, *27*, 946–956. [CrossRef] [PubMed]
34. Iwelunmor, J.; Nwaozuru, U.; Obiezu-Umeh, C.; Uzoaru, F.; Ehiri, J.; Curley, J.; Ezechi, O.; Airhihenbuwa, C.; Ssewamala, F. Is It Time to RE-AIM? A Systematic Review of Economic Empowerment as HIV Prevention Intervention for Adolescent Girls and Young Women in Sub-Saharan Africa Using the RE-AIM Framework. *Implement Sci. Commun.* **2020**, *1*, 53. [CrossRef] [PubMed]
35. Kang, H.S.; De Gagne, J.C.; Son, Y.D.; Chae, S.-M. Completeness of Human Papilloma Virus Vaccination: A Systematic Review. *J. Pediatr. Nurs.* **2018**, *39*, 7–14. [CrossRef]
36. Francis, D.B.; Cates, J.R.; Wagner, K.P.G.; Zola, T.; Fitter, J.E.; Coyne-Beasley, T. Communication Technologies to Improve HPV Vaccination Initiation and Completion: A Systematic Review. *Patient Educ. Couns.* **2017**, *100*, 1280–1286. [CrossRef]
37. Gerend, M.A.; Murdock, C.; Grove, K. An Intervention for Increasing HPV Vaccination on a University Campus. *Vaccine* **2020**, *38*, 725–729. [CrossRef] [PubMed]
38. Kim, M.; Lee, H.; Kiang, P.; Aronowitz, T.; Sheldon, L.K.; Shi, L.; Allison, J.J. A Storytelling Intervention in a Mobile, Web-Based Platform: A Pilot Randomized Controlled Trial to Evaluate the Preliminary Effectiveness to Promote Human Papillomavirus Vaccination in Korean American College Women. *Health Educ. Behav.* **2020**, *47*, 258–263. [CrossRef] [PubMed]
39. Lee, H.Y.; Koopmeiners, J.S.; McHugh, J.; Raveis, V.H.; Ahluwalia, J.S. mHealth Pilot Study: Text Messaging Intervention to Promote HPV Vaccination. *Am. J. Health Behav.* **2016**, *40*, 67–76. [CrossRef] [PubMed]
40. Matheson, E.C.; Derouin, A.; Gagliano, M.; Thompson, J.A.; Blood-Siegfried, J. Increasing HPV Vaccination Series Completion Rates via Text Message Reminders. *J. Pediatr. Health Care* **2014**, *28*, e35–e39. [CrossRef]
41. Mohanty, S.; Leader, A.E.; Gibeau, E.; Johnson, C. Using Facebook to Reach Adolescents for Human Papillomavirus (HPV) Vaccination. *Vaccine* **2018**, *36*, 5955–5961. [CrossRef] [PubMed]
42. Ortiz, R.R.; Shafer, A.; Cates, J.; Coyne-Beasley, T. Development and Evaluation of a Social Media Health Intervention to Improve Adolescents' Knowledge about and Vaccination against the Human Papillomavirus. *Glob. Pediatr. Health* **2018**, *5*, 2333794X18777918. [CrossRef]
43. Patel, A.; Stern, L.; Unger, Z.; Debevec, E.; Roston, A.; Hanover, R.; Morfesis, J. Staying on Track: A Cluster Randomized Controlled Trial of Automated Reminders Aimed at Increasing Human Papillomavirus Vaccine Completion. *Vaccine* **2014**, *32*, 2428–2433. [CrossRef] [PubMed]
44. Piedimonte, S.; Leung, A.; Zakhari, A.; Giordano, C.; Tellier, P.-P.; Lau, S. Impact of an HPV Education and Vaccination Campaign among Canadian University Students. *J. Obstet. Gynaecol. Can.* **2018**, *40*, 440–446. [CrossRef]

45. Rand, C.M.; Brill, H.; Albertin, C.; Humiston, S.G.; Schaffer, S.; Shone, L.P.; Blumkin, A.K.; Szilagyi, P.G. Effectiveness of Centralized Text Message Reminders on Human Papillomavirus Immunization Coverage for Publicly Insured Adolescents. *J. Adolesc. Health* **2015**, *56*, S17–S20. [CrossRef]
46. Rand, C.M.; Vincelli, P.; Goldstein, N.P.N.; Blumkin, A.; Szilagyi, P.G. Effects of Phone and Text Message Reminders on Completion of the Human Papillomavirus Vaccine Series. *J. Adolesc. Health* **2017**, *60*, 113–119. [CrossRef]
47. Richman, A.R.; Torres, E.; Wu, Q.; Carlston, L.; O'Rorke, S.; Moreno, C.; Olsson, J. Text and Email Messaging for Increasing Human Papillomavirus Vaccine Completion among Uninsured or Medicaid-Insured Adolescents in Rural Eastern North Carolina. *J. Health Care Poor Underserved* **2019**, *30*, 1499–1517. [CrossRef]
48. Richman, A.R.; Maddy, L.; Torres, E.; Goldberg, E.J. A Randomized Intervention Study to Evaluate Whether Electronic Messaging Can Increase Human Papillomavirus Vaccine Completion and Knowledge among College Students. *J Am. Coll. Health* **2016**, *64*, 269–278. [CrossRef]
49. Tull, F.; Borg, K.; Knott, C.; Beasley, M.; Halliday, J.; Faulkner, N.; Sutton, K.; Bragge, P. Short Message Service Reminders to Parents for Increasing Adolescent Human Papillomavirus Vaccination Rates in a Secondary School Vaccine Program: A Randomized Control Trial. *J. Adolesc. Health* **2019**, *65*, 116–123. [CrossRef]
50. Chodick, G.; Teper, G.R.; Levi, S.; Kopel, H.; Kleinbort, A.; Khen, E.; Schejter, E.; Shalev, V.; Stein, M.; Lewis, N. The Impact of a Facebook Campaign among Mothers on HPV Vaccine Uptake among Their Daughters: A Randomized Field Study. *Gynecol. Oncol.* **2021**, *160*, 106–111. [CrossRef] [PubMed]
51. Fontenot, H.B.; White, B.P.; Rosenberger, J.G.; Lacasse, H.; Rutirasiri, C.; Mayer, K.H.; Zimet, G. Mobile App Strategy to Facilitate Human Papillomavirus Vaccination among Young Men Who Have Sex with Men: Pilot Intervention Study. *J. Med. Internet Res.* **2020**, *22*, e22878. [CrossRef]
52. Gerend, M.A.; Madkins, K.; Crosby, S.; Korpak, A.K.; Phillips, G.L.; Bass, M.; Houlberg, M.; Mustanski, B. Evaluation of a Text Messaging-Based Human Papillomavirus Vaccination Intervention for Young Sexual Minority Men: Results from a Pilot Randomized Controlled Trial. *Ann. Behav. Med.* **2020**. [CrossRef]
53. White, S.M.; McAuley, E.; Estabrooks, P.A.; Courneya, K.S. Translating Physical Activity Interventions for Breast Cancer Survivors into Practice: An Evaluation of Randomized Controlled Trials. *Ann. Behav. Med.* **2009**, *37*, 10–19. [CrossRef]
54. Gaglio, B.; Shoup, J.A.; Glasgow, R.E. The RE-AIM Framework: A Systematic Review of Use over Time. *Am. J. Public Health* **2013**, *103*, e38–e46. [CrossRef]
55. Dixon, B.E.; Zimet, G.D.; Xiao, S.; Tu, W.; Lindsay, B.; Church, A.; Downs, S.M. An educational intervention to improve HPV vaccination: A cluster randomized trial. *Pediatrics* **2019**, *143*, e20181457. [CrossRef]
56. Rodriguez, S.A.; Roncancio, A.M.; Savas, L.S.; Lopez, D.M.; Vernon, S.W.; Fernandez, M.E. Using Intervention Mapping to Develop and Adapt Two Educational Interventions for Parents to Increase HPV Vaccination Among Hispanic Adolescents. *Front. Public Health* **2018**, *6*, 164. [CrossRef]
57. Watts, L.A.; Joseph, N.; Wallace, M.; Rauh-Hain, J.A.; Muzikansky, A.; Growdon, W.B.; Del Carmen, M.G. HPV vaccine: A comparison of attitudes and behavioral perspectives between Latino and non-Latino women. *Gynecol. Oncol.* **2009**, *112*, 577–582. [CrossRef]
58. Dempsey, A.F.; Zimet, G.D.; Davis, R.L.; Koutsky, L. Factors that are associated with parental acceptance of human papillomavirus vaccines: A randomized intervention study of written information about HPV. *Pediatrics* **2006**, *117*, 1486–1493. [CrossRef]
59. Friedman, L.M.; Furberg, C.D.; DeMets, D.L.; Reboussin, D.M.; Granger, C.B. Issues in Data Analysis. In *Fundamentals of Clinical Trials*; Springer: Berlin/Heidelberg, Germany, 2015.
60. McCoy, C.E. Understanding the Intention-to-Treat Principle in Randomized Controlled Trials. *West. J. Emerg. Med.* **2017**, *18*, 1075–1078. [CrossRef] [PubMed]
61. Hollis, S.; Campbell, F. What Is Meant by Intention to Treat Analysis? Survey of Published Randomised Controlled Trials. *BMJ* **1999**, *319*, 670–674. [CrossRef] [PubMed]
62. Dumville, J.C.; Torgerson, D.J.; Hewitt, C.E. Reporting Attrition in Randomised Controlled Trials. *BMJ* **2006**, *332*, 969–971. [CrossRef]
63. Shanks, C.B.; Harden, S. A Reach, Effectiveness, Adoption, Implementation, Maintenance Evaluation of Weekend Backpack Food Assistance Programs. *Am. J. Health Promot.* **2016**, *30*, 511–520. [CrossRef]
64. Weiss, C.H. *Evaluation: Methods for Studying Programs and Policies*; Oxford University Press: Oxford, UK, 1998.
65. Lipsey, M.; Sechrest, P.; Perrin, E.; Bunker, J. Research Methodology: Strengthening Causal Interpretations of Non-Experimental Data. *Cancer Causes Control* **1990**, *1*, 196.
66. Brazil, K.; Ozer, E.; Cloutier, M.M.; Levine, R.; Stryer, D. From Theory to Practice: Improving the Impact of Health Services Research. *BMC Health Serv. Res.* **2005**, *5*, 1. [CrossRef]
67. Dzewaltowski, D.A.; Estabrooks, P.A.; Glasgow, R.E. The Future of Physical Activity Behavior Change Research: What Is Needed to Improve Translation of Research into Health Promotion Practice? *Exerc. Sport Sci. Rev.* **2004**, *32*, 57–63. [CrossRef] [PubMed]
68. Duggan, M.; Lenhart, A.; Lampe, C.; Ellison, N.B. *Parents and Social Media*; Pew Research Center: Washington, DC, USA, 2015; p. 16.

MDPI
St. Alban-Anlage 66
4052 Basel
Switzerland
Tel. +41 61 683 77 34
Fax +41 61 302 89 18
www.mdpi.com

Vaccines Editorial Office
E-mail: vaccines@mdpi.com
www.mdpi.com/journal/vaccines

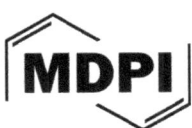

www.ingramcontent.com/pod-product-compliance
Lightning Source LLC
LaVergne TN
LVHW070745100526
838202LV00013B/1307

9 7 8 3 0 3 6 5 5 9 1 7 9